The Streetmedic's Handbook

SECOND EDITION

Owen T. Traynor, M.D. • Thomas Rahilly, Ph.D.

Patrick Coonan, R.N., Ed.D. • Jonathan S. Rubens, Ph.D.

THOMSON

DELMAR LEARNING

Australia Canada Mexico Singapore Spain United Kingdom United States

THOMSON

DELMAR LEARNING

The Streetmedic's Handbook , 2nd Edition
by Owen Traynor, Thomas Rahilly, Patrick Coonan, Jonathan Rubens

Vice President, Health Care Business Unit:
William Brottmiller

Editorial Director:
Cathy L. Esperti

Acquisitions Editor:
Maureen Rosener

Developmental Editor:
Laurie Traver

Marketing Director:
Jennifer McAvey

Marketing Coordinator:
Chris Manion

Production Editor:
Jack Pendleton

Technology Project Manager:
Mary Colleen Liburdi

Library of Congress Cataloging-in-Publication Data

Streetmedic's Handbook / Owen Traynor ... [et al.]. – 2nd ed
p. ; cm.
Includes bibliographical references and index.
ISBN 1-4018-5924-0
1. Medical emergencies–Handbooks, manuals, etc. 2. Emergency medical technicians–Handbooks, manuals, etc. I. Traynor, Owen
[DNLM: 1 Emergency Treatment–methods–Handbooks 2 Emergency Medical Technicians–Handbooks.
WB 39 S915 2004]
RC86.8.S77 2004
616.02'5–dc22
2004062045

NOTICE TO THE READER

TABLE OF CONTENTS

FOREWORD

You have a hard job. As a streetmedic, you face challenges that are unimaginable to most other healthcare professionals. On every call, you are expected to make highly critical decisions with incomplete and often conflicting information. You are placed in highly dynamic and emotional situations and must make high-impact decisions quickly. The patients that you treat represent the entire spectrum of medicine. The decisions that you make have a profound impact on your patient, their family, and their loved ones. While not every call is a matter of life and death, the decisions remain complicated and complex.

I have known Owen Traynor, M.D., for many years and have always been impressed with his dedication to quality prehospital care. In *The Streetmedic's Handbook*, 2nd edition, Dr. Traynor demonstrates his deep respect and appreciation for the difficult job that you do everyday. Along with his exceptional group of contributors, Dr. Traynor draws on his extensive prehospital and emergency medicine experience to develop an easy-to-use, practical resource to help you do your difficult job.

The Streetmedic's Handbook is an extraordinary tool for every EMS practitioner—from student to veteran, from first responder to paramedic. The book is organized in a logical, clear, and concise format. It mirrors the way that experienced practitioners think about prehospital problems and helps you think through the difficult parts of your job. There are many ways that the book can be used. The book helps students and new providers develop an effective strategy for dealing with common and uncommon prehospital situations. Experienced providers will welcome a quick reminder to jog their memory on the way to calls involving infrequent cases. After the initial management of patients, *The Streetmedic's Handbook* can be quickly and discretely consulted to ensure that you have performed a complete assessment and "covered all of the bases" (by the way, physicians do this all the time! What do you think they do when they step out of the exam room?). Finally, *The Streetmedic's Handbook* is a great way to debrief following a call so that you are always better tomorrow than you are today. Whether you use it on the way to a call, during de-briefing, as a periodic study guide, or to help you develop your clinical skills, I am confident that you will find that *The Streetmedic's Handbook* will make your job a little easier.

Not only is your job hard, it is too often thankless. On behalf of the patients who are too sick, injured, frustrated, overwhelmed, sad, mad, confused, drunk, or scared to say so—please allow me to thank you for taking on such an important, rewarding, and difficult job.

Gregg S. Margolis
Associate Director
National Registry of EMTs

PREFACE

Welcome to the second edition of *The Streetmedic's Handbook*!

This book was written to serve as a concise, pocket-size field reference for paramedics and intermediate emergency medical technicians (EMTs). It has also been successfully used during the initial training and continuing education of both paramedics and EMTs.

THE DEVELOPMENT OF THE BOOK

The initial idea for the book developed during medical school. There was a fantastic amount of factual information presented during class. It was challenging to learn the material, but it was even more difficult to organize it in a meaningful way so that it could be applied to the care of a patient. I recognized that this was one of the challenges that I had faced as a paramedic and as an EMS educator as well. Traditionally, EMS students would learn information in a system's approach: cardiovascular, respiratory, musculoskeletal, and so forth. Unfortunately, few patients will offer as a chief complaint, "I am suffering a cardiovascular problem." Rather, their complaint might be, "I am having chest pain." Although it is expected that physicians and EMS professionals will be able to think critically and clinically, little of the educational process focuses on these skills. Fortunately, physicians will spend 2 of their 4 years of medical school in clinical settings, and then at least 3 years in a residency program to hone their clinical skills. EMTs and paramedics will not be that lucky.

THE BOOK'S ORGANIZATION

The Streetmedic's Handbook is organized into four sections. The first section focuses on important and common clinical problems. For example, the chest pain chapter provides a quick discussion of the relevant information needed to evaluate and treat patients who complain of chest pain. Even inexperienced students are able to identify the nature of the patient's complaint and choose the correct chapter. Some 46 presenting problems are covered in the first section of the book.

Each of the chapters in the first section follows a standardized, problem-oriented format, consisting of the following components:

- General statement of the problem

- Thought-provoking questions (with answers) that start the medic thinking while en route to the emergency

- A differential diagnosis of the problem

- A summary of key physical examination findings

- Suggested treatment options

- References for further study

- A space for notes

Section 2 covers special situations and topics. These topics were found to receive little attention in some EMS educational programs. You will find discussions on various topics, including advanced directives, infectious disease exposures, multiple casualty incidents, the approach to pediatric patients, response to terrorism, and capnography.

Section 3 is the procedure section. Common EMS procedures are reviewed. Some of the procedures covered include central venous catheterization, cricothyrotomy, esophageal tracheal combitube insertion, laryngeal mask airway use, intraosseous insertion, and rapid sequence intubation. It is expected that the student or EMS professional has already received instruction in these skills and has been credentialed. The standardized format for chapters in this section includes the following:

- Indications

- Contraindications

- Equipment

- Procedure steps

- Complications

- References for further study

- A space for notes

The final section contains the appendices. Some of the information that may be found here includes summaries of ACLS, BLS, PALS, EMS medications, commonly prescribed medications, and summaries of key weapons of mass destruction agents.

NEW IN THE SECOND EDITION

The first edition was published in 1995. A significant amount of work was done to bring the book into the twenty-first century. Many of the first edition's chapters were entirely rewritten. Several new chapters were added, including rapid sequence intubation, response to terrorism, capnography, the combitube, and the laryngeal mask airway. The book uses the correct terminology required by the current revised National Standard Curricula, and the 2000 American Heart Association Guidelines are employed throughout the book. The references have been updated as well.

THE ELECTRONIC VERSION

Also new to this edition is that the content in this book will be available electronically. It will provide the same ease of use as the printed version and allow for more rapid searching for information. Users can download the content from the Thomson Delmar Learning EMS website into their PDA. Having the book's content available in a PDA will allow medics to quickly search for pertinent information such as specific diagnoses, commonly prescribed medications and ACLS and PALS algorithms when they are en route to calls, on scene with patients, or en route to the hospital. In the increasingly technology-driven world we live in these days, the PDA format allows for emergency personnel to literally have this type of information at their fingertips.

HOW TO USE THE BOOK

Educators may use the book early in the curriculum as a way to prepare students for their field rotations. Because the number of field hours is limited, maximizing the amount of high-level experiences is important. Early in the training program, the book functions as a guidebook to what paramedics do on specific calls. The better the students are prepared for the rotation, the more they will get out of it. Later in the curriculum, students may benefit from an assessment-based management course. *The Streetmedic's Handbook* is a natural fit for these classes. Late in the training program, the book functions as an aid to "putting it all together."

The organization of the book makes it an excellent |tool for guiding continuing education activities, such as call reviews.

The design of the book allows for a quick review while en route to the call. Field personnel may also refer to the book, if needed, while providing care. The medic may also benefit from a postcall review. The provided references can be used as a starting point for further study.

ABOUT THE AUTHORS

Owen T. Traynor, M.D., FAAM, has been active in EMS and emergency medicine since 1978. He has served in many positions, including firefighter/paramedic and captain of the Wantagh, NY, Fire Department, NYC EMS paramedic, EMS instructor and Assistant Chief of the Nassau County EMS Academy, and regional faculty of NYS EMS. Owen graduated from the University of Vermont College of Medicine, the University of Pittsburgh Affiliated Residency in Emergency Medicine, and the University of Pittsburgh EMS Fellowship. During his residency and fellowship training, Dr. Traynor served as an EMS physician responding in a quick-response vehicle to emergencies with the city of Pittsburgh paramedics. He also served as a flight physician with StatMedevac, one of the nation's premier aeromedical transport services. He is currently the medical director for paramedic education at the Center for Emergency Medicine of Western PA, the medical director of the EMS degree program at the University of Pittsburgh School of Health and Rehabilitation Sciences, an EMS medical director for the UPMC Health System, and medical director for several suburban EMS agencies. In addition, Owen is an attending emergency physician and director of EMS at St. Clair Hospital, Pittsburgh, PA.

Dr. Patrick R. Coonan is presently a dean and professor at the School of Nursing at Adelphi University in Garden City, New York. He holds a doctorate in nursing administration and a masters in nursing education from Columbia University, a masters in health care administration from Long Island University, and a bachelors in Nursing from Adelphi University. Previously, he held executive and director of nursing positions in major medical centers and Level 1 trauma centers in the New York metropolitan region. He is a volunteer firefighter and former EMT-CC with the Lynbrook Fire Department in Nassau County, Long Island, New York, for more than 30 years and presently holds the rank of past chief. He has been a New York State regional EMS instructor and an instructor at the Nassau County EMS Academy. Dr. Coonan was also the director of the critical care nurse specialist program at Columbia University before assuming executive nursing positions.

He spent his clinical nursing career in some of the largest and busiest trauma centers and emergency departments in the New York metropolitan region and is well versed in the practice of leadership, management, disaster, and emergency nursing.

Thomas J. Rahilly, Ph.D. is the administrative manager for the Department of Emergency Medicine at North Shore University Hospital, Manhasset, NY, a Level 2 trauma center. He has been involved in EMS for more than 30 years and was one of the first EMT-critical care technicians certified in New York State. Dr. Rahilly has been active in EMS organizations at the federal, state, and local levels and is a past chairman of the New York State EMS Council. He organized the Nassau County EMS Academy, where he was chief for more than fifteen years. Dr. Rahilly is a past chief of the Oyster Bay Fire Department on Long Island and served as the Deputy Executive Director of the New York State Association of Fire Chiefs.

Jonathan S. Rubens, M.D., MHPE, FACEP, FAAEM, a native of New York City, has been practicing emergency medicine for 17 years and is currently vice-president of Regional Emergency Physicians, PA-C in High Point, North Carolina. He is past section-chief of emergency medicine at High Point Regional Health System and has served several state and local EMS agencies in directorship and educator roles. He is also currently the president-elect of the board of directors of the Triad Health Project in Greensboro, North Carolina.

A note from Jonathan: I would like to thank Owen for asking me to be part of this rewarding effort for a second time. I would also like to say a special thank-you to Jeffrey Freeman, R.N., Yvonne A. Rubens, Rosalind R. Newell, Dexter E. Arrington, M.D., Sandra Townsell, R.N., and Mark Gelula, Ph.D., whose encouragement and support played a critical role in my participation in this project.

ACKNOWLEDGMENTS

The authors would like to express their sincere appreciation to:

- The many contributors who provided a wealth of practical information that will make this book a valuable tool for the streetmedic

- The staff of Thomson Delmar Learning, particularly Maureen Rosener, Laurie Traver, Jack Pendleton, Elizabeth Howe, and Mary Colleen Liburdi

- The following manuscript reviewers who provided many thoughtful comments and criticisms:

Reg Allen, B.S., NREMT-P
Paramedic Instructor
Canandaigua EMS
Canandaigua, NY

Ronald R. Bowser, M.B.A., EMTB
Maryland Fire and Rescue Institute
University of Maryland
College Park, MD

Harvey Conner, AS NREMT-P
Professor of EMS
Oklahoma City Community College
Oklahoma City, OK

Joe Ferrell, B.S., NREMT-P
Education Coordinator
Iowa Department of Public Health—Bureau of EMS
Des Moines, IA

Peter C. Flanagan, Jr., NREMT-P
Clinical Assistant Professor of Health Science
Stony Brook University
Stony Brook, NY

Louis Gonzales, B.S., NREMT-P
Clinical Education & Outreach Coordinator
Williamson County EMS
Georgetown, TX
Adjunct Faculty, Department of EMS Professions
Temple College
Temple, TX

Ann Hudgins, R.N., B.S.N., L.P., NREMT-P
Assistant Professor & Paramedic Course Coordinator
UT Southwestern Medical Center at Dallas
Dallas, TX

Steven Pitts, NREMT-P, RRT, FP-C
Program Director, Advanced Life Support
Spokane Community College
Spokane, WA

M. Jane Pollock, EMT-P, CEI, Level II, EMD
Education and Training Specialist
Brody School of Medicine, East Carolina School of
    Medicine,
Emergency Medicine, Division of EMS
Greenville, NC

J. Penny Shutts, AEMT, CIC, NREMT
Educator
Sandy Creek, NY

Paul A. Werfel, NREMT-P
Director, Paramedic Program
Assistant Professor of Clinical Emergency Medicine
Health Science Center
SUNY Stony Brook
Stony Brook, NY

- Our family members and friends who gave us the encouragement and support that was needed to complete this book.

CONTRIBUTORS

THE STREETMEDIC'S HANDBOOK, 2ND EDITION

Michael Baumann, M.D.
Associate Chief, Department of Emergency Medicine,
   Maine Medical Center
Associate Professor of Emergency Medicine
University of Vermont
Associate Medical Director, Lifelight of Maine
Portland, ME

Bernard Beckerman, M.D., FACEP
Department of Emergency Medicine
Huntington Hospital
Huntington, NY

Heidi Betler, NREMT-P
Volunteer Services Coordinator
North Huntingdon Rescue Squad
North Huntingdon, PA

Russell Bradley, M.D.
Emergency Physician
Salt Lake Regional Medical
   Center and VA Medical Center
Adjunct Clinical Faculty
University of Utah
Salt Lake City, UT

Daniel Brooks, M.D.
Assistant Professor of Medical Toxicology
and Emergency Medine
Department of Emergency Medicine
University of Pittsburgh Medical Center
Co-Medical Director, Pittsburgh Poison Center,
Pittsburgh, PA

Michael Cassara, D.O., FACEP
North Shore University Hospital
Assistant Residency Director
Department of Emergency Medicine
Manhasset , NY

Elizabeth Cohn, R.N., NP
Department of Cardiology
North Shore University Hospital
Manhasset, NY

Inspector John Fitzwilliams, B.S., B.A., EMT-CC
Emergency Ambulance Bureau
Nassau County Police Department
Mineola, NY

Gary Goodman, M.D.
Department of Emergency Medicine
North Shore University Hospital
Manhasset, NY

Deepi Goyal, M.D.
Assistant Professor of Emergency Medicine
Mayo Clinic
Rochester, MN

Myles D. Greenberg, M.D.
Clinical Assistant Professor
Department of Emergency Medicine
University of North Carolina School of Medicine
Campus Box 7594
Chapel Hill, NC

Ian Greenwald, M.D.
Assistant Professor of Emergency Medicine
Emory University/Grady Hospital
Atlanta, GA

David Gross, MPAS, PA-C
St. Elizabeth Center
Departments of Orthopedic Surgery
    and Orthopedic Trauma
Youngstown, OH

Micelle Haydel, M.D.
Clinical Assistant Professor and Assistant Residency
    Director
Section of Emergency Medicine
New Orleans, LA

Nora Helfrich, R.N., EMT-P
Tri-community South EMS
Bethel Park, PA

Curtis Judson, M.D.
Mayo Clinic
Rochester, MN

Kenneth Katz, M.D.
Assistant Professor, Medical Toxicology Service
UPMC
Pittsburgh, PA

Robert Kerner, R.N., J.D., CEN
Department of Emergency Medicine
North Shore University Hospital–Syosset
Syosset, NY

Sally Kuzniewski, R.N., M.A., CEN
Department of Surgery
North Shore University Hospital
Manhasset, NY

David LaCovey, EMT-P
EMS Coordinator
Pre-hospital and Emergency Care Services
Children's Hospital of Pittsburgh
Adjunct Instructor, Emergency Medicine Program
School of Health and Rehabilitation Science
University of Pittsburgh
Pittsburgh, PA

Debra Lejeune, M.Ed., NREMT-P
Instructor
University of Pittsburgh
Pittsburgh, PA

Gregg Margolis, M.S., NREMT-P
Associate Director
National Registry of EMTs
Columbus, OH

Kemedy McQuillen, M.D.
Attending Staff, Department of Emergency Medicine
Advocate Christ Medical Center
Oak Lawn, IL

Wanda Millard, M.D.
Department of Emergency Medicine
North Shore University Hospital
Manhasset, NY

Daniel Miller, EMT-P
Operations Manager
SouthBridge Emergency Medical Service
Bridgeville, PA

Michael Nagy, B.S., NREMT-P
Paramedic, Peters Township EMS
McMurray, PA

Thomas Platt, NREMT-P
Assistant Professor and Program Vice Chair
Emergency Medicine Program
University of Pittsburgh School of Health and
    Rehabilitation Sciences
Associate Director Center for Emergency Medicine
    of Western PA

Myron Rickens, EMT-P
Assistant Director, UPMC Prehospital Care Adjunct Facility
University of Pittsburgh
School of Health and Rehabilitation Science
Pittsburgh, PA

Ritu Sahni, M.D., MPH
Assistant Professor of Emergency Medicine
Medical Director, Emergency Communications
    and Transfer Center
Oregon Health and Sciences
Portland, OR

Mark Scheatzle, M.D.
Western Pennsylvania Hospital
Assistant Professor of Emergency Medicine
Department of Emergency Medicine
Pittsburgh, PA

Lawrence Sherman, EMT-CC
Center for Emergency Training and Development
North Shore University Hospital
Manhasset, NY

Steven Shurgot, EMT-P
Operations Director
Eastern Area Prehospital Service
Pittsburgh, PA

Hal A. Skopicki, M.D., Ph.D.
Department of Cardiology
North Shore University Hospital
Manhasset, NY

Andrew William Stern, M.A., MPA, NREMT-P
Senior Paramedic/Flightmedic
CME Coordinator
Town of Colonie Emergency Medical Services
Latham, NY

Walt Stoy, Ph.D., EMT-P
Professor and Director, Emergency Medicine Program
School of Health and Rehabilitation Sciences
Research Professor of Emergency Medicine
School of Medicine Department of Emergency Medicine
University of Pittsburgh
Director, Office of Education and International Emergency
    Medicine
Center for Emergency Medicine
Pittsburgh, PA

Henry Wang, M.D.
Assistant Professor
Department of Emergency Medicine
University of Pittsburgh
Pittsburgh, PA

Mike Yee, B.S., EMT-P
Paramedic Crew Chief, Ret.
EMS Instructor, W. Pa. Center for Emergency
Pittsburgh, PA

SECTION I

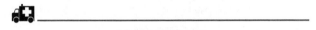

*COMMONLY
ENCOUNTERED
PROBLEMS*

CHAPTER 1

ABDOMINAL PAIN

JONATHAN S. RUBENS, M.D., FACEP
OWEN T. TRAYNOR, M.D.

PRESENTATION

Although most patients with nontraumatic abdominal pain do not have a serious illness, others may harbor a life-threatening illness. The presentation may be subtle or dramatic. Typically the pain is difficult to describe or localize. Abdominal pain can be referred to other locations, such as the chest, shoulders, or back. Many illnesses present in a similar fashion initially.

IMMEDIATE CONCERNS

- ❗ **What is the status of the patient's airway?** Many patients experience nausea and vomiting. They may be at increased risk of aspiration.

- ❗ **What is the patient's hemodynamic status?** Look for and treat if there is evidence of poor perfusion.

- ❗ **Does the patient have a history of an abdominal aortic aneurysm (AAA)?** A leaking or ruptured AAA carries significant mortality. Early recognition and transport to a facility that can surgically manage this disease is recommended.

- ❗ **Is there evidence of peritonitis?** Peritonitis, an inflammatory disorder of the lining of the abdominal cavity, is a life-threatening illness. The causes include infection, perforation, and internal hemorrhage. This patient will likely require surgery or antibiotics. The physical exam may include a tender abdomen with rigidity, guarding, and rebound tenderness. The patient may be hypotensive. Rapid recognition and transport are necessary.

IMPORTANT QUESTIONS

❓ **What is the location of the pain?** The location of the pain can provide clues about the organs affected. Right upper quadrant (RUQ) abdominal pain can be caused by illness of the organs located in that quadrant, such as the liver, gallbladder, and small intestines. Of course, the pain may be referred to a location remote from the illness; for example, the pain from acute cholecystitis, or inflammation of the gallbladder, is often felt at the right shoulder or scapula.

❓ **What was the onset of the pain?** Pain of sudden onset may indicate perforation or obstruction of a hollow organ, or acute aortic dissection or r upture. Diseases associated with an inflammatory process, such as appendicitis, cholecystitis, or diverticulitis, have a gradual onset.

❓ **What is the nature of the pain?** Pain that is crampy or described as coming in waves is known as *colicky pain*. This type of pain often results from the contraction of hollow organs, such as the uterus, gallbladder, ureters, and intestines.

❓ **Has the pain moved or radiated?** There are well-known patterns of movement or radiation that may help suggest a diagnosis. The classic presentation of appendicitis involves periumbilical pain that eventually moves to the right lower abdominal quadrant.

❓ **What are the associated symptoms?** The presence of fever suggests an inflammatory or infectious cause. Melena, hematemesis, or hematochezia suggests bleeding in the gastrointestinal (GI) tract. Dysuria and other urinary symptoms suggest a urologic source. Syncope in an elderly patient suggests a leaking AAA.

❓ **Has the patient had these symptoms before?** The patient may already know the diagnosis.

❓ Could the abdominal pain be caused by nonabdominal pathology? Acute coronary syndromes may cause epigastric pain. Diseases of the lower segments of the lung, such as pulmonary embolism and pneumonia, may refer the pain to the upper abdomen.

❓ What is the past medical history? Patients who have had prior abdominal surgeries are at increased risk of bowel obstructions. Patients with a history of gallstones are at increased risk of cholecystitis. Patient with a history of an AAA are at risk of rupture.

DIFFERENTIAL DIAGNOSIS

Important and common diagnoses are presented here in a regional approach according to the location of the diseased organ. Recognize that many diseases cause pain in several locations.

EPIGASTRIUM

- ***ACUTE CORONARY SYNDROME.*** Pain high in the epigastrium may result from an acute coronary syndrome. Consider this diagnosis for patients over the age of 35 years and those who have a history of coronary artery disease. Acute inferior wall myocardial infarctions also present with prominent GI symptoms, such as nausea and vomiting.

- ***GASTRITIS AND PEPTIC ULCER DISEASE.*** Gastritis is an inflammatory disease of the stomach. Peptic ulcer disease (PUD) involves a distinct defect in the lining of the stomach and duodenum. If unchecked, an ulcer may perforate, leading to peritonitis and shock. Common causes of gastritis and PUD include alcohol use; medications such as aspirin, NSAIDs, and steroids; and *Helicobacter pylori* infection of the gastric mucosa. In hospitalized patients, burns, trauma, and sepsis are known causes. Patients often complain of epigastric burning pain. The pain may be located in either upper abdominal quadrant as well. Heartburn, indigestion, bloating, flatulence, nausea, and vomiting are common symptoms. Determine whether the patient has a history of GI bleeding. The physical examination typically reveals mild epigastric tenderness.

- **PANCREATITIS.**   Alcohol abuse or gallstones cause 75% of all cases of pancreatitis. Patients report severe, persistent, boring epigastric pain that radiates to the back. The pain is often worse in a supine position. Nausea and vomiting are common associated symptoms. Physical findings include abdominal tenderness and, in severe cases, rigidity, guarding, and rebound tenderness. Tachycardia and hypotension may be present. Cullen's sign, periumbilical bluish discoloration, and Turner's sign, a bluish discoloration of the flanks, indicate severe hemorrhagic pancreatitis.

RIGHT UPPER QUADRANT

- **ACUTE CORONARY SYNDROME.**   Discussed above under epigastrium.

- **GASTRITIS AND PEPTIC ULCER DISEASE.**   Discussed above under epigastrium.

- **HEPATITIS.**   Hepatitis is an inflammatory disease of the liver. Its causes include viral infection, alcohol use, and certain drugs and toxins. Most cases are viral. In viral hepatitis, the early symptoms can be mild but include a flulike illness with fever, malaise, nausea, and vomiting. Many patients report a poor appetite. Later symptoms may include RUQ tenderness, jaundice, dark-colored urine, and clay-colored stools. The incubation period can be 2 to several weeks.

- **GALLBLADDER DISEASE. Cholelithiasis**, or gallstones, can cause pain in the RUQ. It usually is described as a dull, aching, continuous pain that may radiate to the right scapula, shoulder, or thoracic spine. The pain often follows a large, fatty meal. It develops over 2 to 3 minutes and lasts 30 minutes to 6 hours. The pain arises when a gallstone attempts to pass through the bile ducts. This process impedes the flow of bile and causes distension of the walls of the ducts and gallbladder spasm. Patients may report anorexia, nausea, and vomiting. These patients are afebrile. Their exam reveals tenderness in the RUQ but no rebound tenderness. **Cholecystitis**, or inflammation of the gallbladder, has a similar presentation. The pain lasts longer—often more than 6 hours. Fever is common. The pain occurs when prolonged bile stasis caused by a stone in the duct leads to increased intraluminal pressure and eventually to inflammation and edema. These patients typically have Murphy's sign, an inspiratory arrest on palpation of the RUQ, caused by an increase in pain as the gallbladder bumps into the examiner's hand. **Cholangitis** is a bacterial infection of the biliary tract associated with fever and chills, RUQ pain, and jaundice. Obstruction of the biliary tree causes bacterial infection and possible sepsis. These patients have RUQ tenderness and often peritoneal signs, such as rebound tenderness, rigidity, and guarding.

- ***PNEUMONIA.*** Consider the diagnosis of pneumonia in patients with a cough, shortness of breath, and upper abdominal pain. Pneumonia in the lower lung may cause referred pain in the abdomen. The physical exam demonstrates abnormal lung sounds and a nontender abdominal exam. Please see chapter 16 for more details.

- ***PULMONARY EMBOLISM.*** Pulmonary embolism may cause referred upper abdominal or lower thoracic back pain. The pain worsens on inspiration. Patients describe the pain as sharp. There are generally few GI symptoms such as nausea, vomiting, or diarrhea. The patient may report dyspnea, pleuritic chest pain, and lower extremity edema. The abdominal exam is unremarkable. There may be few physical findings, as well. The vital signs often reveal mild tachycardia and tachypnea. Many patients have hypoxia. Please see chapter 11 for more details.

LEFT UPPER QUADRANT

- ***ACUTE CORONARY SYNDROME.*** Discussed above under epigastrium.

- ***DISEASES OF THE SPLEEN.*** The most common illness of the spleen is a traumatic rupture of the spleen. Patients with a recent diagnosis of acute mononucleosis may have an enlarged spleen, which puts them at increased risk of rupture after even mild blunt trauma. The patient may complain of left upper quadrant (LUQ) pain, or left shoulder and scapula pain. There can be a significant blood loss, resulting in tachycardia and hypotension. The abdominal exam typically reveals LUQ tenderness. Signs of peritonitis may be present as well. Other nontraumatic disorders of the spleen are uncommon but include splenic infarction and splenic abscess. The exam typically reveals LUQ tenderness.

- ***GASTRITIS AND PEPTIC ULCER DISEASE.*** Discussed above under epigastrium.

- ***PNEUMONIA.*** Discussed above under RUQ.

- ***PULMONARY EMBOLISM.*** Discussed above under RUQ.

PERIUMBILICAL AREA

- ***APPENDICITIS.*** The classic presentation involves periumbilical abdominal pain followed by anorexia and mild fever. The pain eventually moves to the right lower quadrant (RLQ). Many patients report vomiting and either diarrhea or constipation. The location of the pain is quite variable, with many people reporting back or flank pain, testicular pain, suprapubic pain, and even RUQ or left lower quadrant (LLQ) pain. Patients with appendicitis prefer not to move and often walk with a shuffling gait. The exam reveals tenderness, guarding, and rebound tenderness. Look for the following signs: obturator sign, pain on flexion and internal rotation of the right hip; Psoas sign, increased pain on extension of the right hip; and Rovsing's sign, pain in the RLQ on palpation of the LLQ. Elderly patients are more difficult to diagnose before the appendix ruptures because of their more frequent atypical presentations. Pregnant females are difficult to diagnose because the gravid uterus displaces the appendix.

SECTION 1

- ***MESENTERIC ISCHEMIA.*** Poor or absent blood flow through the mesenteric blood vessels that supply the intestines can cause poorly localized, moderate-to-severe abdominal pain. The pain seems out of proportion to the abdominal exam. It is often associated with nausea, vomiting, and diarrhea. The onset can be sudden if caused by an embolism or gradual if caused by thrombosis of the blood vessels. Some patients have a history of intestinal angina—that is, of pain after eating, resolved by vomiting. Necrosis of the intestines can occur in as few as 6 hours. The typical patient is elderly with a history of arrhythmia, valvular heart disease, poorly controlled congestive heart failure (CHF), and prior embolic episodes. The exam reveals abdominal distension and initially only a mildly tender abdomen. Later the abdomen becomes markedly tender. Diffuse peritonitis, shock, and death may occur.

RIGHT LOWER QUADRANT

- ***APPENDICITIS.*** Described under periumbilical area above.

LEFT LOWER QUADRANT

- ***APPENDICITIS.*** Described under periumbilical area above.

- **DIVERTICULITIS.** It is believed that a relatively low-fiber diet causes the formation of firmer stools. Greater colonic muscle contractions are needed to move the stool through the colon. The increased pressure in the colon forces the mucosa and submucosal layers to herniate through the wall of the colon, forming pouches called **diverticula**. This presence of diverticula is called **diverticulosis**. Diverticulosis is usually greatest in the sigmoid and descending colon because the stool is firmer there. Diverticulosis is typically painless. It is often diagnosed by colonoscopy. Diverticulosis may cause painless rectal bleeding or, if inflammation occurs, diverticulitis. Patients with diverticulitis complain of persistent, vague pain in the lower abdomen. Over time, the pain worsens and localizes to the LLQ. Fever, nausea, and poor appetite are common. Patients may report constipation or diarrhea. Urinary frequency may occur if the diverticulitis is adjacent to the bladder. The exam reveals LLQ tenderness and possibly a mass (inflamed colon or abscess). Complications include perforation, abscess, or obstruction.

FLANKS

- **KIDNEY STONES.** Kidney stones are characterized by sudden onset of unilateral crampy pain ranging from the costovertebral angle to the flank and lower abdomen to the suprapubic region. They are often associated with nausea and vomiting. The patient, unable to find a comfortable position, often writhes in pain. Some patients have hematuria. Often there is a prior history of kidney stones. There is no abdominal tenderness. Palpate the abdomen for pulsatile masses. The presence of a pulsatile mass suggests an abnormal aortic aneurysm rather than a kidney stone.

- **PYELONEPHRITIS.** Pyelonephritis is an infection of the upper urinary tract. Patients typically report dysuria, urinary frequency, and urgency. Patients report back pain, flank pain, or abdominal pain. The pain can be unilateral or bilateral. Fever and chills, nausea, vomiting, and malaise are common. The physical exam reveals costovertebral angle tenderness or suprapubic tenderness.

- ***ABDOMINAL AORTIC ANEURYSM.*** Patients may present with a ruptured or unruptured AAA. Those whose AAA has not ruptured may be asymptomatic or complain of back, flank, or abdominal pain. The quality of the pain is variable, either dull, throbbing, or crampy. The physical exam may reveal a nontender pulsatile mass. The femoral and distal pulses in the lower extremities should be present. The absence of the mass on physical exam does not eliminate the diagnosis of AAA. Ruptured or leaking AAAs is a life-threatening emergency. The patient often complains of sudden, severe back, flank, or abdominal pain. The pain can radiate along the path of the aorta to the chest, back, flank, and groin. The classic AAA rupture involves sudden pain, hypotension, and a pulsatile mass. Many patients are initially hypertensive. Some patients may present with syncope. Physical exam findings may include abdominal tenderness, a tender pulsatile mass, and decreased pulses to the lower extremities. The absence of a pulsatile mass does not exclude an AAA. The most common misdiagnoses of a ruptured AAA are kidney stone, diverticulitis, GI bleeding, and lumbosacral strain.

SUPRAPUBIC AREA

- ***APPENDICITIS.*** Described under periumbilical area above.

- ***CYSTITIS.*** Cystitis is defined as a urinary tract infection involving the bladder. Patients complain of dysuria, urinary frequency, and urgency. Fever and suprapubic pain may be present. The physical exam reveals suprapubic tenderness.

- ***PROSTATITIS.*** Prostatitis is an inflammatory disorder of the prostate often caused by a bacterial infection.

These patients complain of dysuria, urinary frequency, and urgency. The pain may be located in the lower back, perineum, suprapubic area, or testicles. Many patients have malaise, fever, chills, and muscle and joint pains. The abdominal exam is unremarkable.

- **SIGMOID DIVERTICULITIS.** See diverticulitis above, under Left Lower Quadrant.

- **URINARY RETENTION.** Patients with urinary retention often present with a history of difficulty voiding. It is usually several hours since they last voided. They may report crampy suprapubic pain. The physical exam often reveals a tender suprapubic mass (bladder). There are many causes of acute urinary retention, including bladder outlet obstruction caused by benign prostatic hypertrophy, prostate cancer, hematuria with blood clots, neurologic disorders, and various medications and anesthetics.

POORLY LOCALIZED PAIN

- **BOWEL OBSTRUCTION.** Bowel obstruction may occur in both the small intestines and the colon. Common causes include adhesions (scar tissue from prior abdominal surgeries), hernias, neoplasms, and strictures from inflammatory bowel disorders. Patients report intermittent abdominal pain that becomes constant. Vomiting is common. Patients are often unable to move their bowels or pass flatus. The physical exam reveals distension and diffuse tenderness. Bowel sounds can be high-pitched and hyperactive. These patients are at increased risk of hypotension and sepsis.

- **GASTROENTERITIS.** Gastroenteritis is a common GI illness causing nausea, vomiting, and diarrhea. Patients report diffuse, crampy abdominal pain. Mild fever, muscle and joint pain, and headache are frequent associated symptoms. Patients are at risk for dehydration and shock. The most common cause of gastroenteritis is a viral infection. Bacterial infections and food poisoning may also cause this disease. The physical exam may reveal mild abdominal tenderness but no evidence of peritonitis.

KEY PHYSICAL EXAMINATION FINDINGS

- ✅ ***Initial assessment.*** Look for alterations in hemodynamic stability.

- ✅ ***Vital signs.*** Although most patients have a normal or slightly elevated heart rate, some may be bradycardic as a result of vagal stimulation. Many patients with an inferior wall myocardial infarction (MI) are bradycardic also. Careful monitoring of the blood pressure (BP) is needed. Patients with ruptured AAAs may be hypertensive initially and hypotensive later.

- ✅ ***Lungs.*** Listen to lung sounds for signs of pneumonia.

- ✅ ***Abdomen.*** Look for evidence of prior surgeries, hernias, and distension. Assess for Cullen's and Turner's sign. Palpate for tenderness and masses. Percussion may help differentiate ascites from distension with air. Be alert for signs of peritonitis.

- ✅ ***Extremities.*** Check for perfusion and equal pulses.

ELECTROCARDIOGRAM

Evaluate for signs of cardiac ischemia or injury.

TREATMENT PLAN

- • ***Patient assessment.*** Perform a rapid and systematic initial assessment and institute treatment as life-threatening problems are discovered. Prompt transport to the appropriate emergency department (ED) is a key intervention. Frequent reassessment of the patient with abdominal pain is necessary because of the potential for worsening. Consider the diagnosis of AAA in all patients over 50 years of age. Consider the diagnosis of appendicitis in all patients with an appendix.

- **Administer O$_2$ and provide ventilatory support** as needed.

  Place the patient in a position of comfort.

- **Monitor the electrocardiogram if ischemia is suspected.**

- **Establish large bore IV** access.

- Consider the following interventions:

  - **Administer 0.9% NaCl or lactated Ringer's fluid resuscitation** if the patient presents with dehydration or shock.

  - **Treat for acute coronary syndrome if present.** See chapter 11.

  - Treat for ruptured AAA if suspected. Establish a second large bore IV. Early notification of the receiving facility to mobilize a vascular surgeon and operating room staff may improve outcome.

  - Frequently reassess the patient's hemodynamic status.

  - Frequently reassess the abdomen.

  - **Transport to the appropriate Emergency Department (ED).** Ensure patient comfort en route.

BIBLIOGRAPHY

Finkel, M. A. (2003). Abdominal pain. In J. J. Schaider, S. R. Hayden, R. Wolfe, R. M. Barkin, & P. Rosen (Eds.), *Rosen & Barkin's 5-minute emergency medicine consult* (2nd ed., pp. 4–7). Philadelphia: Lippincott Williams & Wilkins.

Humphries, R. L., & Russell, J. A. (2004). Abdominal pain. In C. K. Stone & R. L. Humphries (Eds.), *Current emergency diagnosis and treatment* (5th ed., pp. 257–282). New York: McGraw-Hill.

Imperato, J. & Rosen, C. L. (2003). Abdominal aortic aneurysm. In J. J. Schaider, S. R. Hayden, R. Wolfe, R. M. Barkin, & P. Rosen (Eds.), *Rosen & Barkin's 5-minute emergency medicine consult* (2nd ed., pp. 2–3). Philadelphia: Lippincott Williams & Wilkins.

NOTES

_____

_____

_____

_____

_____

_____

_____

_____

_____

_____

_____

_____

_____

_____

_____

_____

_____

_____

_____

_____

SECTION 1

CHAPTER 2

ABDOMINAL AND PELVIC PAIN IN WOMEN

Jonathan S. Rubens, M.D., FACEP
Owen T. Traynor, M.D.

PRESENTATION

This chapter will focus on the care of the female patient with abdominal pain. Chapter 1 focused on nongynecologic causes of abdominal pain. In addition, chapter 32 covers illnesses related to the pregnant patient.

IMMEDIATE CONCERNS

● **What is the status of the patient's airway?** Many patients experience nausea and vomiting. They may be at increased risk of aspiration.

● **What is the patient's hemodynamic status?** Look for and treat if there is evidence of poor perfusion.

● **Might the patient be pregnant?** If the patient is of childbearing age and has a uterus and at least one ovary, pregnancy is possible. A missed or delayed menstrual period indicates a possible pregnancy. If the patient has a positive pregnancy test, find out the due date. Symptoms of an early pregnancy include amenorrhea (absent periods), breast tenderness or tingling, nausea and vomiting, and urinary frequency.

● **Is there evidence of peritonitis?** Peritonitis, an inflammatory disorder of the lining of the abdominal cavity, is a life-threatening illness. The causes include infection, perforation, and internal hemorrhage. This patient will likely require surgery or antibiotics. The physical exam may include a tender abdomen with rigidity, guarding, and rebound tenderness. The patient may be hypotensive. Rapid recognition and transport are necessary.

IMPORTANT QUESTIONS

❓ What is the location of the pain? The location of the pain can provide clues about the organs affected. Pain related to reproductive organs is often found in the lower abdomen or pelvis. Right upper quadrant abdominal pain can be caused by illness of the organs located in that quadrant, such as the liver, gallbladder, and small intestines. Of course, the pain may be referred to a location remote from the illness; for example, the pain from acute cholecystitis, or inflammation of the gallbladder, is often felt at the right shoulder or scapula.

❓ What was the onset of the pain? Pain of sudden onset can indicate perforation or obstruction of a hollow organ, ruptured ovarian cysts, or acute aortic dissection or rupture. Diseases associated with an inflammatory process, such as pelvic inflammatory disease (PID), appendicitis, cholecystitis, or diverticulitis, have a gradual onset.

❓ What is the nature of the pain? Pain that is crampy or described as coming in waves is known as *colicky pain*. This type of pain often results from the contraction of hollow organs, such as the uterus, gallbladder, ureters, and intestines.

❓ Has the pain moved or radiated? There are well-known patterns of movement or radiation that may help suggest a diagnosis. The classic presentation of appendicitis involves periumbilical pain that eventually moves to the right lower abdominal quadrant.

❓ What are the associated symptoms? The presence of fever suggests an inflammatory or infectious cause. Melena, hematemesis, or hematochezia suggests bleeding in the GI tract. Dysuria and other urinary symptoms suggest a urologic source. Syncope in an elderly patient suggests a leaking AAA.

❷ **Has the patient had these symptoms before?** The patient may already know the diagnosis.

❷ **Could the abdominal pain be caused by nonabdominal pathology?** Acute coronary syndromes may cause epigastric pain. Diseases of the lower segments of the lung, such as pulmonary embolism and pneumonia, may refer the pain to the upper abdomen.

❷ **What is the past medical history?** Patients who have had prior abdominal surgeries are at increased risk of bowel obstructions. Those with a history of PID or prior ectopic pregnancies will be at higher risk for an ectopic pregnancy. Patients with a history of gallstones are at increased risk of cholecystitis. Patients with a history of an AAA are at risk of rupture.

DIFFERENTIAL DIAGNOSIS

The differential diagnosis will be primarily limited to diseases specific to women and will be categorized as either in the pregnant patient or the nonpregnant patient. We acknowledge that the pregnancy status of the patient is not always known. Women are also susceptible to many of the illnesses discussed in chapter 1.

THE PREGNANT PATIENT

● *ECTOPIC PREGNANCY.* Ectopic pregnancies are pregnancies that develop outside of the uterus. Most of these pregnancies (approximately 95%) occur in the fallopian tubes. The peak time of diagnosis is between 6 and 9 weeks of gestation. The presentation can be one of profound shock if the tube ruptures. Many presentations are subtle, however. The patients report abdominal pain 95% of the time. The pain is usually poorly localized and on one side only. It can be dull and aching or sharp when the tube ruptures. The abdominal exam can be unremarkable if the tube has not yet ruptured. Often the ectopic pregnancy can masquerade as acute appendicitis, ruptured ovarian cyst, miscarriage, or PID. The risk factors for development of an ectopic pregnancy include a prior ectopic pregnancy, a history of PID, use of an intrauterine device (IUD), use of infertility drugs, and prior gynecologic surgery. In the past, ectopic pregnancies were all treated surgically. However, some can be treated medically using methotrexate.

- **SPONTANEOUS ABORTION.**   This is commonly called a miscarriage. It can be classified as noted below.

  o ***Threatened abortion.*** The patient has not passed the products of conception (POC). Common symptoms include vaginal bleeding, spotting, brownish vaginal discharge, and crampy suprapubic pain. The diagnosis will be made in the ED after evaluation, which includes a pelvic examination, and possibly a pelvic ultrasound. Half of these patients go on to have a normal pregnancy.

  o ***Complete abortion.*** In this case the POC have been passed. The patients commonly report significant suprapubic cramping and vaginal bleeding. Often the symptoms ease after the POC have been passed.

  o ***Incomplete abortion.***   The patient has not expelled the entire POC and complains of moderate to severe suprapubic crampy pain and vaginal bleeding. A pelvic exam and pelvic ultrasound in the ED will help differentiate this from a complete abortion.

  o ***Inevitable abortion.*** This occurs when the pregnancy cannot be salvaged but the POC have not yet been passed. An ED evaluation is necessary to make this diagnosis.

  o ***Missed abortion.*** The missed abortion occurs when there has been death of the fetus without the passage of the POC. The patient usually reports dark vaginal bleeding. A pelvic exam and pelvic ultrasound in the ED will help determine this diagnosis.

o **_Septic abortion._** These patients will report abdominal pain, fever, and vaginal discharge or vaginal bleeding. Their abdominal exam may reveal evidence of peritonitis.

- **HELLP SYNDROME.** HELLP syndrome is a complication of severe eclampsia. It consists of **H**emolysis, **E**levated **Li**ver function tests, and **L**ow **P**latelets. These patients report right upper abdominal pain. In addition, they have the features of preeclampsia and eclampsia—hypertension; edema of the hands, face, and legs; poor urine output; protein in the urine; and possibly seizures. One in three HELLP patients will develop disseminated intravascular coagulation (DIC), a life-threatening disorder characterized by systemic blood clotting followed by severe, uncontrollable bleeding. Hypertension during pregnancy is defined as ≥ 140/90 or an increase of 30/15 from baseline. Treatment is recommended when the BP ≥ 160/100. Magnesium sulfate is the drug of choice for seizure prophylaxis and for severe preeclampsia and eclampsia. Diazepam (Valium) may be used when magnesium fails to control the seizures.

- **ABRUPTIO PLACENTAE.** Abruptio placentae is the separation of the placenta from the uterine wall. It may occur spontaneously or following trauma. It typically occurs after the twentieth week of pregnancy. The patients report vaginal bleeding, uterine cramps, and abdominal pain. Hypotension may occur secondary to blood loss. It is possible that the patient will develop DIC. Abruptio placentae accounts for 15% of fetal deaths and 5% of maternal deaths. It causes approximately 30% of all vaginal bleeding in the last half of pregnancies.

- **PLACENTA PREVIA.** Placenta previa is a common cause (approximately 20% of antepartum bleeding) of bleeding in the second half of pregnancy. Placenta previa is defined as the implantation of the placenta over the cervical os (opening). It may be discovered early in pregnancy on ultrasound. Frequently the placenta may migrate away from the cervical os. The placenta may cover all or part of the os. Patients frequently complain of painless vaginal bleeding. One in five patients will experience uterine cramping. In severe cases, hypotension may occur.

- **NONGYNECOLOGIC CAUSES OF ABDOMINAL OR PELVIC PAIN.**

    o ***Gallbladder disease.***   Gallbladder disease is common during and after pregnancy. See chapter 1 for more details.

    o ***Pulmonary embolism.***   Pregnant women are at increased risk of thromboembolic disorders, such as pulmonary embolism and deep venous thrombosis. Patients may report pleuritic upper abdominal or chest discomfort. See chapter 1 and chapter 11 for more details.

    o ***Appendicitis.***   Pregnant women will have atypical locations for the pain associated with appendicitis because the gravid uterus displaces abdominal organs. See chapter 1 for more details.

    o ***Kidney stones.***   The clinical picture for kidney stones may resemble ectopic pregnancies. See chapter 1 for more details.

    o ***Urinary tract infections and pyelonephritis.***   Urinary tract infections and pyelonephritis are infections of the lower and upper urinary tract. The presence of an infection puts the pregnancy at risk for a miscarriage. Patients typically report dysuria, urinary frequency, and urgency. Patients report back pain, flank pain, or abdominal pain. See chapter 1 for more details.

THE NONPREGNANT PATIENT

These patients are at risk for the illnesses discussed in chapter 1 in addition to some of the illnesses below.

- **GYNECOLOGIC CAUSES.**

    o **_Dysmenorrhea._** Dysmenorrhea is an unusually pain-
    ful menstruation. It typically is found either in ado-
    lescents during their first years of menstruation or in
    women of any age (often caused by endometriosis).
    The pain is described as severe, crampy suprapubic
    pain with an onset just before or at the same time
    as menses. It occurs with every period and can be
    incapacitating for 1 to 2 days. The physical exam
    reveals tenderness over the uterus. Patients are usu-
    ally treated with analgesics.

    o **_Mittelschmerz._** Mittelschmerz is a sudden midcycle
    unilateral pelvic or abdominal pain that is caused by
    the leakage of blood or fluid from the ovary at ovu-
    lation. The pain typically decreases with time. There
    may be tenderness and mild local peritoneal signs.
    There are no systemic signs or symptoms such as
    fever or shock.

    o **_Endometriosis._** Endometrial tissue, normally found
    only within the uterus, may be present outside of the
    uterus. It is responsive to the patient's cyclic hor-
    mones, causing pelvic or back pain, dysmenorrhea
    (painful menses), and dyspareunia (painful sexual
    intercourse). Fifty percent of the patients experience
    a flare-up of symptoms at menses.

    o **_Ovarian cysts._** There are several types of ovar-
    ian cysts. They can occur throughout the life of
    the patient. Patients typically complain of sudden-
    onset unilateral abdominal or pelvic pain. It can
    occur with trauma, intercourse, or a pelvic exam.
    The cysts are typically asymptomatic until they rup-
    ture, bleed, or become infected or twisted (ovarian
    torsion). Rupture can be associated with significant
    bleeding in some cases. The physical exam reveals
    tenderness and sometimes peritonitis. Uncomplicated
    cases require pain medicine and follow-up care.

o **_Ovarian torsion._**   The ovary and its supporting tissue may twist around, causing compromised blood flow. This causes ischemia and, if not rapidly diagnosed and treated, necrosis of the ovary. The ovary is typically enlarged and often has cysts. Ovarian torsion may occur during pregnancy. The patient complains of severe one-sided pain. There is frequent radiation to the back or thigh. Nausea and vomiting are common. Its presentation may be mistaken for renal colic. A surgical intervention is required.

o **_Pelvic inflammatory disease._**   PID is an acute infection of the uterus, fallopian tubes, ovaries, and adjacent tissues. If untreated, it may lead to a tuboovarian abscess. It often develops during or following menses. Patients report fever, bilateral lower abdominal pain, vaginal discharge or bleeding, nausea, and vomiting. The patient may develop inflammation of the capsule of the liver, a condition known as Fitz-Hugh-Curtis syndrome. These patients will have right upper quadrant pleuritic pain and tenderness.

o **_Tuboovarian abscess._**   Tuboovarian abscess is a complication of PID. The abscess often develops when treatment fails to resolve PID. The patient may have a palpable, tender abdominal mass. Peritonitis and sepsis may develop if the abscess ruptures.

o **_Uterine fibroids._**   Uterine fibroids, benign muscular tumors of the uterus, are common. They can cause heavy or irregular menses. They may overgrow their blood supply and become complicated by ischemia, necrosis, and bleeding. Torsion may also occur. Physical exam may reveal an enlarged, irregularly shaped uterus.

• **_NONGYNECOLOGIC CAUSE OF ABDOMINAL OR PELVIC PAIN._**

o **_Gallbladder disease._**   See chapter 1 for more details.

- o ***Pulmonary embolism.*** See chapter 1 and chapter 11 for more details.

- o ***Appendicitis.*** See chapter 1 for more details.

- o ***Kidney stones.*** The clinical picture can resemble ectopic pregnancies or ovarian torsion. See chapter 1 for more details.

- o ***Urinary tract infections and pyelonephritis.*** These are infections of the lower and upper urinary tract. Patients typically report dysuria, urinary frequency, and urgency. Patients report back pain, flank pain, or abdominal pain. See chapter 1 for more details.

KEY PHYSICAL EXAMINATION FINDINGS

- ✔ ***Initial assessment.*** Look for alterations in hemodynamic stability.

- ✔ ***Vital signs.*** Although most patients have a normal or slightly elevated heart rate, some may be bradycardic as a result of vagal stimulation. Be alert for evidence of compensated and uncompensated shock.

- ✔ ***Abdomen.*** Look for evidence of prior surgeries, hernias, and distension. Palpate for tenderness and masses. The pregnant patient may have an enlarged uterus. Be alert for signs of peritonitis—rebound tenderness, guarding, and rigidity.

- ✔ ***Extremities.*** Check for perfusion and equal pulses.

ELECTROCARDIOGRAM

Evaluate for signs of cardiac ischemia or injury.

TREATMENT PLAN

- • ***Patient assessment.*** Perform a rapid and systematic initial assessment and institute treatment as life-threatening problems are discovered. Prompt transport to the appropriate ED is a key intervention. Frequent reassessment of the patient with abdominal pain is necessary because of the potential for worsening. Consider the diagnosis of AAA in all patients over 50 years of age. Consider the diagnosis of appendicitis in all patients with an appendix. Consider the diagnosis of ectopic pregnancy in all women of childbearing age who have a uterus and ovaries.

- **Administer O$_2$ and provide ventilatory support** as needed.

- Place the patient in a position of comfort.

- **Monitor the ECG if ischemia is suspected.**

- **Establish large bore IV** access.

- Consider the following interventions:

  o **Administer 0.9% NaCl or lactated Ringer's fluid resuscitation** if the patient presents with dehydration or shock.

  o **Treat for acute coronary syndrome if present. See chapter 11.**

  o **Treat for ruptured AAA if suspected.** Establish a second large bore IV. Early notification of the receiving facility to mobilize a vascular surgeon and operating room staff may improve outcome.

- Frequently reassess the patient's hemodynamic status.

- Frequently reassess the abdomen.

- **Transport to the appropriate ED.** Ensure patient comfort en route.

SECTION 1

BIBLIOGRAPHY

Berger, K. J. (2003). Ovarian cyst/torsion. In J. J. Schaider, S. R. Hayden, R. Wolfe, R. M. Barkin, & P. Rosen (Eds.), *Rosen & Barkin's 5-minute emergency medical consult* (2nd ed., pp. 782–783). Philadelphia: Lippincott Williams & Wilkins.

Mohler, C. M. (2003). Endometriosis. In J. J. Schaider, S. R. Hayden, R. Wolfe, R. M. Barkin, & P. Rosen (Eds.), *Rosen & Barkin's 5-minute emergency medical consult* (2nd ed., pp. 364–365). Philadelphia: Lippincott Williams & Wilkins.

Ringo, P. M. & M. A. Kaufman (2001). Gynecologic causes of abdominal pain. In A. Harwood Nuss & A. B. Wolfson (Eds.), *The clinical practice of emergency medicine* (3rd ed., pp. 379–383). Philadelphia: Lippincott Williams & Wilkins.

NOTES

_____

_____

_____

_____

_____

_____

_____

_____

_____

_____

_____

_____

_____

_____

_____

CHAPTER 3

ALLERGIC REACTIONS AND ANAPHYLAXIS

Ian B. Greenwald, M.D.

PRESENTATION

Patients with allergic reactions may present with a spectrum of exam findings depending on the severity of the body's allergic response. Minor reactions are typified by diffuse hives and flushing of the skin, whereas more severe reactions are associated with airway swelling, bronchospasm, and possibly hypotension.

IMMEDIATE CONCERNS

❶ **What is the extent of airway involvement?** If the patient demonstrates signs of airway swelling or describes a sensation of difficulty swallowing or breathing, immediate efforts to blunt the patient's allergic response must be taken, including the rapid administration of subcutaneous epinephrine (1:1000), intravenous benadryl, and nebulized albuterol.

❶ **What is the patient's hemodynamic status?** If the patient is hemodynamically unstable, large-bore peripheral access should be obtained and fluid resuscitation initiated. Severe hypotension might require intravenous (IV) epinephrine (1:10,000).

IMPORTANT HISTORY

❼ **Has there been contact or exposure with a suspected allergen?** Patients should be questioned regarding exposure to substances that could have caused the symptoms. Because anaphylaxis is typically an immediate systemic reaction to an exogenous stimulus, the patients can frequently detail the exposure (e.g., bee or wasp sting, food allergy, drug reaction).

❷ **Is there a history of allergic reactions?** If the history is positive, determine the extent of the previous reactions. A previous true anaphylactic reaction should greatly heighten surveillance for airway and hemodynamic compromise. Because of the nature of hypersensitivity reactions, even a minor reaction in the past, might herald a severe impending reaction.

❷ **Is the patient taking any medication?** Patients on beta blockers may be resistant to treatment with epinephrine and may develop refractory hypotension and bradycardia. Glucagon has nonbeta-receptor mediated effects on heart rate and contractility and should be administered in a 1 mg IV bolus dose for patients with hemodynamic or airway compromise.

DIFFERENTIAL DIAGNOSIS

- ***ALLERGIC REACTION.*** An allergic reaction is a mild reaction, caused by histamine release, that does not cause life-threatening hypotension or airway or breathing problems. Itchy rashes and swelling are typical complaints. These reactions develop more gradually than anaphylaxis, making the allergen difficult to identify. The acute treatment may only require antihistamines.

- ***ANAPHYLACTIC REACTION.*** Anaphylactic reaction is a systemic allergic IgE-mediated hypersensitivity reaction, which results in a massive release of histamine from mast cells and basophils.

- ***ANAPHYLACTOID REACTION.*** Anaphylactoid reactions, clinically indistinguishable from true anaphylaxis, occur by a nonantigen/antibody-mediated response. They also result in a massive histamine release.

- ***ASTHMA ATTACK.*** Patients who experience asthma attacks typically have a history of asthma and generally will not be hypotensive. Albuterol and epinephrine may be beneficial therapies.

* ***HEREDITARY OR DRUG-INDUCED ANGIOEDEMA.*** A nonmast cell (nonhistamine-) mediated spectrum of illnesses caused by either a deficiency in a blood protein (C1-inhibitor protein) or an idiopathic reaction to a medication (usually ACE inhibitor or NSAID). There is prominent airway swelling but no other manifestations of an allergic response (i.e., no hives, wheezing, or hypotension).

* ***"RESTAURANT SYNDROMES."*** Certain foods contain histamine-like substances—monosodium glutamate (MSG) in Asian cooking; sulfites in smoked foods; scrombroid, a type of fish—that can trigger diffuse itching and erythema to the skin. These reactions are usually not associated with airway or hemodynamic issues.

SECTION 1

KEY PHYSICAL EXAMINATION FINDINGS

* **Initial assessment.** Look for signs of shock or respiratory distress.

* **Vital signs.** Include pulse oximetry if available.

* **HEENT.** Inspect airway for evidence of edema (including lips, tongue, posterior pharynx).

* **Skin.** Inspect for erythema or hives.

* **Lungs.** Listen for wheezing or diminished breath sounds.

TREATMENT PLAN

* ***Patient assessment.*** Frequent reassessment is necessary because of the risk of airway compromise and hemodynamic instability. Cardiac monitoring should be initiated for patients over the age of 40 who are receiving epinephrine or who have a previous cardiac history.

* **Administer O$_2$ and provide ventilatory support as needed. Consider intubation early.**

- Administer **epinephrine 1:1000 0.3-0.5 mg SQ,** repeated every 10 to 15 minutes, if needed (pediatric dose 0.01 mg/kg, not to exceed 0.5 mg) if the patient is hemodynamically stable, or

- Administer **epinephrine 1:10,000 0.3-0.5 mg IV,** repeated every 5 to 10 minutes, if needed, (pediatric dose 0.01 mg/kg, not to exceed 0.5 mg) if the patient is hemodynamically unstable.

- Hemodynamically unstable patients should be placed in the shock position.

- **Rapidly establish IV access** with large-bore needle and begin fluid resuscitation with 0.9% NaCl or LR.

- Administer diphenhydramine **(Benadryl) 25 to 50 mg slow IV push or IM** injection (pediatric dose 1 to 2 mg/kg IV or IM, not to exceed 50 mg).

- Administer **albuterol 2.5 to 5 mg via nebulizer, may be repeated prn.**

- Administer **methylprednisolone (Solumedrol) 125 mg IVP** (pediatric dose 1 to 2 mg/kg, maximum 125 mg).

- Administer **glucagon 1 to 2 mg IV** if the patient taking beta blockers or calcium channel blockers does not respond to epinephrine.

- **Transport** patient to appropriate ED.

BIBLIOGRAPHY

Atkinson, T. P., & Kaliner, M. A. (1992). Anaphylaxis. *Medical Clinics of North America, 76,* 841–855.

Sean-Xavier, N. (2003). Anaphylaxis. In J. J. Schaider, S. R. Hayden, R. Wolfe, R. M. Barkin, & P. Rosen (Eds.), *Rosen & Barkin's 5-minute emergency medicine consult* (2nd ed., pp. 66–67). Philadelphia: Lippincott Williams & Wilkins.

Winbery, S. L., & Lieberman, P. L. (1995). Anaphylaxis. *Immunology and Allergy Clinics of North America, 15*, 447–475.

NOTES

_____

_____

_____

_____

_____

_____

_____

_____

_____

_____

_____

_____

_____

_____

_____

_____

_____

_____

_____

_____

CHAPTER 4

ALTERED MENTAL STATUS

Owen T. Traynor, M.D.

PRESENTATION

Paramedics are frequently called to care for patients with an altered mental status. At times the cause of the illness will be obvious, as in the case of hypoglycemic patients and those with opiate overdoses, or obscure, as in cases of elderly patients who cannot provide meaningful information about their illness. This chapter focuses primarily on nontraumatic causes of an altered mental status. Head injuries are covered in great detail in chapter 20. Strokes and TIAs are also covered in chapter 10.

IMMEDIATE CONCERNS

❶ **Is the patient's airway secure?** Patients with an altered level of consciousness (LOC) may not be able to protect their airway. In addition, an airway that is not patent may be responsible for the decreased mental status. Basic and advanced airway management may be needed. If the etiology of the altered level of consciousness (LOC) is quickly reversible (as, for example, with hypoglycemia or narcotic overdoses), advanced airway management may not be needed.

❶ **Does the patient have adequate respirations?** Hypoventilation or hypoxia may be either the cause or the sequela of an altered mental status. Supplemental oxygen or advanced airway management should be employed as needed.

❶ **Is there evidence of poor perfusion?** The brain is sensitive to poor perfusion. Treatment for shock should be initiated if there is poor perfusion.

❶ **Is there evidence of trauma?**   Patients who suffer major trauma are likely to require cervical spine immobilization. Advanced airway management and fluid resuscitation may be needed. Expeditious transport to a trauma center is recommended. See chapter 20.

IMPORTANT HISTORY

❷ **Is there a history of diabetes?** Hypoglycemia is one of the most common reasons that diabetic patients require emergency medical services (EMS) assistance. The patient typically has an altered mental status and is diaphoretic. A glucometer reading can confirm the diagnosis. Dextrose containing solutions may be given orally (if the patient is alert enough to drink) or intravenously. If administration of dextrose is not possible, glucagon may be given via IM injection. Hyperglycemia can also cause an altered LOC but is not as quickly remedied. See chapter 14 for further information.

❷ **Is there a possibility of narcotic overdose?**   Patients with narcotic or opiate overdose present with CNS depression—decreased respirations, decreased LOC, often bradycardia and hypotension, and commonly constricted pupils. Naloxone (Narcan) is a competitive antagonist and may reverse the effects of the narcotic. In general, the desired goal is to improve the respiratory rate. Naloxone may precipitate a withdrawal syndrome in narcotic dependent patients. If narcotic dependence is suspected, slowly administer a lower dose of naloxone.

❷ **Is a stroke suspected?**   Although many patients suffering a cerebrovascular accident (CVA) have a normal mental status, some may have an altered LOC. Look for focal neurologic deficits. Typically the deficits are unilateral, not bilateral. If a CVA is suspected, note the time of onset of symptoms or the last time the patient was at usual baseline. Thrombolytic therapy for ischemic strokes must be initiated within 3 hours of onset. See chapter 10.

❷ **Is an acute intracranial hemorrhage suspected?**   The sudden onset of "the worst headache" of the patient's life may indicate an acute subarachnoid hemorrhage. These patients may rapidly deteriorate. Advanced airway management may be required. A computed tomography (CT) scan of the brain is used to make the diagnosis. Neurosurgical intervention may be required. Rapid transport to the appropriate ED is recommended. See chapter 19 for additional details.

❷ **Did the patient have a seizure?**   Witnesses may provide a description of a complex seizure—that is, tonic and clonic motor activity, irregular breathing, incontinence, and a postictal period. The patient may be able to report a past medical history of a seizure disorder. Chapter 37 provides more details regarding seizures. The patient often needs only observation and transport to the appropriate ED. Benzodiazepines, such as diazepam (Valium) or lorazepam (Ativan) may be used if there is status epilepticus or additional seizures.

❷ **Did the patient have a syncopal episode?**   A transient loss of consciousness with full recovery should prompt the consideration of syncope. Discover the circumstances surrounding the event. The physical exam is often unremarkable. Diagnostic tests such as an ECG, glucometer reading, and pulse oximetry should be performed.

❷ **What medications is the patient taking?**   Identifying the medication list may provide clues to the past medical history. Suggest medications as a potential cause of the altered mental status.

❷ **Is substance abuse suspected?**   Alcohol and other drugs may cause an altered mental status. The odor of alcohol on the breath accompanied by slurred speech and ataxia may suggest alcohol intoxication. Be careful, however: People who have alcohol on their breath may harbor another occult illness. Be especially alert for head injuries, hypoglycemia, and hypothermia.

DIFFERENTIAL DIAGNOSIS

- **CENTRAL NERVOUS SYSTEM ETIOLOGIES.**

  o **Acute CVA.** Strokes can be classified as hemorrhagic or ischemic. Typical features include unilateral neurologic deficits. Signs and symptoms can be dynamic. Frequent reassessment is indicated. Make a strong effort to note the time of onset or, if this is not possible, the time the patient was last at baseline. Thrombolytic therapy may only be used if indicated and if the evaluation can be completed within 3 hours of onset. Early notification of the receiving ED can speed the ED evaluation phase. Hypoglycemic patients sometimes present with focal neurologic findings. Perform a blood glucose determination on all patients who have experienced a CVA.

  o **Acute intracranial hemorrhage.** Patients with acute intracranial hemorrhage may bleed from a cerebral aneurysm or an arteriovenous malformation (abnormal tangle of blood vessels). The patient may complain of a severe "thunderclap, worst headache of my life" type of pain often accompanied by nausea and vomiting. Acute intracranial hemorrhage is a life-threatening illness that may rapidly progress. There may be few neurologic deficits initially. Advanced airway management may be needed. Neurosurgical intervention is often needed.

  o **Seizure.** Although there are many etiologies of seizures, the most common is epilepsy. In epilepsy no identifiable cause is identified. Most patients can achieve good control of their seizures by being compliant with their medication regimen. Seizures may occur when the patient's antiseizure medications are subtherapeutic. Seizures may also occur as a component of alcohol withdrawal syndrome. EMS treatment consists of protecting the patient from injury, preventing or treating hypoxia, and observing

FAST exam

the patient's symptoms. Some patients may require benzodiazepines to halt a prolonged seizure or treat recurrent seizures or status epilepticus. Treat hypoglycemia, if present.

o **_Tumors._** Primary or metastatic brain tumors may cause an altered LOC with or without obvious focal neurologic findings. Symptoms may develop as the tumor compresses adjacent tissue or secondary to edema or bleeding of the tumor. Often the patient complains of new onset headaches.

• **_TOXICOLOGIC ETIOLOGIES._** Select toxins are noted below. See chapter 34 for additional toxicology information.

o **_Ethanol and other alcohols._** Ethanol is the most commonly abused alcohol that EMS personnel will confront. Typical clinical features include sedation, slurred speech, and ataxia. Patients can be agitated and uncooperative. The LOC decreases as the blood alcohol level increases. Be alert for other occult illnesses or injuries when considering "obvious" alcohol intoxication.

o **_Opiates/narcotics._** The prototypical EMS opiate overdose occurs with the IV heroin user. The patient has constricted pupils; slow, snoring respirations; and a depressed mental status. At times, drug paraphernalia may be present at the scene. Needle-track marks are common in the habitual user. The goal of naloxone (Narcan) therapy is to improve the respiratory status of the patient. If there are atypical features, such as normal respirations, tachycardia, and hypertension, consider the presence of an additional drug. You may consider withholding the naloxone or giving a reduced dose to prevent waking a potentially agitated or violent patient. Naloxone may induce an acute withdrawal syndrome in dependent patients. Slowly administer a reduced dose when narcotic dependence is suspected.

o **_Carbon monoxide._** Carbon monoxide (CO), a colorless, tasteless gas, can cause an altered mental status. It is present in the environment when there is incomplete combustion. Symptoms increase as CO accumulates in the blood. Remove the patient from the environment as soon as CO poisoning is suspected. High-flow oxygen can significantly increase the elimination of CO from the blood. Patients with a serious illness may benefit from hyperbaric oxygen (HBO). Remember that the pulse oximeter's reading is the sum of the oxygen saturation plus the carbon monoxide saturation. See chapter 40 for information about CO poisoning.

o **_Drug abuse._** Chapter 34 provides a description of common toxidromes, or toxicologic syndromes.

o **_Drug withdrawal syndromes._** Consider a withdrawal syndrome when the patient has a history of substance abuse and presents with agitation, anxiety, tremors, tachycardias, and hypertension after ceasing or cutting back on the substance of abuse. Patients who are withdrawing from ethanol are at increased risk of seizures. See chapter 15.

• *INFECTIOUS ETIOLOGIES.*

o **_Meningitis._** Meningitis is typically a viral or bacterial infection of the meninges. Immunosuppressed patients may be infected by fungi. Patients present with a history of a headache, fever, and possibly nuchal rigidity (a stiff neck). The mental state may become altered as the disease progresses. Meningococcal meningitis, caused by **Neisseria meningitidis** bacteria, is associated with a petechial (small red or purple spots) or purpuric (larger red or purple spots) rash. It can be rapidly fatal, even if treated with IV antibiotics. Infants and the elderly may have less typical presentations.

o **_Encephalitis._** Encephalitis is an inflammation of the brain typically caused by a viral infection, although nonviral etiologies are possible, too. The mortality rate is approximately 10%. The incidence of West Nile virus encephalitis has recently increased in North America. Encephalitis usually begins with a flu-like illness. Patients often have a history of mild headaches, fever, body aches, and poor appetite. The disease may progress to include an altered LOC, worsening headache, vomiting, possible nuchal rigidity, seizures, coma, and death. The diagnosis may be made in the ED after an extensive evaluation.

o **_Sepsis._** Sepsis is defined as a syndrome caused by an infection and associated with a systemic inflammatory response such as fever, hypothermia, altered mental status, tachycardia, tachypnea, hypotension, and poor capillary refill. Patients may require IV fluid resuscitation if in shock and will require antibiotics in the hospital.

• **_PULMONARY ETIOLOGIES._**

o **_Hypoxia._** Many pulmonary diseases can cause hypoxia. Often the addition of supplemental oxygen will improve oxygenation. Nebulized albuterol or Atrovent may be beneficial for bronchospasm.

o **_Hypercapnia._** Patients with chronic obstructive pulmonary disease (COPD) typically develop mildly elevated carbon dioxide (CO_2) levels. This usually causes no harm and is undetectable clinically without measuring end-tidal CO_2 or an arterial blood gas. If the CO_2 levels continue to increase, the patient may become sleepy, which further decreases ventilation. Thus the CO_2 can rapidly increase. Hypoxia will occur as well. This condition can be treated with ventilation.

o **_Acute pulmonary embolism._** Large pulmonary emboli can cause syncope. Hypoxia is often present, too. EMS treatment includes supplemental oxygen and IV fluid resuscitation, if needed. See chapters 11 and 16.

- **METABOLIC ETIOLOGIES.**

  o **Hypoglycemia.** Hypoglycemia is one of the most common causes of altered mental status treated by paramedics. Typically the history reveals a rapid change in mental status in a patient with diabetes. The skin is usually pale and moist. Blood glucose determination confirms the diagnosis. Generally the patient responds rapidly to oral or IV dextrose. Response may be delayed when the patient has experienced a prolonged episode of hypoglycemia. There is a danger of recurrent and resistant hypoglycemia when patients are taking certain oral hypoglycemic agents. Transport to the hospital is recommended. Insulin-dependent patients with diabetes do not typically relapse if they eat a meal after the dextrose is administered. Close supervision and follow-up is needed when patients with diabetes refuse further care and transportation. See chapter 24 for more details.

  o **Hyperglycemia.** The history is one of a gradual onset. Patients with hyperglycemia often report malaise, polyuria, polydipsia, and polyphagia. Hyperglycemia may be the initial presentation for patients with diabetes. See chapter 14.

  o **Electrolyte disorders.** Electrolyte disorders are usually not diagnosed by EMS providers because laboratory analysis of the blood is needed.

  o **Diabetic ketoacidosis and hyperosmolar hyperglycemic syndrome.** Diabetic ketoacidosis and hyperosmolar hyperglycemic syndrome have some of the features of hyperglycemia. EMS treatment involves IV fluid resuscitation. See chapter 14.

  o **Encephalopathy.** Encephalopathy is a progressive syndrome of brain dysfunction. Initially the patient may have a normal mental status but difficulty with memory and concentration. The condition may progress to confusion, impaired ability to perform mental tasks, disorientation, and coma. The many causes of encephalopathy include hypertension, liver disease, and renal failure. EMS care is supportive.

o **_Uremia._** Uremia is a clinical syndrome of metabolic abnormalities associated with electrolyte, fluid, and hormonal imbalances that occur with renal failure. It is more commonly associated with chronic renal failure than acute renal failure. The history is one of progressive decrease in the mental status, culminating in seizures, coma, and death. Patients report nausea, vomiting, anorexia, weakness and fatigue, itchiness, muscle cramps, and thirst. The physical exam can reveal a "uremic frost" on the skin (a fine residue believed to be excreted urea in sweat), a pericardial friction rub if pericarditis is present, and evidence of fluid overload (peripheral edema and possibly pulmonary edema). EMS care is supportive. Dialysis may be required.

o **_Thyroid disorders._** Both hypothyroidism and hyperthyroidism can cause an alteration in mental status. The patient with profound hypothyroidism presents with a history of fatigue, cold intolerance, difficulty with concentration, weight gain, decreased perspiration, decreased appetite, and menstrual irregularities. The physical findings include bradycardia, hypothermia, nonpitting edema, and hypotension. The altered mental status can progress to coma. Hypoglycemia and other electrolyte abnormalities may be present. Patients with severe hyperthyroidism may report palpitations, weight loss, shortness of breath, chest pain, anxiety, and heat intolerance. Physical findings may include fever, tachycardia, hypertension, CHF, tremor, and an altered mental state. Clinical features may suggest the above thyroid problems, and thyroid hormone testing will confirm the diagnosis. The EMS treatment is generally supportive.

- **ENVIRONMENTAL ETIOLOGIES.**

  o **_Heat-related emergencies._** Heat exhaustion and heat stroke are two heat-related emergencies that are associated with an alteration in mental status. Removal to a cooler environment and cooling of the patient are beneficial. Hydration is also beneficial. See chapter 23 for more details.

  o **_Hypothermia._** Changes in mental status become apparent at about 93° F (34° C). See chapter 23.

  o **_Near drowning._** A combination of hypoxia and hypercapnia can lead to a change in mental status. See chapter 31.

- **VASCULAR ETIOLOGIES.**

  o **_Hypertensive encephalopathy._** Hypertensive encephalopathy is an acute, life-threatening alteration in central nervous system (CNS) function caused by hypertension. Common findings include headache, vision changes, altered mental status, and/or neurologic deficits. Although cerebral blood flow remains constant over a wide range of mean arterial blood pressure (MAP) readings, at very high blood pressure levels the cerebral blood flow increases as well. As cerebral blood flow continues to increase, the blood-brain barrier becomes damaged, allowing cerebral edema to develop. This results in decreased blood flow in the brain. Safe reduction in MAP is best accomplished gradually with medications that can be titrated. See chapter 22.

  o **_Hypotension._** The brain is sensitive to the poor perfusion that accompanies hypotension. See chapter 25.

- **_Traumatic etiologies._** Traumatic brain injuries are presented in chapter 20.

SECTION 1

KEY PHYSICAL EXAMINATION FINDINGS

- ✓ ***Initial assessment.*** Look for alterations in mental status, threats to the airway, respiratory compromise, and hemodynamic instability.

- ✓ ***Vital signs.*** Careful monitoring of the vital signs is needed.

- ✓ ***HEENT.*** Examine carefully and note signs of trauma or asymmetry. Examine pupils for responsiveness and equality.

- ✓ ***Neck.*** Assess the neck for trauma. Assess for nuchal rigidity if this is a nontraumatic illness.

- ✓ ***Lungs.*** Listen to lung sounds for signs of pulmonary edema, bronchospasm, or pneumonia.

- ✓ ***Heart.*** Assess for pericardial friction rub.

- ✓ ***Abdomen.*** Assess carefully for masses, tenderness, and peritoneal signs.

- ✓ ***Extremities.*** Assess for edema in the extremities. Check peripheral pulses to equality. Inspect for needle-track marks.

- ✓ ***Skin.*** Assess for rashes.

- ✓ ***Neurologic examination.*** An altered mental status is a sensitive indicator of cerebral perfusion. Assess cranial nerves, and perform a motor and sensory examination. Unilateral deficits may be present in CVAs.

ELECTROCARDIOGRAM

Evaluate for signs of arrhythmias, cardiac ischemia, or injury.

GLUCOMETER

Evaluate for hypoglycemia or hyperglycemia.

PULSE OXIMETER

Evaluate for hypoxia.

TREATMENT PLAN

- ***Patient assessment.*** Perform a rapid and systematic initial assessment, and institute treatment as life-threatening problems are discovered. Prompt transport to the appropriate ED is a key intervention. Frequent reassessment of the patient with an altered mental status is necessary because of the potential for worsening of neurologic status.

GENERAL TREATMENT GUIDELINES

- **Administer O_2 and provide ventilatory support** as needed.

- Elevate the patient's head, unless spinal immobilization is needed, or place the patient in the shock position if shock is present.

- **Monitor the ECG and O_2 saturation. Perform blood glucose determination.**

- **Establish IV** access.

- **Consider the following interventions, if indicated:**

  o **Administer oral glucose** solution in an awake patient with an intact gag reflex.

  o **Administer dextrose 50%, 25 g IV** (pediatric dose, D25 [dilute D50 1:1 with NS or sterile water] 1-2 mL/kg IV, infant dose, D10 [dilute D50 1:4 with NS or sterile water] 2-4 mL/kg IV). The dose may be repeated if there is insufficient improvement.

  o **Administer glucagon 1 mg IM** (pediatric dose 0.1 mg/kg IM, maximum 1 mg) if there is no IV access. Repeat the dose in 10 to 30 minutes if needed. As mental status improves, you may give an oral glucose solution.

- **Naloxone (Narcan) 0.4-2 mg IV,** IM or SC (pediatric dose, 0.01 mg/kg IV, IM, or SC, maximum 2 mg). The dose may be repeated as necessary.

- Frequently reassess the patient's airway and hemodynamic and neurologic status.

- **Transport to the appropriate ED.** Ensure patient comfort en route.

DIAGNOSIS-SPECIFIC TREATMENT GUIDELINES

- Acute CVA. See chapter 10.

- Acute intracranial hemorrhage. See chapter 10.

- Seizures. See chapter 37.

- Carbon monoxide poisoning. See chapter 40.

- Drug withdrawal syndromes. See chapter 15.

- Sepsis. See chapter 38.

- Hyperglycemia. See chapter 14.

- Heat-related emergencies. See chapter 23.

- Hypothermia. See chapter 26.

- Hypertensive encephalopathy. See chapter 22.

- Hypotension. See chapter 25.

- Traumatic head injuries. See chapter 20.

BIBLIOGRAPHY

Bhatia, K., & Brown, D. F. (2003). Altered mental status. In J. J. Schaider, S. R. Hayden, R. Wolfe, R. M. Barkin, & P. Rosen (Eds.), *Rosen & Barkin's 5-minute emergency medical consult* (2nd ed., pp. 52–53). Philadelphia: Lippincott Williams & Wilkins.

Kelley, S.D., & Saperston, A. (2004). Coma. In C. K. Stone & R. L. Humphries (Eds.), *Current emergency diagnosis and treatment* (5th ed., pp. 311–331). New York: McGraw-Hill.

Seip, R. A., Martin, M. L., & Thomas, S. H. (2001). Approach to coma and transient loss of consciousness. In A. Harwood-Nuss, A. B. Wolfson, C. H. Linden, S. M. Shepard, & P. H. Stencklyft (Eds.), *The clinical practice of emergency medicine* (3rd ed., pp. 31–35). Philadelphia: Lippincott Williams & Wilkins.

NOTES

SECTION 1

CHAPTER 5

BITES, STINGS, AND ENVENOMATIONS

Kenneth D. Katz, M.D.

PRESENTATION

The envenomated patient may present in many ways, but most commonly there is a history of a witnessed bite or sting with ensuing clinical effects. Depending on the particular toxin involved, the patient may experience signs and symptoms ranging from mild (e.g., localized pain, swelling, bleeding) to life-threatening (e.g., profuse bleeding, hypotension, shock, anaphylaxis, and airway compromise)

IMMEDIATE CONCERNS

❶ **Is there immediate danger to the patient or prehospital personnel?**   Sometimes, the venomous creature may still be present when rescuers arrive. Prehospital personnel should ensure that the scene is secured before rescue is attempted. In no instance should a snake be captured or killed for identification purposes. Furthermore, decapitated snakes may still envenomate.

❶ **Is the airway patent, and what is the hemodynamic status?**   Regardless of the specific envenomation, patients presenting in extremis with respiratory compromise or cardiovascular instability require immediate resuscitation. Standard treatment of hemorrhage, shock, anaphylaxis, or respiratory failure should be initiated.

IMPORTANT HISTORY

❷ **What toxin is involved?**   Usually, the patient or witness can identify the particular insect or animal involved. If not, the environment or locale in which the patient is found may offer diagnostic clues.

❷ **Is there associated trauma or environmental exposure?** Patients may also experience associated trauma or environmental exposure during or after envenomation (e.g., hypothermia, drowning).

❷ **What is the medical history?** It is important to determine whether the patient has been previously envenomated, and, if so, what reaction occurred (e.g., anaphylaxis). Any pulmonary, cardiovascular, or allergic disease (e.g., asthma, angina) should be noted.

❷ **What are the patient's medications, allergies?** What is the tetanus status? A medication list should be procured, highlighting antihypertensives (especially beta blockers), cardiovascular drugs (e.g., nitroglycerin, warfarin), and allergy agents and bronchodilators. Patient allergies and tetanus immunization should be recorded.

DIFFERENTIAL DIAGNOSIS

- **CROTALINAE *SNAKE BITES.*** *Crotalinae* snakes, which include rattlesnakes, copperheads, and cottonmouths, live in many regions of the U.S. Envenomation is characterized by a exquisitely painful bite with fang marks, localized bleeding, swelling, ecchymosis, and tissue necrosis. Patients may experience nausea, vomiting, or hypotension. Shock, anaphylaxis, and disseminated intravascular coagulation (DIC), a condition resulting from the massive consumption of clotting factors that leads to uncontrolled bleeding, are rare.

- **LATRODECTUS *SPIDER BITES.*** The *Latrodectus* genus includes the black widow spider. The spiders are found in many regions of the U.S. and live in dark areas such as barns and woodpiles. Patients present with a painful, erythematous papule (small raised bump) with visible punctum (puncture site). Signs and symptoms of significant envenomation may include nausea, vomiting, diaphoresis, salivation, muscle spasm and rigidity, premature labor, and severe hypertension.

- **CENTRUROIDES *SCORPION STINGS*.** The bark scorpion, or *Centruroides* scorpion, is found in the Southwest U.S., and its sting usually causes only localized pain *without a visible wound*. However, tapping the involved area elicits pain ("tap sign"). Severe systemic manifestations are usually seen in either children or elderly people and include fasciculations, cranial nerve dysfunction, difficulty swallowing, and hypersalivation.

- **HYMENOPTERA *STINGS*.** Members of the *Hymenoptera* order include bees, hornets, wasps, yellow jackets, and fire ants. Patients may present in several ways: with a localized, erythematous papule; a generalized urticarial rash; anaphylaxis; or rhabdomyolysis (multiple stings). Stingers may be found embedded in the skin. Found in the Southwest U.S., "Africanized bees" ("killer bees") are more aggressive, frequently swarm, and chase victims compared with typical *Hymenoptera*.

- **COELENTERATA *STINGS*.** Members of the *Coelenterata* phylum include jellyfish, anemones, and corals. Victims commonly develop a localized, painful papule. However, moderate to severe envenomations (e.g., from box jellyfish, Portuguese Man of War) can result in skin necrosis, muscle spasm, delirium, convulsions, anaphylaxis, and cardiovascular collapse. Drowning may co mpound the clinical situation.

- ***STINGRAY ENVENOMATIONS*.** Found in warm waters, the stingray is the most commonly implicated fish involved in human envenomations. A venomous spine is jabbed into the victim, creating both a toxic and traumatic wound. Patients experience localized pain, bleeding, and edema with a strong propensity for bacterial infection. A spine may be embedded in the wound. Severe systemic manifestations may include nausea, diaphoresis, syncope, muscle cramps, paralysis, and cardiac arrhythmias.

- **SCORPAENIDAE *STINGS*.** Members of the *Scorpaenidae* family include the scorpionfish, lionfish, zebrafish, and stonefish. Beautiful warm-water bottom-dwellers, these fish possess venomous spines that can cause mild (e.g., lionfish), moderate (e.g., scorpionfish), or severe (e.g., stonefish) envenomation. Common clinical manifestations include intense localized pain, erythema, and vesicle formation. Severe envenomations may involve nausea, vomiting, diaphoresis, delirium, seizures, hypertension, and cardiopulmonary arrest.

KEY PHYSICAL EXAMINATION FINDINGS

SECTION 1

- ⊘ **Initial assessment.**   Note presence of shock, anaphylaxis, or severe bleeding.

- ⊘ **Vital signs.**   Pay close attention to pulse, blood pressure, and pulse oximetry.

- ⊘ **HEENT.**   Examine for oropharyngeal swelling, loss of pharyngeal control, hypersalivation, or stridor.

- ⊘ **Chest.**   Note presence of prolonged expiratory phase, wheezing, or poor air movement.

- ⊘ **Extremities.**   Check for bleeding, wounds, presence of venom apparatus, or trauma.

- ⊘ **Skin.**   Note presence of hives, erythema, cyanosis, or mottling.

TREATMENT PLAN

- *Patient assessment.*   The envenomated patient requires frequent reassessment because of the potential for rapid, progressive clinical deterioration. All patients with severe bleeding, shock, anaphylaxis, or respiratory compromise should be treated aggressively with standard measures. Medical command and regional poison center should **always** be consulted for specific treatment recommendations; it is beyond the scope of this chapter to address all possible clinical scenarios, especially with such varied toxins.

CRITICALLY ILL PATIENTS

- **Administer 100% O$_2$ and provide ventilatory support** as needed.

- **Establish large-bore IV access** and administer normal saline solution (NSS) or lactated Ringer's (LR) solution for hypotension.

- **Control profuse bleeding.**

- **Treat anaphylaxis** with epinephrine and antihistamines. See chapter 3.

- **Address environmental exposure or associated trauma.**

- **Transport rapidly** to emergency facility for definitive therapy (e.g., antivenom).

NON CRITICALLY ILL PATIENTS

In general, most mildly envenomated patients require only local wound care, mild analgesia, and transport to an emergency facility. Some specific points are addressed below.

- **Crotalinae.** Elevate the extremity. Do not use tourniquets, suction kit, ice, or electricity.

- **Latrodectus.** Administer analgesia and sedatives for pain and muscle spasm. Calcium gluconate is ineffective.

- **Centruroides.** Apply cool compresses. Avoid use of analgesia or sedation in patients with any potential for respiratory compromise (e.g., hypersalivation, loss of pharyngeal control). These agents may depress respiratory drive and cause apnea.

- **Hymenoptera.** Apply cool compresses, remove stingers, and administer antihistamines for pruritis.

- **Coelenterates.** Local application of 5% acetic acid (vinegar) may inactivate the toxin and provide analgesia.

- **Stingray/Scorpaenidae.** Local application of nonscalding hot water (upper limit 45° C) can inactivate the heat-labile toxin and provide comfort.

BIBLIOGRAPHY

Auerbach, P. S. (2001). Envenomation by aquatic-invertebrates. In P. S. Auerbach (Ed.), Wilderness medicine (pp. 1454–1471 and pp. 1488–1497). Philadelphia: Mosby.

Auerbach, P. S., Donner, H. J., & Weiss, E. A. (2003). Bites and stings from arthropods. In P. S. Auerbach, H. S. Donner, & E. A. Weiss, Field guide to wilderness medicine (pp. 272–275 and pp. 294–296). Philadelphia: Mosby.

Hahn, I. H., & Lewin, N. A. (2002). Arthropods. In L. R. Goldfrank, N. E. Flomenbaum, N. A. Lewin, M. A. Howland, R. S. Hoffman, & L. S. Nelson (Eds.), Goldfrank's toxicologic emergencies (pp. 1574–1577). New York: McGraw-Hill.

Norris, R. L., & Bush, S. P. (2001). North American venomous reptile bites. In P. S. Auerbach (Ed.), Wilderness medicine (pp. 896–922). Philadelphia: Mosby.

SECTION 1

NOTES

_____

_____

_____

_____

_____

_____

_____

_____

CHAPTER 6

BRADYCARDIA

Owen T. Traynor, M.D.

PRESENTATION

The adult patient with a pulse rate of less than 60 bpm may be considered bradycardic. Bradycardia may be a normal physiologic finding, as in the well-conditioned athlete, or pathologic, causing syncope, hypotension, or heart failure.

IMMEDIATE CONCERNS

❶ **What is the patient's hemodynamic status?** If the patient is hemodynamically unstable, immediate resuscitation is warranted, including oxygen administration, IV access, IV medications, and possibly pacing. Patients with bradycardia caused by central nervous system (CNS) injury and increased intracranial pressure (ICP) may need to be hyperventilated.

IMPORTANT HISTORY

❷ **Is the patient symptomatic?** Bradycardia may lead to inadequate cardiac output, resulting in the following common complaints: chest pain, dyspnea, fatigue, syncope, dizziness, and neurologic deficits. Chest pain may be either the result of a myocardial infarction (MI), which may be causing the bradycardia, or the consequence of poor coronary perfusion caused by the bradycardia. Asymptomatic patients require less aggressive immediate therapy.

❷ **Is the patient taking any medication?** Many medications, particularly beta-adrenergic blockers, calcium channel blockers, clonidine, and antiarrhythmic agents such as digitalis, can cause bradycardia.

❷ **Is there a history of hypothyroidism?** The thyroid hormones must be present in sufficient amounts for the hormones of the sympathetic nervous system to function properly. Therefore hypothyroidism may lead to bradycardia.

❷ **Is the patient hypothermic?** Hypothermia can cause conduction abnormalities and myocardial irritability (see chapter 26).

❷ **Does the patient have a pacemaker?** Pacemakers are often implanted to treat bradycardias and heart blocks. Pacemaker failure may lead to the return of the rhythm disturbance.

DIFFERENTIAL DIAGNOSIS

- *SINUS BRADYCARDIA.* Sinus bradycardia can result from increased vagal tone, decreased sympathetic tone, and pathologic changes to the sinus node. It may occur in the well-trained athlete also. Increased ICP, cervical tumors, mediastinal tumors, hypothyroidism, hypothermia, severe hypoxia, and certain medications (see previous discussion) can cause sinus bradycardia as well. Sinus bradycardia occurs in 10% to 15% of patients with acute MI and more commonly in inferior wall MIs than in anterior wall MIs. It is usually transient. Sinus bradycardia has been noted during reperfusion with thrombolytics.

- *SINUS PAUSE OR ARREST.* Sinus pause or arrest is identified by a pause in the sinus rhythm. The PP interval of the pause is not a multiple of the PP interval of the underlying sinus rhythm. It may result in episodes of ventricular asystole if no latent pacemakers initiate an escape rhythm. These are usually of little significance unless there are no escape beats.

- **SINOATRIAL EXIT BLOCK PAUSE.** Sinoatrial exit block pause occurs secondary to the absence of the normally expected P wave. The duration of the pause is a multiple of the PP interval of the underlying sinus rhythm. It is usually transient and of little significance.

- **WANDERING ATRIAL PACEMAKER.** A wandering atrial pacemaker results in the transfer of the dominant pacemaker focus from the SA node to other supraventricular pacemaker sites with the next highest level of automaticity. Characterized by more than two P wave morphologies, it can be normal in young, healthy athletes. Persistence of atrioventricular (AV) junctional rhythms for extended periods may indicate underlying heart disease. Treatment is usually not necessary.

- **HYPERSENSITIVE CAROTID SINUS SYNDROME.** Hypersensitive carotid sinus syndrome develops as a result of direct pressure or extension on the carotid sinus from head turning, neck tension, or tight collars and can cause syncope by stimulation of a hypersensitive carotid sinus. The syndrome is usually characterized by asystole secondary to cessation of atrial activity from sinus exit block or sinus arrest. AV blocks may also occur. There are two types:

  o **Cardioinhibitory carotid sinus hypersensitivity,** characterized by periods of asystole

  o **Vasodepressor carotid sinus hypersensitivity,** characterized by a decrease in the systolic BP of 50 mm Hg or more without associated cardiac slowing, or a decrease in the systolic BP of 30 mm Hg or with cardiac slowing

- **SICK SINUS SYNDROME** is a sinoatrial (SA) node abnormality that includes persistent spontaneous inappropriate sinus bradycardia, episodes of sinus arrest or sinus exit block, a combination of SA or AV node conduction anomalies, or an alteration of periods of paroxysmal atrial tachycardias with slow atrial and ventricular rhythms. This is also known as the bradycardia tachycardia syndrome.

- **AV BLOCKS**

  o **First degree AV block**—Each P wave is conducted. The PR interval is greater than 0.20 seconds. Increased vagal tone or an acceleration of the atrial rate may convert first degree AV block into second degree AV block type I.

  o **Second degree AV block type I**—PR intervals increase until a P wave is not conducted. Second degree AV block type I with normal QRS complexes is not likely to progress to complete heart block.

  o **Second degree AV block type II**—P waves are not consistently conducted; however, PR intervals are constant. Second degree AV block type II may progress to complete heart block. In the context of an anterior wall MI, second degree AV block type II may require either temporary or permanent pacing. It is associated with increased mortality, generally the result of pump failure.

  o **Third degree AV block**—No atrial activity is conducted to the ventricles. The most common causes in adults are drug toxicity and coronary artery disease.

KEY PHYSICAL EXAMINATION FINDINGS

✓ *Initial assessment.* Look for signs of shock.

✓ *Vital signs.* Assess for hypotension. The presence of hypertension and bradycardia in a patient with an altered mental state may indicate increasing ICP and CNS injury.

✓ *Lungs.* Listen for rales, which, if present, indicate CHF.

✓ *Heart.* Listen for gallop rhythm.

✓ *Mental status.* Monitor mental status; inadequate perfusion can cause an altered mental status.

ELECTROCARDIOGRAM

The ECG is an important diagnostic tool that will help determine therapy.

SECTION 1

TREATMENT PLAN

- *Patient assessment.* Frequent reassessment of the patient is necessary because of the potential for a worsening of hemodynamic status and CHF. Cardiac monitoring is necessary. Be prepared: The potential for cardiac arrest exists. Treat for an MI if the bradycardia is occurring in the context of a myocardial infarction.

HEMODYNAMICALLY STABLE PATIENT

- Administer O_2 and **provide ventilatory support** as needed.

- Have an external pacemaker standing by.

- **Transport to appropriate ED.** Continue to reassess the patient's ECG and hemodynamic status.

- Ensure patient comfort en route.

HEMODYNAMICALLY UNSTABLE PATIENT

- Administer O_2 and **provide ventilatory support** as needed. Monitor O_2 saturation with pulse oximetry if available.

- Place patient in the **supine position with legs elevated** unless pulmonary edema is present.

- Establish **IV access** with 0.9% NaCL or LR.

First line therapy includes

- **Atropine 0.5 to 1.0 mg IV bolus.** Dosage may be repeated every 3 to 5 minutes as needed to a maximum dose of 0.04 mg/kg.

- **Transcutaneous pacing (TCP).** Use sedation as needed. Do not delay TCP in symptomatic patients to establish IV access or to wait for atropine to work.

Consider the following options when the above therapies are ineffective:

- **Dopamine, 5 to 20 µg/kg** per minute infusion

  or

- **Epinephrine, 2 to 10 µg** per minute infusion

- **Transport to appropriate ED.** Continue to reassess the patient's ECG and hemodynamic status.

PATIENTS WITH BRADYCARDIA SECONDARY TO CNS INJURY

See chapter 20.

HYPOTHERMIC PATIENTS WITH BRADYCARDIA

- Treat as a hypothermic patient (see chapter 26).

NOTE: Use extreme caution when using lidocaine in the presence of bradycardia. Use of lidocaine in the presence of a ventricular escape rhythm may lead to asystole.

BIBLIOGRAPHY

Hazinski, M. F., R. O. Cummins, & J. M. Field (Eds.) (2000), *2000 Handbook of Emergency Cardiovascular Care for Healthcare Providers,* Dallas TX: American Heart Association.

McKay, M. P., Bradyarrhythmias. In J. J. Schaider, S. R. Hayden, R. Wolfe, R. M. Barkin, & P. Rosen (Eds.), *Rosen & Barkin's 5-Minute Emergency Medicine Consult,* (2nd ed., pp. 160–161), Philadelphia: Lippincott Williams & Wilkins.

NOTES

_____

_____

_____

_____

CHAPTER 7

BURNS

Michael Baumann, M.D.

PRESENTATION

The patient with burns may present in many different ways, depending on the type of burn severity and complexity of the burn injury. Burns may be chemical or thermal and range from a superficial burn (i.e., first degree such as sunburn), which results only in mild discomfort, to a full-thickness burn (third degree), which results in large amounts of charred and destroyed tissue. Initial attention should be directed to the systemic care of the burn patient.

IMMEDIATE CONCERNS

● **Is the scene safe?** Do not become a patient yourself. Watch for unsafe situations at the scene of chemical accidents and fires. Contact support agencies, such as the fire department, police department, and utility companies, if such services are required.

● **Stop the burning process!** The patient with thermal burns is best cooled only in the first minutes after injury. After several minutes the burn is not advancing, and excessively cooling the patient may cause profound hypothermia. Hypothermia is dangerous because it shifts the patient's metabolism to a catabolic metabolism, one in which tissues are being broken down to create heat to warm the patient, leading to an increased mortality.

● **What is the patient's airway and respiratory status?** If the patient has been exposed to fire or smoke, ensure adequate ventilation and oxygenation. The most immediate threat to life is inhalation injury. These injuries are secondary to superheated gas, steam, smoke, or other toxic fumes. The diagnosis is made on clinical criteria. Airway management is the priority with any patient. Carbon monoxide and other products of combustion can impair oxygenation; high-flow oxygen is indicated.

● **Is the patient hemodynamically stable?** Large burns can cause significant loss of blood volume. In addition, severely burned patients may have other serious injuries that may cause hypovolemic shock. A large-bore IV fluid infusion can help prevent hemodynamic compromise.

IMPORTANT HISTORY

❷ **Did the patient lose consciousness?** This finding along with the physical findings of circumoral burns; intraoral burns; singed facial hair; singed nasal hair; and the development of hoarseness, wheezing, dyspnea, a rasping cough, or hemoptysis leads to a diagnosis of a probable pulmonary injury. Other indicators of pulmonary injury include history of burning in an enclosed space. Early recognition is important, because pulmonary injury may lead to a significant oxygenation-perfusion defect and complete respiratory failure. In general, 95% of patients with inhalation injuries have associated burns of the neck and face. However, the presence of these injuries does not mean that the patient necessarily has an inhalation injury.

❷ **What is the history of the event?** Burns caused by a wide variety of agents have the same effect on the layers of the skin but are approached differently in treatment. The extent and ultimate depth of burn depends on both the nature and the length of exposure. This is especially true for chemical burns.

❷ **What is the patient's chief complaint?** It may not be the burn. Do not let a surface burn distract from a thorough search for other injuries. Obtain a complete medical history, and perform a thorough physical examination.

❷ **Were there other hazardous conditions?** Fire, steam, and many chemicals or vapors can cause inhalation injury in addition to a surface burn. In addition, there may be substantial risk of exposure to hazardous materials, placing healthcare workers at risk. Electrical injury can cause minor damage to the body surface, but extensive tissue destruction as well as fractures occur below the surface.

❷ **Does the patient have any underlying medical problems?** Chronic illnesses, specifically heart, kidney disease, diabetes mellitus, and pulmonary problems, can complicate the course of the patient's recuperation. Other pertinent data should be gathered, including age, weight, height, previous state of health, and medication history.

DIFFERENTIAL DIAGNOSIS

DEPTH OF BURNS

- *SUPERFICIAL (FIRST DEGREE).* These burns cause reddened, painful skin.

- *PARTIAL THICKNESS (SECOND DEGREE).* These burns are of partial thickness and involve the presence of blisters and destruction of the epidermis and dermal layers. Skin is moist and mottled.

- *FULL THICKNESS (THIRD DEGREE).* These burns involve the destruction of all layers of skin down to subcutaneous layer. Skin may be leathery, charred, and anesthetic (loss of sensation).

ETIOLOGY OF BURNS

- *CHEMICAL.* Many chemicals cause tissue destruction. Make an attempt to bring the name of the causative agent to the hospital because this information can affect treatment decisions.

- *THERMAL.* Thermal burns can be caused by any heat source: sun, stove, open flame, steam, or hot liquids.

- *ELECTRICAL.* Many sources exist for electrical burns, from household current to lightning. Electrical burns often cause severe muscle damage, resulting in rhabdomyolysis. Renal failure, secondary to the presence of muscle breakdown products in the blood, is a significant risk. Aggressive IV hydration may help limit or prevent renal failure.

- *RADIATION.* Radiation burns may not show as an external injury. These patients may present with myriad complaints and are very difficult to diagnose unless the patient gives a history of exposure to radiation or radioactive materials.

SEVERITY OF BURNS

- *CRITICAL BURNS*

    o Covering more than 25% of the body surface area (BSA)

    o Third degree burns covering more than 10% BSA

    o Respiratory burns

    o Burns of face, hands, feet, genitalia

    o Electric burns, deep chemical burns

    o In patients with underlying chronic disease

    o Complicated by major injury

NOTE: The extent of a burn may be determined by using the "Rule of Nines." Lund and Browder charts may be found in Appendix G.

KEY PHYSICAL EXAMINATION FINDINGS

- **Initial Assessment.** Form an initial impression of the stability of the patient, and decide whether the patient needs expedited transport. Ensure the airway is patent, and assess whether the airway is injured in any way

SECTION 1

that may cause it to become compromised. Evaluate the oxygenation status of the patient, checking pulse oximetry, work of breathing, and breath sounds. Assess the circulatory status for signs of shock, and ensure that no other injuries are contributing to the patient's status.

✅ ***Vital signs.*** Check for orthostatic vital signs owing to fluid loss. Watch for hypothermia.

✅ ***HEENT.*** Look for signs of inhalation injury: soot, burns, swelling, discoloration around or in the nares or mouth, and chemical burns to the eyes.

✅ ***Neck.*** Check for circumferential burns.

✅ ***Cardiac status.*** Monitor victims of electrical injury. These patients can have abnormal cardiac rhythms that often respond readily to intervention.

✅ ***Lungs.*** Assess breath sounds for pulmonary edema or pneumothorax.

✅ ***Skin.*** Assess skin for depth, extent, and presence of critical burns. Use the rule of nines to estimate the extent of the burn.

✅ ***Extremities.*** Check for circumferential burns, fractures, soft tissue injuries, and distal pulses.

TREATMENT PLAN

• ***Patient assessment.*** Frequent reassessment is necessary because of the potential for airway compromise and massive fluid loss. Life-threatening conditions often coexist with a large burn, including arrhythmias; long bone fractures, particularly in electrical injury; and hypovolemia in patients with extensive thermal injury. Consequently, every patient with burns warrants a complete examination and frequent reassessment. Although minor burns are usually considered a low-priority injury, burns in young and elderly patients are associated with increased morbidity and mortality.

- Provide general management of burn wounds:

    o **Put out the fire.** Remove the causative agent.

    o **Safeguard the airway,** and watch for clues to airway compromise.

    o **Provide ventilatory support.** Give high-flow oxygen, and monitor O_2 saturation with pulse oximetry if available.

    o **Ensure circulation.** Establish **large-bore IV** with **0.9% NaCl or LR.** Burn patients suffer increased loss of body fluids; therefore, they require large volumes of IV rehydration. The Parkland formula specifies that 4 cc/kg/% BSA burned of either LR or 0.9% NaCl be infused during the first 24 hours. Usually half of this amount is given during the first 8 hours, and the second half is given during the remaining 16 hours.

NOTE: Avoid insertion of the IV catheter through the burn site. Fluid resuscitation, however, is an essential component of burn care, and insertion of an IV catheter may, of necessity, be through burned tissue.

    o **Pain management.** Burns cause extreme pain, and patients often require large amounts of pain medicine. Start with morphine sulfate 2 to 4 mg IV and repeat as necessary for pain control.

    o Treat the burns, covering them with clean or sterile dressings. Because excessive use of moist dressings may cause hypothermia, it is recommended that their use be limited.

    o Remove jewelry, and elevate the patient's extremities.

    o Splint fractures.

    o Keep patient warm.

SECTION 1

- Add for electrical burns:

    o Monitor cardiac rhythm.

- Add for chemical burns:

    o Remove clothes. Promptly remove chemical from contact with skin. Dry chemicals should be brushed away and then copiously irrigated with water.

- Special cases:

    o Dry lime: brush off first, then irrigate with water.

    o Hydrofluoric acid: Hydrofluoric acid is the ingredient in some cleaning and stripping products. It can cause extensive tissue damage without any change in appearance of the skin. Because tissue damage continues without appropriate treatment, these patients should be transported quickly.

BIBLIOGRAPHY

Danks, R. R. (2003). Burn management: A comprehensive review of the epidemiology and treatment of burn victims. *Journal of EMS, 28,* 118–139.

Eldrich, R. F., Bailey, T. L., & Bill, T. J. (2002). Chemical burns. In J. A. Marx, R. S. Hockberger, & R. M. Walls (Eds.) *Rosen's Emergency medicine* (5th ed., 802–814 and 814–822). St. Louis, MO: Mosby.

Schwartz, L. R., & Chenicheri, B. (2000). Thermal burns. In J. E. Tintinalli, E. Ruiz, & R. L. Krome (Eds.), *Emergency medicine: A comprehensive study guide* (5th ed., 1281–1286). New York: McGraw-Hill.

NOTES

_____

_____

_____

CHAPTER 8

CARDIAC ARREST: ADULT

Thomas Platt, NREMT-P

PRESENTATION

By definition, patients who have experienced cardiac arrest are unresponsive, apneic, and pulseless. Several etiologies may cause this event, including lack of oxygenation, loss of oxygen-carrying capacity, failure of the heart as an adequate pump, and failure of the central nervous system.

IMMEDIATE CONCERNS

❶ **Is CPR indicated?** Cardiopulmonary resuscitation (CPR) is indicated for all patients who are apneic and pulseless if there are no contraindications. Contraindications include obvious mortal injury, the presence of rigor mortis or extreme areas of dependent lividity, and a legal living will or Do Not Resuscitate (DNR) order, which expresses the patient's wishes that CPR not be performed.

❶ **Is CPR being performed adequately?** Ensure that satisfactory compressions and ventilations are being performed. Poorly performed CPR does not facilitate the delivery of oxygen or medications.

❶ **Is the patient in ventricular fibrillation (VF) or ventricular tachycardia (VT) without a pulse?** After responsiveness is determined and the airway opened, a rapid assessment for the presence of VF or pulseless VT is critical. The sooner that the patient is defibrillated, the more likely it is that defibrillation will be successful. The "quick-look" survey is performed by applying the defibrillator paddles or pads to the patient's chest immediately. If a defibrillator is not available, chest compressions and ventilation should be initiated until the defibrillator is available. Perform a precordial thump in a witnessed arrest if a defibrillator is not immediately available. Following the diagnosis of the rhythm and defibrillation (when indicated), the next concerns are to place an airway device as soon as possible and to obtain vascular access. Confirm and secure the airway device. Primary and secondary confirmation is recommended. Use a commercial device to secure the advanced airway device. Some experts recommend placing a cervical collar and securing the patient to a long spine board to reduce endotracheal tube migration during movement of the patient.

❶ **Was the cardiac arrest caused by trauma or blood loss?** It is important to determine whether this event is primarily cardiac or if it is the result of traumatic injuries. The management of traumatic arrest differs from that of a primary cardiac event. Arrests caused by blood loss or secondary to trauma generally require fluid resuscitation and surgical intervention. An additional concern is hypothermia. The management of patients with hypothermia also differs (see chapter 26).

IMPORTANT HISTORY

❷ **Is CPR being performed adequately?** The importance of all healthcare providers having adequate knowledge and practice in the skills of basic life support (BLS) cannot be overemphasized. Without adequate ventilation and artificial circulation, the patient has no chance of survival.

DIFFERENTIAL DIAGNOSIS

Once the initial treatment priorities have been accomplished, it is important to determine the patient's rhythm and perfusion status. Identify and treat potentially treatable causes of the cardiac arrest (5 Hs and Ts).

- **H**ypovolemia

- **H**ypoxia

- **H**ydrogen ions (acidosis)

- **H**yperkalemia/hypokalemia

- **H**ypothermia

- **T**ablets (overdoses)

- **T**amponade (cardiac)

- **T**ension pneumothorax

- **T**hrombosis (acute coronary syndromes)

- **T**hrombosis (acute pulmonary embolism)

Be sure to frequently reassess for return of pulses. It is especially important to check central pulses every time the ECG changes. It is common for the ECG to change during the resuscitation.

KEY PHYSICAL EXAMINATION FINDINGS

✅ ***Initial Assessment.*** Assess the patient who is apneic and pulseless according to the criteria presented in the universal algorithm for adults.

TREATMENT PLAN

- ***Patient assessment.*** Remember to frequently reassess the patient. Any change in the patient's perfusion status or rhythm will require a change in algorithms. Always treat the patient, not the monitor.

- ***The team leader.*** If there is more than one EMS crew (i.e., BLS and advanced life support (ALS)) on the scene or multiple rescuers are present, identify a team leader early during the resuscitation effort. This person will facilitate the interventions to be followed. The team leader is responsible for interpreting the rhythms, assigning tasks to other members of the team, directing management, and anticipating changes.

- ***Communications.*** Along with the following standing orders, consultation with the medical control physician for guidance and institution of additional orders, including transportation or termination of resuscitation orders, may prove valuable in the care of the patient in cardiac arrest.

- **The algorithmic approach.** When using the American Heart Association (AHA) algorithms a number of assumptions are made: The condition in the algorithm persists, the patient remains apneic and pulseless, and compressions and ventilations are continued throughout the resuscitation effort. The use of algorithms is to aid in treating the patient; they cannot replace clinical judgment.

- **Termination of resuscitation efforts.**   Paramedics may consider termination of resuscitation efforts if the patient shows no response to therapy after an adequate trial of satisfactory advanced cardiac life support (ACLS) and BLS. Consultation with a medical command physician may be required.

THE UNIVERSAL ALGORITHM FOR ADULTS

The universal algorithm for adults provides the recommended initial approach to care of the adult patient who may require ACLS interventions. In this chapter, only those patients in cardiac arrest are considered. Please refer to the appropriate chapters for information regarding the treatment of patients with arrhythmias, pulmonary edema, myocardial infarction, hypotension, or shock.

- Assess responsiveness: The responsive patient requires observation and treatment as indicated by his or her condition.

- Assess for respiratory and cardiac arrest and perform CPR, if indicated, until a defibrillator is available. Be sure to protect the cervical spine if indicated.

- Perform a "quick-look" and assess rhythm. If VF or pulseless VT is present, perform the interventions listed in the following ventricular fibrillation and pulseless ventricular tachycardia algorithm. If there is electrical activity on the monitor and no pulse is present, perform the interventions listed in the pulseless electrical activity (PEA) algorithm. If asystole is found, perform the interventions listed in the asystole algorithm.

VENTRICULAR FIBRILLATION AND PULSELESS VENTRICULAR TACHYCARDIA

The majority of cardiac arrest patients present in VF or VT. This, coupled with the fact that most of the survivors of sudden death are those patients who respond to interventions in this sequence, makes it imperative that the paramedic understand the algorithm presented here.

* **Assess for respiratory and cardiac arrest** and perform CPR until a defibrillator is available.

* **Perform a "quick-look"** and assess rhythm.

* **Defibrillate at 200 joules** (or equivalent biphasic energy level) if VF or pulseless VT.

* Assess rhythm.

NOTE: If defibrillation is effective and patient reverts to VF or VT, subsequent defibrillation should be performed, starting at the dose that was previously effective.

* If VF or VT persists, **defibrillate at 200 to 300 joules** (or equivalent biphasic energy level).

* Assess rhythm.

* If VF or VT persists, **defibrillate at 360 joules** (or equivalent biphasic energy level).

* Assess pulse and rhythm, keeping in mind that a change in pulse or rhythm will change the algorithm.

* Continue CPR.

- Place an advanced airway device as soon as possible. Confirm its placement using primary and secondary means. Secure it with a commercial device.

- **Obtain vascular access** by the IV route.

- As soon as vascular access is obtained, administer **epinephrine** (1:10,000), **1 mg IV bolus;** repeat every 3 to 5 minutes. Epinephrine may be administered via the endotracheal route at 2 to 2.5 times the usual dose using appropriate dosage of epinephrine (1:1000) in sterile water or 0.9% NaCl to limit the fluid down the tube to no more than 10 ml at a time. When epinephrine is used, it should be repeated at 3- to 5-minute intervals in a drug-shock pattern. An alternative to the initial dosing of epinephrine is **vasopressin 40 units IV**. The AHA recommends a single dose only because of its long half life. Consider beginning epinephrine 1 mg IV therapy 20 minutes after the vasopressin dose.

- **Defibrillate at 360 joules** (or equivalent biphasic energy level).

- Assess pulse and rhythm, keeping in mind that a change in pulse or rhythm will change the algorithm. If there has been no change in VF or VT, the patient is considered to be in refractory VF or VT. The following antifibrillatory agents should be employed in a drug-shock, drug-shock pattern, and the patient should be defibrillated at 360 joules 30 to 60 seconds after administration of each medication. The current guidelines recommend that we use only a single antiarrhythmic agent, if possible. Use of multiple antiarrhythmic agents may actually be proarrhythmic.

- **Administer amiodarone, 300 mg IV bolus.** This drug may be repeated every 3 to 5 minutes at a dose of 150 mg. The maximum dose is 2.2 grams in 24 hours.

- **Administer lidocaine, 1.5 mg/kg IV.** This dose may be repeated in 3 to 5 minutes. The maximum dose is 3 mg/kg.

If the maximum dose is reached, an additional 0.5 mg/kg can be administered but not more often than every 8 to 10 minutes.

- **Administer procainamide, 20 to 30 mg/min** to a maximum total dose of 17 mg/kg. An acceptable method in cardiac arrest is 100 mg IV bolus every 5 minutes.

- If hypomagnesemia is known or clinically suspected, **administer magnesium sulfate, 1 to 2 grams IV.**

- Should the patient's rhythm convert to a supraventricular rhythm after a defibrillation, an antifibrillatory agent should be employed to prevent recurrence. If no antifibrillatory agent has been given previously, give lidocaine, 1.0 to 1.5 mg/kg, followed by a lidocaine infusion at the rate of 2 to 4 mg/minute. The infusion dosage should be cut in half in patients in shock with hepatic dysfunction or in patients older than 70 years of age. If antifibrillatory agents have already been given, the patient should receive a maintenance infusion of whatever drug was helpful during defibrillation—lidocaine, 2 to 4 mg per minute; amiodarone, 0.5 to 1 mg per minute; or procainamide, 1 to 4 mg per minute.

PULSELESS ELECTRICAL ACTIVITY (PEA)

Pulseless electrical activity includes electromechanical dissociation (EMD), pseudo-EMD, idioventricular rhythms, bradyasystolic rhythms, and postdefibrillation idioventricular rhythms.

- Continue **CPR** as initiated in the AHA universal algorithm.

- Place an advanced airway device as soon as possible. Confirm its placement using primary and secondary means. Secure it with a commercial device.

- Consider possible causes and therapy:

    o **H**ypovolemia. Begin fluid resuscitation.

    o **H**ypoxia. Continue oxygenation.

o **H**ydrogen ions (acidosis). Improve perfusion and ventilation. Consider sodium bicarbonate IV.

o **H**yperkalemia/hypokalemia. If hyperkalemia is suspected (patients in end-stage renal failure who have missed dialysis): Calcium chloride 500 to 1000 mg IV; Sodium bicarbonate, 50 to 100 mEq IV.

o **H**ypothermia. See chapter 26.

o **T**ablets (overdoses). Beta blocker and calcium channel overdoses may be treated with glucagon IV. Tricyclic antidepressant (TCA) overdose may be treated with IV 0.9% NaCl or sodium bicarbonate IV.

o **T**amponade (cardiac). Provide fluid resuscitation and rapid transport for pericardiocentesis.

o **T**ension pneumothorax. Perform needle chest decompression.

o **T**hrombosis (acute coronary syndromes). Provide rapid transport for revascularization.

o **T**hrombosis (acute pulmonary embolism). Provide fluid resuscitation and rapid transport for thrombolytics or surgery.

• **Administer epinephrine** (1:10,000), **1 mg IV;** repeat every 3 to 5 minutes. Epinephrine may be given via the endotracheal route at 2 to 2.5 times the usual dose, diluted in 10 ml of either 0.9% NaCl or sterile water. When epinephrine is repeated, it may be given at the initial dose or at higher doses (up to 1.0 mg/kg or 5 mg). Remember to administer 20 to 30 ml of fluid and to perform effective CPR for 30 to 60 seconds after each medication bolus.

• **If patient is experiencing bradycardia, administer atropine, 1 mg IV push.** Dosage may be repeated every 3 to 5 minutes (maximum total dose: 0.04 mg/kg or 3 mg); remember to follow the IV bolus recommendations previously mentioned. Atropine may be given via the endotracheal route at 2 to 2.5 times the usual dose, diluted in 10 ml of either 0.9% NaCl or sterile water.

ASYSTOLE ALGORITHM

- Continue **CPR** as initiated in the AHA universal algorithm.

- Place an advanced airway device as soon as possible. Confirm its placement using primary and secondary means. Secure it with a commercial device.

- Consider possible causes and therapy:

  o **H**ypovolemia. Begin fluid resuscitation.

  o **H**ypoxia. Continue oxygenation.

  o **H**ydrogen ions (acidosis). Improve perfusion and ventilation. Consider sodium bicarbonate IV.

  o **H**yperkalemia/hypokalemia. If hyperkalemia is suspected (patients with end-stage renal failure who have missed dialysis): Calcium chloride, 500 to 1000 mg IV; Sodium bicarbonate, 50 to 100 mEq IV.

  o **H**ypothermia. See chapter 26.

  o **T**ablets (overdoses). Beta blocker and calcium channel overdoses may be treated with glucagon IV. TCA overdose may be treated with IV 0.9% NaCl or sodium bicarbonate IV.

  o **T**amponade (cardiac). Provide fluid resuscitation and rapid transport for pericardiocentesis.

  o **T**ension pneumothorax. Perform needle chest decompression.

  o **T**hrombosis (acute coronary syndromes). Provide rapid transport for revascularization.

  o **T**hrombosis (acute pulmonary embolism). Fluid resuscitation and rapid transport for thrombolytics or surgery.

- **Consider the immediate use of transcutaneous pacing.** Remember that the earlier the pacemaker is applied, the greater the chance of obtaining capture.

- **Administer epinephrine** (1:10,000), **1 mg IV;** repeat every 3 to 5 minutes. Epinephrine may be given via the endotracheal route at 2 to 2.5 times the usual dose, diluted in 10 ml of either 0.9% NaCl or sterile water. When epinephrine is repeated, it may be given at the initial dose or at higher doses (up to 1.0 mg/kg or 5 mg). Remember to administer 20 to 30 ml of fluid and to perform effective CPR for 30 to 60 seconds after each medication bolus.

- **Administer atropine, 1 mg IV push.** Dosage may be repeated every 3 to 5 minutes (maximum total dose: 0.04 mg/kg or 4 mg); remember to follow the IV bolus recommendations previously mentioned. Atropine may be given via the endotracheal route at 2 to 2.5 times the usual dose, diluted in 10 ml of either 0.9% NaCl or sterile water.

- If patient remains asystolic, after successful intubation and adequate ventilations and initial medications, and if reversible causes cannot be found, consider termination of efforts in consultation with the medical control physician.

BIBLIOGRAPHY

American Heart Association. (2003). *ACLS provider manual.* Dallas, TX: American Heart Association.

American Heart Association. (2003). *ACLS experienced provider manual.* Dallas, TX: American Heart Association.

American Heart Association. (2003). *Handbook of emergency cardiovascular care for healthcare providers.* Dallas, TX: American Heart Association.

Mistovich, J. J., R. W. Benner, & G. S. Margolis (2004). *Prehospital advanced cardiac life support.* Upper Saddle River, NJ: Prentice-Hall.

CHAPTER 9

CARDIAC ARREST: PEDIATRICS

David LaCovey, EMT-P

PRESENTATION

Cardiac arrest in children is a rare event. Unlike the adult patient who may experience a sudden cardiac event, in children cardiac arrest is often a late secondary event. It usually results from progressive hypoxic or ischemic events, shock, CNS dysfunction, or a combination of any of the above. Cardiac arrest in children is usually preceded by cardiopulmonary failure. Bradypnea and agonal respirations with bradycardia and poor perfusion signal impending arrest. Recognition and appropriate management can often reverse the condition and keep a child from progressing to cardiac arrest. Although less common in children than adults, sudden cardiac arrest does occur in children.

IMMEDIATE CONCERNS

❶ **Is resuscitation indicated?** Prehospital care providers are encouraged to begin full resuscitative measures in all pediatric patients who are found to be apneic and pulseless unless the following exists: valid DNR order; obvious mortal injury; or signs of irreversible death, such as rigor mortis, decapitation, or dependent lividity.

❶ **Is ventilatory support needed?** Airway management and ventilatory support are the hallmark of pediatric resuscitation. Children who are apneic or bradypneic or who have clinical signs of poor oxygenation (cyanosis) and ventilation (absent or diminished lung sounds) need to be ventilated with a bag-valve-mask (BVM) device. Care should be taken during BVM ventilation to ensure that the appropriate size bag and mask device (minimum of

450-500 ml), BVM mask, ventilation volume (just enough tidal volume to cause visible chest rise), and inspiratory time of 1 to 1.5 seconds is used to minimize gastric inflation.

❶ **Are chest compressions needed?** Chest compressions coordinated with ventilations should be initiated in an infant or child who is being ventilated and either has no pulse or has a pulse rate of less than 60 with signs of poor perfusion (unresponsiveness, apnea or agonal respirations, absent peripheral pulses, and hypotension).

❶ **Is the patient in ventricular fibrillation (VF) or pulseless ventricular tachycardia (VT)?** Perform a "quick look." Defibrillate immediately if the patient is in VF or has VT without a pulse. Use pediatric paddles if the patient is under 1 year of age or weighs less than 10 kg. If the pediatric paddles are not immediately available, or the patient is older than 1 year and weighs less than 10 kg and is too small for adult paddles to make full skin contact, then the patient can be turned on one side and the paddles placed in an anterior/posterior position with the child sandwiched between the two paddles.

IMPORTANT HISTORY

❷ **Is there a history of congenital disease?** Congenital heart disease occurs in up to 1% of births. Although most of these defects are not life-threatening, some may have serious consequences. The most common defects involve the heart valves, the myocardium, and the major blood vessels. One way to classify these defects is to identify them as either cyanotic or noncyanotic congenital heart defects. Those with cyanotic congenital heart disease have less ability to compensate for other illnesses and can become quite ill with illnesses that are considered mild or moderate in severity for healthy children. These patients are also more likely to exhibit cardiac dysrrythmias such as VF, VT, or other arrest rhythms associated with the adult resuscitation.

❓ **Has the cardiac arrest been caused by trauma or blood loss?** It is important to determine whether this event is primarily cardiac/respiratory or whether it results from trauma. The management of a traumatic arrest differs from the management of a medical arrest. One must be cognizant of concerns with cervical spine stability when managing the patient's airway and assessment of those conditions that may interfere with a successful resuscitation, such as pneumothorax, tension pneumothorax, and hypovolemia. Arrests caused by blood loss or trauma generally require fluid resuscitation (20 ml/kg, 10 ml/kg if there is a history of heart disease) and possibly surgical intervention (see chapter 28). The management of a hypothermic arrest differs as well (see chapter 26). The patient should also be transported to an appropriate trauma center where specialty care is available.

❓ **Is the child taking any medications?** Most children will not be taking any medication; however, any medications taken may provide clues to past medical history or the possibility of medication side effects. Also, assess the possibility that the patient may have ingested someone else's (e.g., a parent's or grandparent's) medications. Consultation with medical command may assist with the determination of additional medications that might need to be administered during the resuscitation.

❓ **Has the patient been ill recently?** Attempt to discover the illness leading to the cardiac arrest. Recall that cardiopulmonary arrest in pediatric patients is not usually caused by heart disease. Infectious disease, traumatic injuries, airway obstructions, seizures, and metabolic problems are more common than a primary cardiac arrest. Although initial resuscitation priorities will likely not change, fluid may need to be administered to a patient with a history of vomiting and diarrhea, and glucose to a patient who is hypoglycemic.

DIFFERENTIAL DIAGNOSIS

After the initial treatment priorities have been established, it is important to determine the patient's rhythm and
perfusion status. Be sure to assess for pulses whenever
there may be a perfusing rhythm on the ECG monitor. Remember to treat the patient and not the monitor. If there
is a change in the rhythm, check for a pulse. A variety of
rhythms may be present. It is important that you have the
ability to interpret electrocardiograms (ECGs) rapidly. This
ability combined with the knowledge of the AHA's Pediatric
Advanced Life Support (PALS) algorithms, will allow you to
make a diagnosis and follow the correct treatment plan.

KEY PHYSICAL EXAMINATION FINDINGS

✔ *Initial assessment.*   Quickly assess the patient who is
  apneic and pulseless to determine whether cardiac arrest
  has occurred.

TREATMENT PLAN

- *Patient assessment.*   Frequent reassessment of the
  pediatric patient is critical during resuscitation. You need
  to ensure that the chest compressions and ventilations
  are effective. Any change in the patient's rhythm or perfusion status will require a change in the algorithm that you
  are using.

- *Communication.*   Protocols and standing orders are
  useful in giving guidance during the initial minutes of
  resuscitation. However, communication with medical
  command is important to aid treatment decisions beyond
  the scope of an algorithm.

- *Medication administration.*   Drug dosage calculations
  during pediatric resuscitation are based on the patient's
  weight. This requires the rescuer to accurately determine
  the patient's weight and then perform a dose calculation
  based on the patient's weight. This need for mental calculation significantly increases the likelihood of a dosing

error during pediatric resuscitation. Therefore, it is recommended that rescuers use either a length-based type of resuscitation tape or some other chart or card that calculates the appropriate drug dose based on the patient's weight. The parent or guardian may be able to provide the correct weight. Ideally, medication should be given either via the IV or IO route. However, prior to IV or IO access, epinephrine, lidocaine, atropine, and naloxone may be given via the tracheal tube. Currently, epinephrine is the only drug that has a specific tracheal tube dose (0.1mg/kg of 1:1000 solution). If lidocaine, atropine, or naloxone is given via the tracheal route, the dose should be 2 to 2.5 times the IV or IO dose. Regardless of the medication, it should be diluted with either normal saline or sterile water to obtain a total volume of up to 5 ml and followed with 5 manual ventilations.

- ***The algorithmic approach.*** When the PALS algorithms are used, a number of assumptions are made: The condition in the algorithm persists, the patient remains apneic and pulseless, and adequate chest compressions and ventilation with 100% oxygen are continued throughout the resuscitation. Algorithms were developed to aid in the treatment of certain conditions and should not take the place of clinical judgment.

PULSELESS ARREST ALGORITHM: ASYSTOLE

Asystole is the most common observed rhythm in infants and children presenting in out-of-hospital cardiac arrest. The etiology of the arrest is almost always a combination of hypoxia and ischemia. Unfortunately, the prognosis for intact neurologic survival is poor. Despite that, patients who receive prompt bystander CPR with prompt advanced life support (ALS) are most likely to survive.

- Determine pulselessness and no signs of circulation, and **begin CPR.**

- **Confirm asystole** in more than one lead.

- **Perform endotracheal intubation** if skilled in pediatric intubation.

- Obtain vascular access by the IV or IO route.

- Administer **epinephrine (1:10,000) 0.01 mg/kg (0.1 mL/kg) either IV or IO;** repeat every 3 to 5 minutes. The same dose of epinephrine is recommended for the second and subsequent doses for unresponsive asystolic and pulseless arrest. Higher doses of epinephrine (0.1 to 0.2 mg/kg) may be considered for special resuscitation circumstances that suggest a catecholamine-resistant condition (e.g., anaphylaxis, known alpha or beta blocker overdose, severe sepsis). Epinephrine may be given via the tracheal tube. The dose is 0.1 mg/kg (0.1 mL/kg) of a 1:1,000 solution. The epinephrine should be diluted with enough normal saline or sterile water to obtain a total volume of at least 5 mL and should be followed with 5 manual ventilations.

- Identify and treat potential reversible causes:

  o **Hypoxemia:** Ensure that the patient is being oxygenated and ventilated with 100% oxygen.

  o **Hypovolemia:** Provide a rapid 20 ml/kg of isotonic crystalloid solution.

  o **Hypothermia:** may require rapid rewarming (see chapter 26).

  o **Hyperkalemia/hypokalemia and metabolic disorders:** Consider calcium chloride and sodium bicarbonate for hyperkalemia; ensure adequate ventilation.

  o **Tension pneumothorax:** Perform needle decompression.

  o **Tamponade:** Transport immediately.

  o **Toxins/poisonings/drugs** may require specific therapies and rapid transport.

  o **Thromboembolism:** Provide rapid transport.

- **Consider transport.** The determination of when to begin transport depends on the clinical circumstances of the resuscitation, system protocol, or medical direction. Once the airway has been secured (via BVM ventilation or tracheal intubation), IV access has been established, and epinephrine has been administered, initiation of transport to the hospital should be considered. Some EMS systems permit termination of resuscitation efforts when the patient is normothermic and has not responded to a satisfactory trial of PALS and BLS.

PULSELESS ARREST ALGORITHM:
PULSELESS ELECTRICAL ACTIVITY

Pulseless electrical activity (PEA) is a rhythmic display of electrical activity other than VF or VT that does not produce a palpable pulse. Although the outcome is usually poor, PEA may be reversible if identified and treated early. Many causes of PEA involve obstruction of venous return to the heart or hypovolemia. Unfortunately, unless a specific cause can be identified and treated, the rhythm will likely degenerate quickly into an agonal ventricular rhythm or asystole.

- Determine pulselessness, and **begin CPR.**

- **Perform endotracheal intubation** if skilled in pediatric intubation.

- Obtain vascular access by the IV or IO route.

- Administer **epinephrine (1:10,000) 0.01 mg/kg (0.1 mL/ kg) either IV or IO;** repeat every 3 to 5 minutes. The same dose of epinephrine is recommended for the second and subsequent doses for unresponsive asystolic and pulseless arrest. Higher doses of epinephrine (0.1 to 0.2 mg/ kg) may be considered for special resuscitation circumstances that suggest a catecholamine-resistant condition (e.g., anaphylaxis, known alpha or beta blocker overdose, severe sepsis). Epinephrine may be given via the tracheal tube. The dose is 0.1 mg/kg (0.1 mL/kg) of a 1:1,000 solution. The epinephrine should be diluted with enough normal saline or sterile water to obtain a total volume of at least 5 mL and should be followed with 5 manual ventilations.

- Identify and treat potential reversible causes:

  o **Hypoxemia:** Ensure that the patient is being oxygenated and ventilated with 100% oxygen.

  o **Hypovolemia:** Provide a rapid 20 ml/kg of isotonic crystalloid solution.

  o **Hypothermia** may require rapid rewarming (see chapter 26).

  o **Hyperkalemia/hypokalemia and metabolic disorders:** Consider calcium chloride and sodium bicarbonate for hyperkalemia; ensure adequate ventilation.

  o **Tension pneumothorax:** Perform needle decompression.

  o **Tamponade:** Transport immediately.

  o **Toxins/poisonings/drugs** may require specific therapies and rapid transport.

  o **Thromboembolism:** Provide rapid transport.

- **Consider transport.** The determination of when to begin transport depends on the clinical circumstances of the resuscitation, system protocol, or medical direction. Once the airway has been secured (via BVM ventilation or tracheal intubation), IV access has been established, and epinephrine has been administered, initiation of transport to the hospital should be considered. Some EMS systems permit termination of resuscitation efforts when the patient is normothermic and has not responded to a satisfactory trial of PALS and basic life support (BLS).

VENTRICULAR FIBRILLATION AND PULSELESS
VENTRICULAR TACHYCARDIA

VF and VT are uncommon terminal events in the pediatric population. Although they are thought to occur more frequently than previously suspected, VT or VF is documented in only about 10% of children in whom a terminal rhythm is recorded. One should suspect VF or pulseless VT if there is a history of sudden collapse, electrocution, drowning, or trauma. As with the adult patient, survival decreases with increasing time to defibrillation. When there is a history of sudden collapse, every attempt should be made to determine the underlying rhythm as quickly as possible. Recent advances in AED pad technology have led to the development of pads that can be used in children between 1 year (10 kg) and 8 years (25 kg), and responders may find patients connected to an AED upon their arrival.

- Determine pulselessness, and **begin CPR.**

- **Identify VF or pulseless VT** as quickly as possible.

- **Defibrillate at 2 joules/kg** (maximum dose of 200 joules). NOTE: Pediatric size paddles should be used in patients younger than 1 year of age who weigh less than 10 kg. Adult paddles should be used in patients older than one year who weigh more than 10 kg. If adult-sized paddles do not allow for full skin contact when utilizing the anterior paddle placement is used for the small child, use an anterior/posterior paddle placement.

- **Reassess rhythm.**

- **Defibrillate at 4 joules/kg** (maximum dose of 360 joules) if the VF or pulseless VT persists.

- **Reassess rhythm.**

- **Defibrillate at 4 joules/kg** (maximum dose of 360 joules) if the VF or pulseless VT persists.

- **Reassess pulse and rhythm,** keeping in mind that a change in pulse or rhythm will dictate a change in algorithm.

- **Continue CPR.**

- **Perform endotracheal intubation** if skilled in pediatric intubation.

- Administer **epinephrine (1:10,000) 0.01 mg/kg (0.1 mL/ kg) either IV or IO;** repeat every 3 to 5 minutes. The same dose of epinephrine is recommended for the second and subsequent doses. Higher doses of epinephrine (0.1 to 0.2 mg/kg) may be considered for special resuscitation circumstances that suggest a catecholamine-resistant condition (e.g., anaphylaxis, known alpha or beta blocker overdose, severe sepsis). Epinephrine may be given via the tracheal tube. The dose is 0.1 mg/kg (0.1 mL/kg) of a 1:1,000 solution. The epinephrine should be diluted with enough normal saline or sterile water to obtain a total volume of at least 5 mL and should be followed with 5 manual ventilations.

- Assess pulse and rhythm, if VF or VT is evident. Defibrillate at 4 joules/kg. Note that defibrillation should occur within 30 to 60 seconds after each medication. Follow the pattern of shock-drug-CPR-shock (repeat) or drug-CPR-shock-shock-shock (repeat).

- Reassess pulse and rhythm after each intervention or rhythm change.

- Administer an antiarrhythmic agent. Note that any of the following antiarrhythmics may be used during shock-resistant VF or pulseless VT. Selection should be based on patient presentation and consultation with medical command.

o **Amiodarone 5 mg/kg rapid bolus either IV or IO.** Repeat dose of 5 mg/kg may be given to a maximum daily dose of 15 mg/kg. Amiodarone should not be administered concurrently with any other agent that prolongs the QT interval (e.g., procainamide).

o **Lidocaine 1 mg/kg bolus either IV, IO, or ET.** Dosage may be repeated in 5 to 15 minutes with a total dose of 3 mg/kg. It is recommended that a lidocaine infusion follow a bolus of lidocaine of 20 to 50 μcg/kg per minute. The infusion should begin within 15 minutes of a bolus. If more than 15 minutes has elapsed between the last bolus and the start of the infusion, then a second bolus of 0.5 to 1 mg/kg may be given to restore therapeutic concentrations.

o **Administer magnesium sulfate 25 to 50 mg/kg up to 2 g IV/IO** over 10 to 20 minutes for the treatment of torsades de pointes or hypomagnesemia.

• Reassess pulse and rhythm. If no response:

o Identify and treat potential reversible causes:

  • **Hypoxemia:** Ensure that the patient is being oxygenated and ventilated with 100% oxygen.

  • **Hypovolemia:** Provide a rapid 20 ml/kg of isotonic crystalloid solution.

  • **Hypothermia** may require rapid rewarming (see chapter 26).

  • **Hyperkalemia/hypokalemia and metabolic disorders:** Consider calcium chloride and sodium bicarbonate for hyperkalemia; ensure adequate ventilation.

  • **Tension pneumothorax:** Perform needle decompression.

  • **Tamponade:** Transport immediately.

- **Toxins/poisonings/drugs** may require specific therapies and rapid transport.

- **Thromboembolism:** Provide rapid transport.

- **Consider transport.** The determination of when to begin transport depends on the clinical circumstances of the resuscitation, system protocol, or medical direction. Once the airway has been secured (via BVM ventilation or tracheal intubation), IV access has been established, and epinephrine has been administered, initiation of transport to the hospital should be considered. Some EMS systems permit termination of resuscitation efforts when the patient is normothermic and has not responded to a satisfactory trial of PALS and BLS.

TERMINATION OF RESUSCITATION

No single factor is predictive of outcome of a resuscitation event. History has shown us that pediatric patients in cardiac arrest in the field usually do not respond to our resuscitative efforts. Generally, if a child has had no return of spontaneous circulation after 30 minutes of resuscitative efforts, if there are no mitigating factors such as profound prearrest hypothermia (e.g., submersion in icy water) and a young age, and if potential reversible causes (the 4 Hs and 4 Ts) have been addressed, then termination of resuscitative efforts can be considered. However, if at any time during resuscitation spontaneous circulation of any duration returns, then it may be appropriate to consider extending the resuscitative efforts. Most EMS systems will transport the patient to the hospital and allow the decision to terminate resuscitation to be made by the doctor in the emergency room.

SUPPORTING THE PROVIDER

The death of a child can have a profound impact on healthcare providers. Healthcare providers often view a failed resuscitation as a personal or professional failure.

This perception often leads to a feeling of guilt or remorse even when the medical care was perfect. Because of these feelings, it is important that an EMS system have established policies and procedures to address the providers' needs.

INTUBATION AND VASCULAR ACCESS

- Prehospital pediatric intubation has been a subject much discussion in the last few years. The frequency of pediatric intubation is significantly less than that of adult intubation. Studies have shown success rates ranging from 50% to 78%. A study by Gausche et al. showed no improvement in survival or neurologic outcome of intubated pediatric patients versus those who received BVM ventilation in an urban EMS system with short transport times.

- Intubation should be based on provider training and skill level, transport time to the hospital, availability of the appropriate equipment, and comfort level of the provider.

- Determining appropriate tube and blade size is best accomplished by using a length-based tape system, PALS reference card (comes with the Pediatric Advanced Life Support Textbook), or other similar reference card.

- Secondary confirmation devices (such as end-tidal CO_2 detector or capnography) must be used to assist in determination of correct tube position. The pediatric end-tidal CO_2 detector should be used for any patient weighing less than 15 kg, and the adult size should be used for anyone weighing more than 15 kg.

- The detector may be left in circuit <u>IF</u> the correct size of detector is used and it does not get wet. If an adult-size detector is used for someone weighing less than 15 kg, it should not be left in the respiratory circuit because of excessive dead air space.

- The esophageal detector bulb or syringe is contraindicated for use in children under 20 kg.

- Once tube position has been confirmed, many people find that stabilization of the patient's head using either a cervical collar or towels and immobilization of the patient to a spine board help limit head movement and thus tube movement.

- Remember to frequently reassess tube position during the resuscitation.

- Intraosseous (IO) infusion is often the best route for vascular access during pediatric resuscitation, and there is no age limit for its use. IO infusion is contraindicated in patients with lower extremity deformity in the same bone as the insertion site.

- The needle should be inserted at either a 90-degree angle or with the needle angled away from the joint. A firm twisting motion should be used to advance the needle into the bone. Successful placement of the IO needle can be determined by either the aspiration of bone marrow or by infusing 10 ml of normal saline without resistance or swelling of the calf of the leg in which the needle has been placed.

- All medication that can be given intravenously can be infused via the IO route. All medications should be followed by a saline flush of at least 5 ml of normal saline. The fluid used during resuscitation should be either normal saline or Ringer's lactate.

BIBLIOGRAPHY

American Academy of Pediatrics. (2000). *Pediatric education for prehospital professionals.* Sudbury, MA: Jones and Bartlett.

American Heart Association. (2002). *Textbook of pediatric advanced life support.* Dallas, TX: Author.

Markenson, DS, ed. *Pediatric emergency care.* Paramus, NJ: Brady.

CHAPTER 10

CEREBROVASCULAR ACCIDENTS AND TRANSIENT ISCHEMIC ATTACKS

Russell Bradley, M.D.
Owen T. Traynor, M.D.

PRESENTATION

A stroke, or cerebral vascular accident (CVA), is a sudden neurologic injury related to impaired cerebral blood flow. In essence, it is a closed head injury. A transient ischemic attack (TIA) resembles a stroke in presentation, but the symptoms last less than 24 hours. For all intents and purposes, a TIA must be treated in the prehospital arena in the same way as a stroke.

It is useful to divide strokes into two major categories: ischemic and hemorrhagic. Although there is no way to distinguish between hemorrhagic and ischemic strokes on the street, a hemorrhagic stroke is more likely to involve an altered level of consciousness or a severe headache that may rapidly progress to stupor or unconsciousness. A hemorrhagic stroke can occur secondary to trauma, either to the head or the body. Ischemic strokes are usually a result of either local clotting (thrombosis) of a blood vessel or blockage caused by the blood vessel becoming plugged by material (an embolus) that comes from elsewhere in the body. Hemorrhagic strokes result from bleeding either directly into the brain tissue or outside of the brain into the cerebrospinal fluid.

Strokes present according to which area of the brain is inadequately perfused. Symptoms include the following:

- Paralysis or weakness of a lower limb, upper limb, one whole side of the body, or one or both sides of the face

- Altered mental state, includ ing impaired judgment, insight, and memory

- Sensory deficits of the body or the face: numbness, pain, pins and needles, loss of pain, or temperature sensation

- Clumsiness and impaired gait

- Blindness in half of the visual field or in just one eye

- Pinpoint, dilated, or unequal pupils

- Aphasia: inappropriate use of language, poor understanding of language, difficulty finding words

- Dysarthria: slurred speech, difficulty with pronunciation

- Vertigo: the feeling of spinning or dizziness

- Syncope, loss of consciousness, coma

- Vomiting

- Headache

- Bowel and bladder incontinence

- Seizures

- Impaired or absent gag reflex

- Abnormal respiratory patterns, including respiratory arrest

Be aware that strokes may occur either suddenly or with a slow, insidious onset. If the patient is found at some point hours to days after the stroke, the presenting picture might also include dehydration and hypothermia.

IMMEDIATE CONCERNS

❶ What is the status of the patient's airway?   A depressed mental status with or without an intact gag reflex can increase the risk of aspiration. If the airway is not patent or the patient is unconscious, intubation may be warranted. Placing the patient in the coma position can help decrease the aspiration risk.

● **Are the patient's respirations effective?** Injury to the respiratory centers of the brain can cause an altered respiratory pattern and ineffective ventilations. At the very least, supplemental oxygen should be administered. Intubation may be required.

● **Is the patient hemodynamically stable?** Circulatory collapse might occur secondary to disruption of the autonomic nervous system. Oxygen should be administered, and a saline lock established unless the patient exhibits signs of shock.

● **Is the patient hypoglycemic?** Blood glucose should be evaluated, and dextrose should be given if the blood glucose level is low. If glucose evaluation is not possible, glucose should be given only to diabetic patients in whom hypoglycemia is clinically suspected.

● **When did the symptoms begin?** The time of onset of symptoms is important because patients with ischemic strokes may qualify for thrombolytic therapy if their ED evaluation can be completed within 3 hours of the onset of symptoms. Postthrombolytic intracranial hemorrhage increases with time after symptom onset. Thrombolytics are contraindicated after 3 hours because of a dramatic increase in intracranial bleeding. Paramedics should make a strong effort to determine the time of onset. If this cannot be determined, find out when the patient was last known to be okay. If the patient's presentation is within 3 hours of onset, efforts should be made to expedite transport.

● **What is the patient's neurologic status?** It is imperative that the paramedic assess the patient's level of consciousness, score on the Glasgow Coma Scale, pupillary reaction, gross motor and sensory status, facial asymmetry, and the ability to speak and walk on the scene, given that the examination might markedly change. If the patient presents with seizures, management should follow the guidelines discussed in chapter 37.

IMPORTANT HISTORY

❷ **Does the patient have any risk factors for cerebrovascular disease?**   These risk factors are the same as for cardiovascular disease and include a history of smoking, elevated cholesterol levels, hypertension, and diabetes mellitus and a family history. Both diabetes and hypertension predispose a person to stroke through their deleterious effects on the small blood vessels of the brain.

❷ **Has the patient ever had a CVA or TIA before?**   People who have a previous history of CVA or TIA are at increased risk for further episodes.

❷ **Is there any history of cardiac disease or cardiac arrhythmias?** Patients with heart disease are at higher risk for the development of a thrombus (clot) in the heart that may become dislodged, enter the blood circulation as an embolus, and travel to the brain to cause a stroke. Patients with chronic atrial fibrillation and those with prosthetic heart valves are often anticoagulated with warfarin (Coumadin) to decrease the risk of embolization. In the first 2 months after an acute myocardial infarction (AMI), the risk of stroke is 13 times greater than in people without recent AMIs. Patients with strokes are often found to have underlying "silent" myocardial infarction (MI). A stroke may result from the low-flow state in the peri-MI period.

❷ **Is there any history of alcohol or drug abuse?**   Intravenous drug usage can cause bacterial colonization of the heart valves, and the bacteria have the potential to break off in clumps and form emboli. Cocaine can cause marked elevation in blood pressure, bursting cerebral blood vessels and causing hemorrhagic stroke. Alcohol lowers the seizure threshold, making seizures more likely, and withdrawal from alcohol can also cause seizures.

❷ What medications is the patient taking? Oral anticoagulants, such as warfarin, can increase the risk of intracranial hemorrhage. Oral contraceptives also increase
the risk of stroke because of the increased risk of clot formation. Nonsteroidal anti-inflammatory agents (NSAIDs),
through their antiplatelet properties, can make a hemorrhagic stroke bleed more actively.

DIFFERENTIAL DIAGNOSIS

ISCHEMIC STROKE

Current AHA guidelines recommend treatment of
ischemic strokes with thrombolytic agents if they present
within 3 hours of onset and there are no contraindications.
Although this is a level I recommendation, the AHA's stron-
gest recommendation, some physicians, including the Canadian Association of Emergency Physicians (CAEP) and
the American College of Emergency Physicians (ACEP),
do not believe there is sufficient data to support this therapy as a standard of care. Although this is a controversial
therapy, paramedics should continue to act in support of
the patient's best interest, promptly recognizing the CVA,
notifying receiving facilities early, and promptly transporting the patient. Decisions regarding thrombolytics can be
made in the ED after further evaluation.

- **Local thrombosis** of cerebral or neck vasculature causes
  approximately 50% of all strokes. Diseases that predispose people to this type of stroke include hypertension,
  diabetes, polycythemia vera, sickle cell anemia, collagen
  vascular diseases, arteritis, and migraine headaches.
  Trauma can cause ascending aortic dissection and
  cerebral artery dissection, both of which lead to thrombus formation. Pregnancy can lead to a hypercoagulable
  state and therefore predispose someone to thrombus
  formation.

- **Embolic obstruction** accounts for another 33% of all ischemic strokes. The majority of emboli arise from a source

in the heart. One quarter of all brain infarcts in patients younger than 40 years of age are secondary to cardiogenic emboli. The following diseases predispose the patient to development of an intracardiac clot and subsequent potential embolization: MI, atrial fibrillation, alcoholic cardiomyopathy, congestive heart failure, bacterial endocarditis, and any valvular disease or valvular prostheses. IV drug abuse can lead to bacterial endocarditis.

HEMORRHAGIC STROKE

- **Spontaneous intracerebral hemorrhage** is responsible for 8% to 11% of all acute strokes. The bleeding forms a hematoma that causes local tissue injury, decreased tissue perfusion, and an increase in intracerebral pressure. Predisposing conditions include hypertension, arteriovenous malformations (AVMs), and tumors. Other factors that can lead to hemorrhage include cocaine use, oral contraceptives, and anticoagulant and antiplatelet agents.

- **Arteriovenous malformations** (AVMs) are tangles of connections between arteries and veins and are usually present from birth. The walls of these connections are abnormally thin and grow thinner with advancing age. They are often the cause of intracerebral hemorrhages in patients between the ages of 10 and 30 years. Because there is usually a family history with the disease, ask whether other family members might have had the same symptoms.

- **Brain tumors** are often first indicated by a stroke, in which the tumor has eroded into a blood vessel, causing bleeding. Find out whether any other area of the body has had tumors because this could indicate a metastatic tumor.

- **Subarachnoid hemorrhage** is caused by a leakage of blood into the subarachnoid space (between the brain and the first layer of surrounding membrane). These are most commonly caused by the rupture of an aneurysm. An aneurysm is a localized ballooning of a blood vessel in which the wall is weakened for some reason. Five percent of the general population have these aneurysms.

TRANSIENT ISCHEMIC ATTACKS

By definition TIAs are neurologic deficits that resolve within 24 hours. They are usually short-lived events and can occur many times within 24 hours in a waxing and waning fashion. They are caused by a momentary lack of blood flow to some area of the brain, followed by the return of blood to that area. They are serious events and often indicate impending stroke.

Many other disease states mimic CVAs, including the postictal state of a seizure disorder, hypoglycemia or hyperglycemia in diabetes mellitus, migraine headaches, multiple sclerosis, and toxic ingestions.

ELECTROCARDIOGRAM

All patients who have experienced a CVA or TIA should receive cardiac monitoring. Cardiac monitoring may suggest evidence of possible MI as well as dysrhythmias that may be causing inadequate cardiac output and, therefore, inadequate cerebral blood flow.

BLOOD GLUCOSE DETERMINATION

Checking of serum glucose readings in patients suspected of an acute CVA is recommended. Hypoglycemia can, in some patients, mimic an acute stroke.

KEY PHYSICAL EXAMINATION FINDINGS

- ✓ ***Initial assessment.*** Look for compromised airway, ineffective breathing, and signs of shock.

- ✓ ***Vital signs.*** Note the presence of hypertension, bradycardia, and an altered mental state because these conditions may indicate rising intracranial pressure.

✅ ***Neurologic examination.*** Assess mental status, pupillary responses, facial asymmetry, and motor and sensory status. Perform a prehospital stroke scale. The Cincinnati Prehospital Stroke Scale, recommended by the AHA, is reproduced below.

> **1. Facial droop.** Have the patient smile or show his or her teeth. An abnormal finding is when one side of the patient's face does not move as well as the other.
>
> **2. Arm drift.** Have the patient close his or her eyes and extend both arms straight out with palms up for 10 seconds. An abnormal finding is when one arm does not move or one arm drifts compared with the other.
>
> **3. Abnormal speech.** Have the patient say, "You can't teach an old dog new tricks." An abnormal finding is if the patient slurs words, uses the wrong words, or cannot speak.

✅ ***HEENT.*** Look for head or neck trauma, pupil asymmetry, and facial asymmetry. Check for blindness. Listen for carotid bruits.

✅ ***Lungs.*** Listen for rales that may suggest CHF and, therefore, a cardiac-related cause of the stroke.

✅ ***Extremities.*** Look for any gross motor and sensory deficits. Check for a Babinski reflex by rubbing a firm, but not sharp, object along the lateral edge of the sole of the patient's foot from the heel to the ball of the foot and then across the ball to the medial edge of the foot. The reflex is positive when the initial movement of the great toe is upward, thus indicating a neurologic injury in either the spinal cord or brain. A Babinski reflex may be normal in children.

TREATMENT PLAN

- *Patient assessment.* Perform rapid and systematic primary survey initially and institute therapy as life-threatening problems are discovered. Early notification of the receiving hospital of the acute CVA can help mobilize resources inside the hospital. This preparation can result in a significant reduction in delays in both diagnosis and treatment, which is critical when patients present less than 3 hours after symptom onset. Frequent reassessment of the patient with a CVA or TIA is necessary because of the potential for worsening of the neurologic status.

- Administer **O₂** and **provide ventilatory support,** including endotracheal intubation as indicated.

- Place patient in the **semiFowler or Fowler position.** The coma position is also useful to reduce the aspiration risk in patients with a compromised gag reflex or depressed consciousness.

- **Establish IV access** with a saline lock, 0.9% NaCl, or LR as needed.

- If the patient has an altered mental status and opiate overdose is suspected, consider the administration of the following agents:

  o **Naloxone** (Narcan) **0.4 to 2.0 mg IV bolus.** Dosage may be repeated in 2 to 3 minutes.

  o **Dextrose 50%, 25 g IV** if the patient is hypoglycemic or if hypoglycemia is suspected in a patient with diabetes. It is best to use serum glucose determination to guide the administration of dextrose to patients who may be suffering a CVA. Hyperglycemia has been associated with poor outcomes in acute CVA.

- **Treat symptomatic arrhythmias** as indicated. See chapters 6 and 44 for specific options.

- **Treat nonlife-threatening injuries** as appropriate (i.e., control bleeding, splint fractures).

- **Transport to appropriate ED,** and ensure patient comfort en route.

BIBLIOGRAPHY

The American Heart Association in collaboration with the International Liason Committee on Resuscitation Part 7: The Age of Reperfusion. *Circulation, 102* (Suppl. 1), 204–216.

Hoffman, J. R. (2000, September). Should physicians give tPA to patients with acute ischemic stroke? Against: and just what is the emperor of stroke wearing? *Western Journal of Medicine, 173:* 148–149.

Robinson, D. J. (2000, September). Should physicians give tPA to patients with acute ischemic stroke? For: thrombo-lytics in stroke: whose risk is it anyway? *Western Journal of Medicine, 173:* 148–149.

Scott, P. A., W. G. Barsan (2001). Cerebrovascular Disease. In A. Harwood-Nuss, A. B. Wolfson, C. H. Linden, S. M. Shepard, P. H. Stenklyft (Eds.), *The Clinical Practice of Emergency Medicine*, (3rd ed., pp. 983–994). Philadelphia: Lippincott Williams & Wilkins.

NOTES

_____

_____

_____

_____

_____

_____

CHAPTER 11

CHEST PAIN

Ritu Sahni, M.D., M.P.H.

PRESENTATION

The patient experiencing chest pain can present in a variety of ways, with a wide range of symptoms—from the healthy 20-year-old patient with a sharp chest pain to the elderly cardiac patient with a crushing chest pain and new-onset congestive heart failure. The diagnosis of acute myocardial infarction (AMI) is easy to make when a patient presents with the classic symptoms: crushing retrosternal chest pain that is unrelieved by nitroglycerin, ECG changes, dyspnea, and diaphoresis accompanied by a known history of heart disease; however, one must not overlook the patient who presents with an atypical story. National statistics show that 5% of all AMIs are actually misdiagnosed, and the patient is discharged from the ED. Misdiagnosis of AMI results in the most malpractice dollars spent. Given the difficulty in diagnosing the nonclassical AMI, it is imperative that all patients with chest pain be evaluated in the ED. At the very least, these patients should receive O_2 and ECG monitoring and have IV access established. It is prudent to err on the side of treatment rather than allow the patient with cardiac chest pain to go untreated. The medical control physician can be a valuable consultant for the field EMS provider faced with this diagnostic dilemma.

IMMEDIATE CONCERNS

❶ **Is the patient hemodynamically stable?** Airway, breathing, and circulation should be assessed in all patients. The airway should be secured and fluid resuscitation initiated if the patient is showing signs of shock.

❗ **All chest pain is cardiac until proven otherwise.** All patients who complain of chest pain should be monitored, given oxygen therapy, and have an IV started immediately.

IMPORTANT HISTORY

❓ **What is the quality of the pain?** The quality of the patient's pain and its sources can give you an indication as to the underlying cause. Cardiac pain is often described as a pressure or crushing sensation on the chest. A sharp, knifelike pain is more likely to be musculoskeletal or pleuritic, whereas a burning midepigastric pain can indicate gastrointestinal (GI) distress. Keep in mind, however, that cardiac pain can and will present in any of these fashions.

❓ **Does the pain radiate?** Cardiac pain can radiate into both arms, the neck, jaw, and back. A tearing sensation that is felt into the middle of the back is a hallmark for thoracic aortic dissection.

❓ **What is the timing of the pain?** Angina pain generally lasts less than 15 minutes, whereas chest pain from MI can last longer than 30 minutes, at rest, without relief. Chest pain lasting for days is generally not cardiac in origin.

❓ **Are there any associated symptoms?** Vagal stimulation caused by an acute MI or unstable angina can cause nausea, vomiting, and diaphoresis. Patients with CHF, MI, or angina often have difficulty breathing. Of course, chest pain associated with a pulmonary etiology may also cause shortness of breath.

❓ **Is there a history of similar chest pain, heart disease, or other medical problems?** Often, patients with a history of heart disease know what their cardiac chest pain normally feels like. They will usually be able to indicate any change from previous patterns of pain and other related symptoms. During the history, it is important to find risk factors for heart disease, such as diabetes and hypercholesterolemia. It is also helpful to note that not all patients with AMI exhibit the classic signs and symptoms. Diabetic patients, for example, are notorious for presenting with MI in an atypical manner, including silent MI. Elderly patients are less likely to present with chest pain. Women are more likely than men to have atypical presentations for cardiac ischemia. Other complaints, such as malaise, hypotension, altered mental status, and stroke, become more common indicators of cardiac-related emergencies.

❷ Is thrombolytic therapy indicated? Thrombolytic therapy has been shown to limit infarct size and to reduce both morbidity and mortality. Thrombolytic therapy is indicated for all AMI patients with ST-segment elevations who present within 6 hours of the onset of symptoms, if there are no contraindications. There is some evidence that patients who are up to 24 hours out may also benefit from the use of thrombolytics. Patients with the most to gain are those with an anterior wall MI, but some positive results have been seen in patients with inferior wall MIs as well. Because the benefit of thrombolytics decreases with time, the patient must be promptly transported to the ED if thrombolytic agents are not available in the prehospital phase. Some researchers have suggested that percutaneous coronary intervention (PCI) is superior to thrombolytics.

❷ Are thrombolytic agents contraindicated? The AHA recommends this prehospital tool to determine who may have a contraindication to thrombolytics. This tool serves to shorten the decision time for reperfusion therapy once the patient arrives in the ED. A sample thrombolytic checklist is on page 104. The following are absolute contra-indications to thrombolytic therapy: GI bleeding; prolonged (greater than 1 minute) or traumatic CPR; recent (less than 2 months) history of intracranial or intraspinal surgery or trauma; intracranial neoplasm, atrioventricular malformation, or aneurysm; and history of a previous hemorrhagic CVA. The relative contra-indications are recent (less than 10 days) trauma or surgery, poorly controlled severe hypertension, active peptic ulcer disease, previous CVA, known bleeding disorder, hepatic insufficiency, hemorrhagic retinopathy, and pregnancy.

❷ What medications does the patient take? This information can often provide a good clue as to the exact nature of the patient's past history, especially when the patient is a poor historian.

❷ **Does the patient have any allergies?** Many patients report an aspirin allergy. On further questioning, that allergy is often manifested as GI upset or even peptic ulcer disease. In addition, they may state that they are not to take aspirin because of blood thinners. The only absolute contraindication to aspirin therapy in acute coronary syndromes is a true allergic reaction to salicylates.

DIFFERENTIAL DIAGNOSIS

There are many different organ systems represented in the chest and each one is a possible source of chest discomfort.

CARDIAC DISEASE

*   ***ANGINA***.   Angina is often described as a pressure type of pain that is brought on by exertion and that resolves after 10 to 15 minutes of rest and one or two sublingual nitroglycerin doses.

    o   ***Acute coronary syndrome (ACS).*** The concept of an acute coronary syndrome reflects the idea that patients with coronary atherosclerosis have a progressive disease. The clinical spectrum of ACS include unstable angina, non-Q-wave MI, and Q-wave MI.

    o   ***Unstable Angina.*** Unstable angina is characterized by a change in the pattern of angina, such as an increase in the severity of pain, an increase in the frequency of pain, a change in nitroglycerin requirements, or new-onset angina.

    o   ***AMI (non-Q-wave MI and Q-wave MI).*** This most often occurs at rest and the pain usually lasts for longer than 30 minutes. It is most often characterized by a severe, crushing substernal chest pain that is unrelieved by sublingual nitroglycerin. Many times, it is accompanied by severe nausea, vomiting, or diaphoresis. It is important to note that an AMI can have multiple types of presentation and can even be silent. Q-wave MIs are characterized by the appearance of Q-waves in the ECG. This occurs when an occlusive thrombus is present in a coronary artery for a prolonged time, resulting in transmural myocardial necrosis. Non-Q-wave MIs result from a partially occluding thrombus or an intermittently occlusive thrombus, resulting in necrosis of a portion of the myocardial wall. A Q-wave does not appear on the ECG. Q-waves, like other ECG abnormalities associated with cardiac ischemia, may be absent on the initial 12 lead ECG. Serial ECGs may be needed before the ischemia is revealed.

- ***PERICARDITIS OR PERICARDIAL TAMPONADE***. This pain is usually sharp, retrosternal, and radiating into the jaw. It often has a viral etiology, and patients may have a history of recent viral syndrome. At other times there is a pericardial effusion, which is detectable on ultrasound. On cardiac examination, many of these patients will have a pericardial friction rub, narrowing pulse pressure, and jugular venous distension (JVD). The ECG is typically abnormal in pericarditis. The most common abnormalities are nonspecific ST segment and T-wave abnormalities. These changes are dynamic, changing over time. PR segment depression is highly suggestive of pericarditis.

PULMONARY DISEASE

- ***PULMONARY EMBOLUS.*** Pulmonary embolus represents a serious, life-threatening disease that most often manifests as acute shortness of breath with tachycardia. Some patients may also complain of a pleuritic type of chest pain, reproducible with palpation, and increased pain on inspiration. Common symptoms include chest pain in 88% of patients, dyspnea in 84% of patients, and cough in 53% of patients. Common physical findings include tachypnea (respiratory rate greater than 16) in 92% of patients, tachycardia (heart rate greater than 100 bpm) in 44% of patients, and temperature greater than 100° F in 43% of patients. Risk factors of pulmonary embolism include a history of atrial fibrillation, obesity, pregnancy, prolonged immobilization, posttrauma, oral contraceptive use, recent hospitalization, postsurgery, and cancer.

- ***ASTHMA OR CHRONIC OBSTRUCTIVE PULMONARY DISEASE.*** The shortness of breath experienced by asthmatics is often described as a tightness similar to cardiac chest pain. The history of onset and duration are key points in the history.

- ***SPONTANEOUS PNEUMOTHORAX.*** A sudden onset of chest pain with shortness of breath may also be a spontaneous pneumothorax. These patients are usually tall, thin, relatively healthy men. People with asthma are also at increased risk for pneumothorax.

AORTA

- ***ACUTE AORTIC DISSECTION.*** Acute aortic dissection is often described as a tearing chest pain that radiates into the back. Most of these patients are hypertensive and can have a marked difference in blood pressure in both arms. This is a surgical emergency.

- ***RUPTURED AORTIC ANEURYSM.*** The majority of aneurysms are abdominal and produce abdominal or lower back pain. However, there are occasional thoracic aneurysms that may leak. Their presentation is usually similar to that of an aortic dissection. This is also a surgical emergency, and some of these patients may become acutely hypotensive.

GASTROINTESTINAL

- ***GASTROESOPHAGEAL REFLUX OR HIATAL HERNIA.*** Gastroesophageal reflux or hiatal hernia pain that can closely mimic cardiac chest pain. Often there is a history of the pain occurring for days to months to years. These patients, however, should be treated as cardiac patients until proven otherwise. It is also important to note that patients with cardiac disease experience relief of symptoms after being given a "GI cocktail," a combination of antacid, viscous lidocaine, barbiturate, and antispasmodic agents.

- ***ESOPHAGEAL SPASM.*** Esophageal spasm is a diagnosis of exclusion that is generally reached after a full workup and most often given to relatively young, healthy people with an unexplained source of chest pain. This pain can actually resolve with sublingual nitroglycerin. This diagnosis should never be considered as a working diagnosis in transport, and these patients should be treated like all other patients with chest pain.

CHEST WALL PAIN

- ***TRAUMA.*** Rib fractures and bruises secondary to trauma can cause a sharp chest wall pain that is reproducible on palpation. It is also important to consider traumatic visceral injuries, such as pulmonary or cardiac contusion, if the mechanism is suggestive. Also remember that trauma patients can still have AMIs.

KEY PHYSICAL EXAMINATION FINDINGS

- ✓ ***Initial assessment.*** Assess airway and breathing and look for signs of cardiogenic shock.
- ✓ ***Vital signs.*** Measure blood pressure in both arms.
- ✓ ***Neck.*** Check for JVD, which can be a sign of CHF, pericardial tamponade, or tension pneumothorax.
- ✓ ***Lungs.*** Assess for signs of CHF (i.e., crackles at the bases). Also listen for an absence of breath sounds, indicating pneumothorax.
- ✓ ***Cardiac examination.*** Listen for a friction rub, indicative of pericarditis, or an S_3 or S_4, another sign of CHF.
- ✓ ***Abdomen.*** Palpate the abdomen for a pulsatile mass, indicative of an abdominal aortic aneurysm.
- ✓ ***Extremities.*** Check for evidence of peripheral edema, a sign of CHF. Assess peripheral pulses.

ELECTROCARDIOGRAM

- ***12-lead ECG.*** Obtain a 12-lead ECG as soon as possible. The findings can help triage the patient into the categories below. Emergent therapy in the hospital, including revascularization as well as admission to critical care or intermediate care beds, will be based on these categories.

o ***ST elevation-AMI.*** There is ST elevation or new or presumably new left bundle branch block (LBBB).

o ***High-risk unstable angina/non-ST-elevation AMI.*** There is ST depression or dynamic T-wave inversion.

o ***Intermediate/low-risk unstable angina.*** The ECG is nondiagnostic. There are no changes in the ST segment or T-waves.

SAMPLE THROMBOLYTIC ELIGIBILITY CHECK LIST

Consideration of thrombolytic use requires that the first 4 items below be checked *Yes*.

	Yes	No
ECG evidence of myocardial infraction: > 1 mm ST elevation in > 2 contiguous inferior leads; > 2 mm ST elevation in > 2 contiguous anterior leads; new left bundle branch block.	❏	__
Ongoing Chest discomfort (> 30 minutes and < 12 hours)	❏	__
Pain unresponsive to NTG	❏	__
Age > 35 or > 40, if female	❏	__

Thrombolytic use requires that all remaining items be checked *No*.

	Yes	No
History of CVA, brain aneurysm, tumor	__	❏
Known bleeding disorder	__	❏
Active internal bleeding in past 2 to 4 weeks	__	❏
Surgery or trauma in past 3 weeks	__	❏
Terminal illness	__	❏
Significant liver disease, kindney failure	__	❏
Use of anticoagulants	__	❏
Prolonged CPR in last 2 weeks (> 10 min)	__	❏
Systolic BP > 180 mm Hg	__	❏
Diastolic BP > 110	__	❏
Pregnant?	__	❏
Diabetes with eye problems	__	❏

TREATMENT PLAN FOR PATIENTS WITH CHEST PAIN CONSISTENT WITH AMI

- ***Patient assessment.*** Reassess patient frequently because of the potential for a worsening of the hemodynamic status, CHF, or life-threatening arrhythmia. Cardiac monitoring is necessary. Be prepared—a high potential for cardiac arrest exists. Rapid but safe transport to the ED is an important component of care, and short scene times are essential if thrombolytic therapy is to be effective.

- Administer **O₂, provide ventilatory support** as needed, and monitor O₂ saturation by pulse oximetry if available.

- **Monitor the ECG** and obtain a **12-lead ECG.**

- Give aspirin 160 mg to 325 mg po. It is preferred that this be chewed and swallowed.

- **Establish IV access** with a saline lock.

- Give **nitroglycerin, 1/150 grain (0.4 mg) SL** (for systolic BP greater than 90 mm Hg). Dosage may be repeated every 5 minutes.

- **Complete thrombolytic eligibility checklist.**

- If nitroglycerin has been ineffective, give **morphine sulfate 2 to 5 mg IV** (for systolic BP greater than 90 mm Hg). Dosage may be repeated every 5 minutes as needed.

- Consider the use of IV beta blockers. These medications have been shown to reduce infarct size as well as medium- and long-term complications. The most commonly used beta blocker is metoprolol, 5 mg IV every 5 minutes x 3. Hold for HR < 60, SBP < 110, second- or third-degree heart block, or signs of CHF.

- If local protocol allows, consider taking the acute MI patient directly to a hospital that provides emergency angioplasty, known as percutaneous coronary intervention (PCI). Current AHA guidelines state that a slight delay in order to perform PCI is equivalent to thrombolytics.

Recent literature suggests that emergent PCI, if readily available, is superior to thrombolytics.

- If prehospital thrombolytic therapy is available, appropriate, and not contraindicated, use the following agents:

Retaplase (Retevase) 10 U IV over 2 minutes. Repeat once in 30 minutes.

Tenectaplase (TNKase) Administer IV over 5 seconds.

Patient weight (kg)	Patient weight (lbs)	Tenecteplase (mg)	Volume of Tenecteplase (mL)
< 60	< 132	30	6
≥ 60 to < 70	≥ 132 to < 154	35	7
≥ 70 to < 80	≥ 154 to < 176	40	8
≥ 80 to < 90	≥ 176 to < 198	45	9
≥ 90	≥ 198	50	10

- **Treat symptomatic arrhythmias as indicated.** See chapters 6 and 44 for specific options.

- **Treat cardiogenic shock** as described in chapter 38.

- **If pulmonary edema is present, give furosemide (Lasix), 40 to 80 mg IV** (pediatric dose: 1 to 3 mg/kg IV).

BIBLIOGRAPHY

Aufderheide, T. P., W. J. Brady, W. B. Gibler (2002). Acute Ischemic Coronary Syndromes. In J. A. Marx (Ed.) *Rosen's Emergency Medicine: Concepts and clinical practice.* (5th ed., pp. 1112–1152). St. Louis, MO: Mosby.

Crocco T. J., M. R. Sayre, & T. P. Aufderheide (2002). Prehospital Triage of Chest Pain Patients. *Prehospital Emergency Care, 6:* pp. 224–228.

Cummins, R. O., (2001). (Ed.) *ACLS Provider Manual.* Dallas, TX: American Heart Association.

Schneider, S. M. & J. L. Syrett (2002). Chest Pain. In: A. E. Kuehl (Ed.) Prehospital Systems and Medical Oversight. (3rd ed., pp. 672–682). Dubuque, IA: Kemdall/Hunt.

CHAPTER 12

CHILD ABUSE

Nora Helfrich, R.N., EMT-P

PRESENTATION

Experts classify child abuse into four overlapping categories—physical abuse, sexual abuse, psychological abuse, and neglect. This chapter focuses primarily on physical abuse. Approximately 40% of the incidents reported to child protective services are substantiated. More than 150,000 children are seriously injured annually, with 1,100 deaths. Children's hospitals report that 25% to 35% of their traumatic deaths are caused by abuse.

IMMEDIATE CONCERNS

❗ **Is there evidence of a life-threatening injury?** Most of the immediately life-threatening injuries involve head and abdominal injuries and burns. Treatment priorities are the same as with any patient who has experienced critical trauma.

IMPORTANT HISTORY

❓ **What is the mechanism of injury?** Common historical characteristics of suspected child abuse include a mechanism of injury that is inconsistent with the injuries found, changing histories of the present illness, and unexplained or poorly explained injuries.

❓ **Was there a delay in seeking care?** A delayed presentation is common in child abuse cases. A parent who appears to be more concerned about the reason that the ambulance has been called than about the nature of the child's injury is also suspicious.

❓ Is there a history of domestic violence in the home? In up to 50% of cases of severe child abuse there is a history of domestic violence. Other risk factors for child abuse include poverty, maternal depression, parental psychiatric disease, substance abuse, and single parenthood. Male children and children 4 years of age or younger are at higher risk of abuse. Although risk factor evaluation is helpful in predicting at-risk populations, it is less helpful in individual cases.

DIFFERENTIAL DIAGNOSIS

- **ABDOMINAL TRAUMA.** Abdominal trauma is the second leading cause of death in abused children. Abdominal trauma may be present without visible external signs or history. Signs and symptoms include repeated vomiting, abdominal pain, abdominal distension, burning on voiding, and presence of blood in urine or in diapers. Have a high index of suspicion for these injuries in a child with GI symptoms and other evidence of abuse.

- **BURNS.** Burns are the third leading cause of death in abused children. Of children whose burns require medical attention, an estimated 40% will eventually be killed by their abuser if returned home. The shape or pattern of the burn may suggest a nonaccidental cause. Cigarette burns typically are rounded, of uniform size, and deep. Abusive contact burns are often found on the face and the dorsum of the hands and feet—unusual locations for accidental burns. Nonaccidental hot water immersion burns are typically bilateral and symmetrical, with well-demarcated lines, and no apparent splash marks. Often there is sparing of the burns in flexion creases as the child flexes his limbs to avoid injury. Children younger than 2 years of age are probably not capable of entering a tub and turning a rotary handle.

- **BRUISES.** Bruises are the most frequent injuries inflicted on the abused child. Often there are bruises in different stages of healing. The pattern of the bruise may indicate that a weapon was used. Bruises present on the face, genitals, buttocks, and inner aspects of thighs and arms are common in the abused child. Bruises are not common in the nonambulating infant. Accidental bruises are not typically found on both the front and the back or both the right and the left sides.

- **HEAD TRAUMA.** Intentional head trauma (IHT) is the leading cause of child abuse deaths. Some evidence suggests that these injuries can be occult in children younger than 1 year of age. Lethargy, irritability, unexplained vomiting, apnea, coma, convulsions, and seizures are common signs and symptoms of head trauma. There may be "no history of trauma" from the abuser.

- **SHAKEN BABY SYNDROME.** Shaken baby syndrome (SBS) is caused by the violent shaking of a young infant. The resulting injuries include retinal hemorrhages and intracranial injuries such as subdural hematomas, diffuse axonal injury, and cerebral edema. Often there are anterior and posterior rib fractures as well as long bone fractures.

- **SKELETAL INJURIES.** Very few young children are able to generate the force needed to break large bones. Unless there is a significant mechanism of injury, skull, rib, and long bone fractures suggest abuse. These fractures can be caused by twisting, pulling, jerking, or wringing of the child's arms or legs. Dislocations and injuries to the cervical spine and neck are common abuse injuries. Some studies reveal that up to 30% of childhood fractures may be caused by abuse, with nearly 75% of all fractures in those younger than 1 year of age attributed to abuse.

KEY PHYSICAL EXAMINATION FINDINGS

✔ **Initial assessment.** The goal of the initial assessment is to identify and immediately correct life-threatening patient conditions. Include an assessment of the environment and other potential victims.

SECTION 1

- ✅ ***Vital signs.*** Watch for hemodynamic instability and poor perfusion.

- ✅ ***HEENT.*** Assess for head trauma. Protect the cervical spine as necessary.

- ✅ ***Chest.*** Palpate for rib fractures.

- ✅ ***Abdomen.*** Look for abdominal tenderness, distension, and hypoactive bowel sounds. External injuries may be absent.

- ✅ ***Orthopedic exam.*** Assess for difficulty or pain on movement of extremities, inability to bear weight, and deformity from twisting, pulling, jerking, or wringing. Look for bruises or burns on inner or posterior aspects of extremities.

- ✅ ***Neurologic exam.*** A thorough neurologic exam may help detect an occult CNS injury.

TREATMENT PLAN

GENERAL TREATMENT GUIDELINES:
HEMODYNAMICALLY STABLE PATIENT

- **Administer O$_2$ and provide ventilatory support** as needed. Protect cervical spine as indicated.

- **Treat nonlife-threatening injuries as appropriate** (e.g., control bleeding, splint fractures).

- **Transport to the appropriate ED.** Ensure patient comfort en route.

GENERAL TREATMENT GUIDELINES:
HEMODYNAMICALLY UNSTABLE PATIENT

- **Administer O$_2$ and provide ventilatory support** as needed. Protect cervical spine as indicated.

- **Place the patient in the shock position.**

- **Establish large-bore IV/IO access with NS or LR at 20 mL/kg.**

- **Rapid transport to the appropriate ED. Do not needlessly delay patient transport—expedite transport.**

- **Treat nonlife-threatening injuries as appropriate** (e.g., control bleeding, splint fractures).

- **Supporting documentation.** All suspected cases of child abuse must be investigated. Clear and accurate descriptions of the home environment, a history, and statements made by the patient and caregivers may prove invaluable. Be sure to quote directly all key statements. Use lay terms when describing injuries.

- **Mandatory reporting.** All 50 states have passed laws regarding the mandatory reporting of suspected child abuse by healthcare workers. Although legal requirements may vary, report your findings to the receiving facility and to either the local police or the designated child protection agency.

BIBLIOGRAPHY

Barkin, S. (2003). Abuse, pediatric (nonaccidental trauma, NAT). In J. J. Schaider, S. R. Hayden, R. Wolfe, R. M. Barkin, & P. Rosen (Eds.), *Rosen & Barkin's 5-minute emergency medicine consult* (2nd ed., pp. 22–23). Philadelphia: Lippincott Williams & Wilkins.

Ricci, L. R. & A. S. Botash (n.d.) Child abuse. The eMedicine web page. Retrieved December 12, 2003, at http://www.emedicine.com/emerg/topic368.htm.

NOTES

_____

_____

_____

CHAPTER 13

CROUP, EPIGLOTTITIS, AND PEDIATRIC RESPIRATORY DISTRESS

Owen T. Traynor, M.D.
Patrick R. Coonan, R.N., Ed.D.

PRESENTATION

Respiratory complaints are a common cause of pediatric emergencies. Some young infants may be troubled only by nasal congestion whereas others can experience airway obstruction caused by foreign bodies, croup, and epiglottitis. Bronchospasm from asthma is not uncommon. Infectious causes of respiratory illness include bronchiolitis and pneumonia. Nonpulmonary causes of labored breathing, such as arrhythmias, diabetic ketoacidosis, abdominal pain, and seizures, may be present. This chapter focuses on respiratory diseases in pediatric patients.

IMMEDIATE CONCERNS

❶ **Is there an abnormal mental status?** The brain is very sensitive to hypoxia. Patients with an altered mental state are at increased risk of aspiration.

❶ **Is the patient's airway patent and stable?** Neonates are obligate nasal breathers, so secretions in the nose serve as an easily treated obstruction. A bulb syringe can be used to clear the obstruction. In other cases, simple techniques can be used to open the airway. Caution should be used when epiglottitis is suspected. No inspection or manipulation of the airway should be performed unless endotracheal intubation is necessary.

❶ **Are the respirations adequate?**   The patient's breathing must be observed while his or her chest is visualized. Typically the patient's respiratory rate increases with distress. Pediatric patients often have retractions as well. Apply supplemental oxygen and assist respirations if necessary.

❶ **Is the patient hypoxic?**   Signs of hypoxia include an altered mental status, tachycardia or bradycardia, tachypnea or bradypnea, and cyanosis. Continuous pulse oximetry should be initiated in pediatric patients with respiratory distress. Apply supplemental oxygen in all dyspneic patients regardless of the room air oxygen saturation.

❶ **Are there abnormal respiratory sounds?**   Stridor indicates upper airway obstruction. Wheezing may indicate bronchospasm or a foreign body aspiration. Rales or rhonchi may indicate pneumonia or CHF. Respiratory sounds are easily transmitted in pediatric patients, making it difficult, at times, to accurately determine their location.

SECTION 1

IMPORTANT HISTORY

❷ **Does the patient have a history of respiratory or cardiac disease?**   Many children with special needs live in our communities. The parents or guardians are usually experienced caregivers who can provide expert level guidance to the EMS provider. Illnesses such as asthma are not uncommon in children.

❷ **What was the onset of the respiratory distress?**   Acute onset distress is found in foreign body aspiration and bronchospasm. Gradual onset is more typical of respiratory infections. Epiglottitis typically develops over 6 to 24 hours. Croup gradually develops over 1 or 2 days and suddenly worsens.

❷ **Does the patient have a fever?**   The presence of a fever may indicate an infectious process. Fever also increases the respiratory rate.

❷   **Does the patient have a sore throat?**   Patients with epiglottitis typically report a sore throat and high fever. They sit forward and drool, preferring not to swallow their saliva. They may experience respiratory distress. Patients with a peritonsillar abscess or retropharyngeal abscess may have a similar presentation.

❷   **Are there any associated symptoms?**   Fever suggests an infectious cause. Poor feeding and decreased activity level are part of many illnesses, particularly in young children.

DIFFERENTIAL DIAGNOSIS

UPPER AIRWAY DISEASE

* *UPPER RESPIRATORY INFECTION.* An upper respiratory infection (URI) is better known as the common cold. Patients develop a watery nasal discharge that later becomes thicker and may be associated with fever. Patients commonly report sneezing and coughing. Neonates and young infants have the greatest trouble with URIs. The physical exam reveals nasal congestion and discharge. There is no evidence of hypoxia. No specific EMS treatment is needed. Provide supplemental oxygen if the patient is experiencing respiratory distress.

* *ANAPHYLAXIS.* Anaphylaxis, a severe allergic reaction, may cause swelling of the upper airway and acute bronchospasm. Patients often have hives, too. Stridor may be present with upper airway obstruction. Wheezing is found with bronchospasm. Treatment with epinephrine may be required. Antihistamines are commonly used for less severe reactions. Beta-agonists such as albuterol are often used to treat bronchospasm. See chapter 3 for further details.

* *CROUP.* Croup is a viral illness characterized by mild cold symptoms initially, followed by a seal-bark cough and stridor. It is a viral illness that causes inflammation

and edema in the region of the larynx, trachea, and bronchioles. It is the stridor and barking cough that usually initiates EMS contact. The patient is typically 6 months to 3 years of age. Physical findings include stridor, retractions, occasionally wheezing, and, if the disease is severe, hypoxia and an altered mental state. EMS treatment consists of humidified oxygen, nebulized racemic epinephrine, or l-epinephrine. Dexamethasone (Decadron) is given orally or via intramuscular (IM) injection to counter the airway inflammation. Its effects take many hours to become clinically apparent.

- **EPIGLOTTITIS.** Epiglottitis is an acute bacterial infection involving the epiglottis and the surrounding tissues. The incidence has decreased dramatically following immunization against the organism that caused the majority of cases. The peak incidence is from 2 to 6 years of age. The patient appears ill, with a high fever (> 101.1° F, 38.4° C). The patient assumes a sniffing position. Symptoms include a sore throat, drooling, and a muffled voice. There may be subtle stridor and progressive respiratory distress. Efforts must be made not to upset the patient because agitation may result in rapid deterioration. The child should be transported with the parent. The parent should administer blow-by supplemental oxygen. Nebulized epinephrine may be used as a temporizing measure if it does not cause distress to the patient. Intubation may be difficult and therefore should be avoided in the prehospital environment, if possible. Ventilating the patient is usually possible, although endotracheal intubation is not. Notify the receiving hospital early so that staff may prepare to address the difficult airway.

- **PERITONSILLAR AND RETROPHARYNGEAL ABSCESS.** Peritonsillar abscess is a complication of pharyngitis. An abscess forms in the deep tissues around a tonsil. Patients report a sore throat, unilateral ear pain, fever, a muffled voice, and a sensation of fullness in the pharynx. Its greatest incidence is in teens and young adults.

Physical findings include a large, bulging tonsil; deviation of the uvula; and cervical adenopathy. No stridor or abnormal breath sounds are usually present. Retropharyngeal abscess occurs in younger patients, ages 6 months to 4 years. The abscess develops behind the pharynx in a potential space that is anterior to the vertebrae and extends in to the mediastinum. These patients have recently experienced pharyngitis or an ear infection. They are febrile and often drooling. They report neck pain and sore throat. Physical findings include a muffled voice, pain on movement of the neck, cervical adenopathy, and a bulging pharynx. EMS care includes gentle transport with the parent, continuous pulse oximetry, supplemental oxygen, and having suction equipment and intubation equipment at the ready.

LOWER AIRWAY DISEASE

- **PNEUMONIA.**   Pneumonia is an inflammation of the lung tissue with congestion, cough, and fever. It is commonly caused by bacterial or viral infection. The presentation varies by age. Typical features include fever, cough, tachycardia, tachypnea, hypoxia, retractions, and malaise. Infants may exhibit listlessness, poor feeding, grunting respirations, vomiting, nasal flaring, and wheezing. Older children may report pleuritic chest pain and a productive cough. The physical exam may reveal decreased breath sounds, rales, wheezes, and a dull percussion note. EMS treatment typically involves supplemental oxygen and IV hydration if dehydration or shock is present. Albuterol may be used for bronchospasm.

- **BRONCHIOLITIS.**   Bronchiolitis is an acute inflammatory disease of the upper and lower airways that causes bronchoconstriction and inflammation of the airways. Respiratory syncytial virus (RSV) causes most of the cases. The disease occurs in patients younger than 2 years of age. The clinical features include fever, cough, nasal congestion, wheezing, rales, hypoxia, nasal flaring, retractions, and grunting respirations. Apnea spells occur in those younger than 6 months. EMS treatment includes supplemental oxygen and a trial of nebulized albuterol. Studies have failed to demonstrate effectiveness of beta-agonists, steroids, or nebulized racemic epinephrine.

- *ASTHMA.* Asthma is an episodic inflammatory disease that causes bronchospasm and wheezing. In addition to bronchoconstriction, mucosal edema and mucus plugging are present. Chronic treatment focuses on the prevention of attacks through the use of inhaled steroids and other medications. Acute attacks are treated with inhaled beta-agonists as a rescue intervention. Clinical features of an acute attack include tachypnea, wheezing, respiratory distress, tachycardia, and cough. The physical exam reveals poor airflow, prolonged expiration, and wheezes. EMS treatment includes supplemental oxygen, nebulized beta-agonists, and, in some systems, corticosteroids.

SECTION 1

KEY PHYSICAL EXAMINATION FINDINGS

- ✅ *Initial assessment.* Look for alterations in mental status, threats to the airway, respiratory compromise, and hemodynamic instability.

- ✅ *Vital signs.* Careful monitoring of the vital signs is needed. Check temperature, if possible.

- ✅ *HEENT.* Examine carefully and note signs of swelling, redness, or unusual warmth. Look for pharyngeal exudate, erythema, or tonsillar enlargement. Do not inspect the airway of pediatric patients suspected of having epiglottitis.

- ✅ *Neck.* Assess for cervical adenopathy and stridor.

- ✅ *Lungs.* Listen to lung sounds for signs of bronchospasm or pneumonia. Percuss for areas of consolidation (dull percussion notes).

- ✅ *Chest.* Assess for retractions and respiratory accessory muscle use.

- ✅ ***Extremities.*** Assess nail beds for cyanosis and capillary refill.

- ✅ ***Skin.*** Assess for rashes.

- ✅ ***Neurologic examination.*** An altered mental status can be a sign of hypoxia, infection, or sepsis.

ELECTROCARDIOGRAM

Evaluate ECG results for signs of arrhythmias in tachycardic or bradycardic patients.

GLUCOMETER

Evaluate serum glucose if mental status is altered and hypoglycemia or hyperglycemia is suspected.

PULSE OXIMETER

Evaluate for hypoxia.

TREATMENT PLAN

- ***Patient assessment.*** Perform a rapid and systematic initial assessment, and institute treatment as life-threatening problems are discovered. Prompt transport of seriously ill or unstable patients to the appropriate ED is a key intervention. Frequent reassessment of patients with an altered mental status or respiratory distress is necessary because of the potential for worsening of their condition.

- **Administer O$_2$ and provide ventilatory support** as needed.

- Place the patient in a **head-elevated position** or position of comfort.

- **Monitor the ECG and O$_2$** saturation of all unstable patients and those at risk of becoming unstable.

- Consider the following interventions for bronchospasm:

o **Albuterol** 0.15 mg/kg nebulized, maximum 5 mg. The dose may be repeated as necessary .

o **Ipratropium bromide (Atrovent)** age < 12 years: 1/2 unit dose (1.25 ml (250 µg) of a 0.2% solution) nebulized. Age >12 years: 1/2 to 1 unit dose (1.25 ml (250 µg) to 2.5 ml (500 µg) of a 0.2% solution) nebulized. Repeated in 4 to 6 hours, if needed.

o **Epinephrine** 0.01 mg/kg SC, maximum 0.3 to 0.5 mg. The dose may be repeated in 20 minutes, if needed.

o **Terbutaline** age > 6 years: 5 to 10 µg/kg SC. Maximum single dose 0.4 mg. The dose may be repeated once in 15 to 50 minutes if improvement is insufficient.

- Consider the following interventions for croup:

  o Racemic epinephrine 2.25%, 0.25 to 5 ml in 2.5 ml NS nebulized.

  o Epinephrine 1:1000, 5 ml nebulized.

  o Dexamethasone (decadron) 0.6 mg/kg IM/PO for croup. Maximum dose is 10 mg.

- Consider the following interventions for anaphylaxis:

  o **Epinephrine 1:1000** 0.01 mg/kg SC, max 0.5 in ml. The dose may be repeated in 10 to 15 minutes.

  o **Epinephrine 1:10,000** 0.01 mg/kg, not to exceed 0.5 mg, if the patient is hemodynamically unstable. The dose may be repeated in 5 to 10 minutes.

  o **Diphenhydramine (Benadryl)** 1 mg/kg IV/IM, maximum 50 mg.

  o **Methylprednisolone (Solumedrol)** 2mg/kg IV—not to exceed 125 mg IV.

- Perform frequent reassessment. Respiratory distress may worsen.

- **Transport to the appropriate ED**. Ensure patient comfort enroute.

BIBLIOGRAPHY

Duffy, S. J. (2003). Epiglottitis, pediatric. In J. J. Schaider, S. R. Hayden, R. Wolfe, R. M. Barkin, & P. Rosen (Eds.), *Rosen & Barkin's 5-minute emergency medicine consult* (2nd ed., pp. 374–375). Philadelphia: Lippincott Williams & Wilkins.

Humphries, R. L., K. D. Bricking, & T. M. Huhn (2004). Pediatric emergencies. In C. K. Stone & R. L. Humphries (Eds.), *Current emergency diagnosis and treatment* (5th ed., pp. 1050–1059). New York: McGraw Hill.

Steele, D. (2003). Croup. In J. J. Schaider, S. R. Hayden, R. Wolfe, R. M. Barkin, & P. Rosen (Eds.), *Rosen & Barkin's 5-minute emergency medicine consult* (2nd ed., pp. 274–275). Philadelphia: Lippincott Williams & Wilkins.

NOTES

_____

_____

_____

_____

_____

_____

_____

_____

_____

CHAPTER 14

DIABETIC KETOACIDOSIS AND HYPERGLYCEMIA

Owen T. Traynor, M.D.

PRESENTATION

Patients with hyperglycemia or diabetic ketoacidosis (DKA) often present with malaise and signs of dehydration. When the disease is severe, patients have an altered mental status, signs of shock, and potentially life-threatening electrolyte and metabolic abnormalities. A related disorder, hyperosmolar hyperglycemic nonketotic syndrome (HHNS), also is associated with elevated glucose levels and severe dehydration. DKA is more common in type I diabetics, whereas HHNS is more common in type II diabetics.

IMMEDIATE CONCERNS

● **What is the patient's level of consciousness?** Mental status provides a good index of severity. The alert patient with normal vital signs who provides a coherent history of frequent urination, increased thirst, and mild nausea should obviously be treated differently than the patient who is comatose and hypotensive. The airway may also be at risk in the patient with an altered mental state.

● **What is the patient's hemodynamic status?** Patients with DKA and HHN can have significant fluid deficits as a result of urination and vomiting. Aggressive resuscitation with intravenous fluids (preferably normal saline or lactated Ringer's solution) may be needed.

● **Are there tall peaked T-waves on the patient's ECG?** Hyperglycemic patients may be acidotic. Severe acidosis can lead to hyperkalemia (elevated serum potassium). Other ECG abnormalities that may be seen include a wide QRS, loss of p-waves, and a sine-wave configuration of the ECG. Eventually, ventricular fibrillation and asystole may occur. Hyperkalemia may be treated with calcium chloride, beta-agonists, sodium bicarbonate, and diuretics.

IMPORTANT HISTORY

❓ **Does the patient have a history of diabetes?** Patients with type I (insulin-dependent) diabetes may suffer from hyperglycemia when they are noncompliant with their insulin and diet regimen. The initial presentation of some patients with undiagnosed diabetes is hyperglycemia or DKA.

❓ **Has the patient been ill recently?** Other factors, such as sepsis, acute illness, myocardial infarction, and glucocorticoid steroid use, can cause hyperglycemia.

❓ **Has the patient been having symptoms associated with hyperglycemia?** Once blood glucose levels rise above 180 mg/dL, many patients experience frequent urination, thirst, and hunger.

❓ **How long has the patient been sick?** DKA typically has a quicker onset than HHNS (1 or 2 days versus days or weeks).

❓ **When was the patient's last meal?** The hyperglycemia may be caused by a recent meal.

❓ **Are there any new medications?** Diuretics and steroids, as well as anticonvulsants such as phenytoin and some blood pressure medications, can precipitate HHNS.

DIFFERENTIAL DIAGNOSIS

• **TYPE I DIABETES.** Patients with type I diabetes require insulin (even when not eating). The onset of diabetes occurs when the patient is a child or young adult. Patients with type I diabetes are at risk of DKA.

- **TYPE II DIABETES.** Patients with type II diabetes typically have the onset of diabetes during adulthood. They are often obese. They are managed with oral agents primarily, although some patients use insulin as well. These patients are more likely to develop HHS than DKA.

- **DIABETIC KETOACIDOSIS.** DKA is defined by blood sugar levels that are greater than 300 mg/dL, ketones in the blood or urine, and a low serum pH (< 7.30). Patients with DKA have an insulin deficiency that prevents glucose metabolism, leading to hyperglycemia, diuresis, and fat metabolism. Metabolism of fats yields ketoacids. Dehydration, electrolyte abnormalities, and metabolic acidosis result. Many patients have GI symptoms such as abdominal pain, nausea, and vomiting. A patient with DKA may report polydipsia, polyphagia, and polyuria. Kussmaul respirations and a fruity breath odor may be apparent. In severe cases the patient has an altered mental state. If untreated, shock, severe hyperkalemia and acidosis, altered mental status, and death may occur. These patients often require more than 5 liters of IV fluids.

- **GESTATIONAL DIABETES.** Glucose intolerance can occur during pregnancy, leading to gestational diabetes.

- **HYPEROSMOLAR HYPERGLYCEMIC SYNDROME.** Patients with HHNS have sufficient insulin to prevent the metabolism of fats and the production of ketones. The typical patient is elderly. Many are nursing home residents. There may be no history of diabetes. Typically an infection is the acute stressor that leads to HHNS. Other physiologic stresses include acute MI, CVA, and trauma. Medications have also been implicated. HHNS develops over several days to weeks. The patient typically appears ill and has an altered mental status on presentation. Kussmaul respirations are not common. Abdominal pain is unusual. Any abdominal pain must be considered as

SECTION 1

part of the precipitating illness. Elderly patients can have atypical presentations of appendicitis and cholecystitis. HHNS patients will have greater fluid deficits than DKA patients. The average HHNS patient may require 9 L of IV fluids.

- **POSTPRANDIAL HYPERGLYCEMIA.** Postprandial hyperglycemia is the hyperglycemia that occurs transiently after meals.

- **ACUTE STRESS REACTION.** The stress of an acute severe illness (sepsis, acute MI, shock, trauma) can cause hyperglycemia.

- **MEDICATION-INDUCED HYPERGLYCEMIA.** Certain medications such as glucocorticoid steroids and thiazide diuretics may cause hyperglycemia.

- **OTHER SOURCES.** Exogenous glucose load, pancreatic disease, and Cushing's syndrome are infrequent causes of hyperglycemia.

- **SPURIOUS HYPERGLYCEMIA.** Repeat testing if the patient lacks signs and symptoms of hyperglycemia.

KEY PHYSICAL EXAMINATION FINDINGS

- ✅ **Initial assessment.** Look for signs of shock, hypovolemia, and altered mental status.

- ✅ **Vital signs.** Look for tachycardia, tachypnea, and hypotension. Patients with DKA often develop severe acidosis and compensate for this by increasing their respiratory rate. Kussmaul's respirations are the deep, sighing, rapid breaths characteristic of this response.

- ✅ **HEENT.** Note any fruity, sweet, or acetone-like odor on the breath characteristic of ketoacidosis. Examine the oral mucosa for signs of dehydration.

- ✅ **Lungs.** Listen for signs of pneumonia that may have precipitated the current illness. Evaluate the depth and quality of respirations.

⊘ ***Abdomen.*** Evaluate for tenderness and peritoneal signs.

⊘ ***Neurologic examination.*** Evaluate mental status and look for signs of focal weakness or paralysis.

GLUCOMETER

The glucometer will reveal hyperglycemia.

ELECTROCARDIOGRAM

The ECG may reveal evidence of ischemia or hyperkalemia. Early ECG features of hyperkalemia include tall, peaked T-waves. Higher levels of potassium cause prolongation of the PR interval and the QRS-complex. Still higher levels cause a biphasic (sine wave–like) QRS. Ventricular fibrillation and asystole may follow. Common arrhythmias associated with hyperkalemia include sinus bradycardia, sinus arrest, first-degree arteriovenous block and junctional and idioventricular rhythms.

TREATMENT PLAN

* **Administer O$_2$** and provide ventilatory support as needed.

* Draw a red-top tube for pretreatment glucose reading if a glucometer is not available.

* **Establish large-bore IV access,** and begin IV fluid resuscitation with 0.9%NaCL or LR.

* Consider the following interventions if hyperkalemia is suspected:

  o Calcium chloride 8 to 16 mg/kg (usually 500 to 1000 mg) slow IV.

  o Sodium bicarbonate 1 mEq/kg IV.

  o Albuterol 2.5 mg nebulized.

* **Transport to appropriate ED.** Do not needlessly delay patient transport—expedite transport. Ensure patient comfort en route.

BIBLIOGRAPHY

Chiasson, J. L., et al. (2003). Diagnosis and treatment of diabetic ketoacidosis and the hyperglycemic hyperosmolar state. *Canadian Medical Association Journal 168,* 859–866, 2003.

Ferri, F. (2004). *Practical guide to the care of the medical patient,* (6th ed.). St. Louis, MO: Mosby.

Goldman, L., & J. C. Bennett (Eds.). (2000). Cecil textbook of medicine (21st ed.). Philadelphia: W. B. Saunders.

Kitabchi, A. E., et al. (2001). Management of hyperglycemic crises in patients with diabetes. *Diabetes Care 24,* 131–153, 2001.

Marx, J., et al. (Eds.) (2002). *Rosen's emergency medicine: concepts and clinical practice* (5th ed.). St. Louis, MO: Mosby.

NOTES

_____

_____

_____

_____

_____

_____

_____

_____

_____

_____

_____

_____

CHAPTER 15

DRUG WITHDRAWAL SYNDROME

Hal A. Skopicki, M.D., Ph.D.
Elizabeth Cohn, R.N., N.P.

PRESENTATION

Drug withdrawal syndromes occur when addicted patients reduce or discontinue using the drug to which they are addicted. Common syndromes include alcohol, opiate, benzodiazepine, and stimulant withdrawal syndromes. Withdrawal syndrome may occur when prescribed drugs are discontinued as well. Often the withdrawing patient is anxious, tachycardic, hypertensive, and diaphoretic and complains of nausea and vomiting. In some cases, withdrawal can be life-threatening. It can be difficult to distinguish acute withdrawal from other illnesses.

IMMEDIATE CONCERNS

- **Does the patient have an altered mental status?** Some withdrawal syndromes can cause an altered mental state, including alcohol and benzodiazepine withdrawal. Many other illness and head injuries may be responsible as well.

- **Is the airway patent and safe?** Nausea and vomiting are common during withdrawal. The airway may be at risk.

- **Is there evidence of respiratory distress?** Respiratory distress is not a common element of withdrawal syndromes. Patients may have anxiety, which can lead to mild tachypnea.

● **Is the patient hemodynamically stable?** Autonomic instability is common and is typically manifested by tachycardia and hypertension. Some patients may have orthostatic hypotension. Barbiturate withdrawal may cause hypotension.

IMPORTANT HISTORY

● **Has the patient had a seizure?** Withdrawal seizures occur with alcohol, benzodiazepine, and barbiturate withdrawal. Seizures may indicate severe withdrawal and warn of a potentially life-threatening course. See chapter 37.

● **Has the patient been febrile?** Fever is not a presenting feature of most drug withdrawal syndromes but may occur in life-threatening cases of benzodiazepine withdrawal. Hyperthermia can occur as a result of stimulant drug use, as well as other illnesses, including infection. See chapter 23.

● **Does the patient have a history of substance abuse?** Ask specifically about past drug use in a nonjudgmental manner. Diagnosing a drug withdrawal syndrome is difficult with no history of drug or alcohol abuse. Find out about the frequency of use, the amount of use, and the duration of use.

● **When was the last use of the drug?** Withdrawal symptoms can occur within 6 to 8 hours of decreasing alcohol use. Opiate withdrawal can begin within 4 to 8 hours for heroin and within 36 to 72 hours for methadone. Benzodiazepine withdrawal symptom onset is variable, with onset within 24 hours for alprazolam (Xanax) or as late as 1 week for diazepam (Valium). The symptoms can persist for weeks.

● **Does the patient report drug craving?** Drug craving is an early symptom of withdrawal.

● **Has the patient had withdrawal before?** Some believe that there is a phenomenon known as kindling, in which prior episodes of withdrawal promote more serious subsequent withdrawal. Certainly a prior history of severe withdrawal should alert the paramedic of the potential for a serious current illness.

❷ Has there been any change in medications recently? Not all withdrawal syndromes are caused by withdrawal from illegal drugs. Look specifically for changes in opiate analgesics, benzodiazepines, sedatives, psychiatric medications, and antihypertensive agents.

DIFFERENTIAL DIAGNOSIS

WITHDRAWAL SYNDROMES

* ***ALCOHOL WITHDRAWAL SYNDROME.*** Alcohol withdrawal syndrome can begin as early as 6 hours after the last drink. It can last about 5 days. Symptoms include anxiety, agitation, depression, tremors, anorexia, insomnia, nausea, and vomiting. Seizures may occur in 5% to 25% of patients. The peak time for seizures is between 13 and 24 hours after the last drink; however, seizures may occur up to 96 hours after cessation. A severe form of withdrawal is marked by delirium tremens (DTs). Patients with the DTs have severe sympathetic instability (tachycardia, hypertension) with tremors, altered mental status, and fever. DTs usually begin about 48 to 72 hours after the final drink. The mortality rate for DTs is 10% to 15%. Physical exam findings include tachycardia, hypertension, tremors, diaphoresis, flushed skin, and hyperreflexia. The Clinical Institute Withdrawal Assessment of Alcohol Scale, Revised (CIWA-Ar; see appendix L) is a tool used to assess the severity of alcohol withdrawal. Scores lower than 8 indicate mild or minimal withdrawal. Scores greater than 8 and equal to or less than 15 indicate moderate withdrawal. Scores greater than 15 indicate severe withdrawal and impending DTs. EMS care includes seizure precautions, ECG monitoring, and treatment of hypoglycemia, if present. Treatment of the DTs involves intravenous (IV) benzodiazepines.

- ***BENZODIAZEPINE WITHDRAWAL SYNDROME.*** Benzodiazepine withdrawal has a similar presentation to alcohol withdrawal. Symptom onset is variable, with onset within 24 hours for alprazolam (Xanax) or as late as 1 week for diazepam (Valium). The symptoms can persist for weeks. An acute withdrawal can be precipitated by flumazenil (Romazicon). The symptoms are those of autonomic instability and CNS stimulation. Patients report anxiety, nausea, vomiting, diaphoresis, insomnia, palpitations, and tremor. Initial physical findings include tachycardia and hypertension. Later the patient can develop hypotension, hyperthermia, and seizures. EMS treatment is typically supportive. IV benzodiazepines may be used if there is a significant withdrawal syndrome.

- ***OPIATE WITHDRAWAL SYNDROME.*** Withdrawal symptoms for patients addicted to opiates begin typically at about the time the next dose is due. Heroin withdrawal begins 4 to 8 hours after the last dose. The symptoms peak at 36 to 72 hours and may persist up to 7 to 10 days. The administration of naloxone (Narcan) can precipitate an acute withdrawal syndrome. Typical withdrawal symptoms include anxiety, restlessness, lacrimation, runny nose, dilated pupils, and piloerection. Myalgias, abdominal cramps, nausea, and vomiting follow. Intense drug craving is reported. EMS care is supportive.

- ***BARBITURATE WITHDRAWAL SYNDROME.*** Barbiturate withdrawal syndrome involves anxiety, insomnia, diaphoresis, nausea, and vomiting. Physical findings include tachycardia, confusion, hypotension, and seizures. EMS care is supportive.

OTHER SOURCES OF DELIRIUM

- ***CENTRAL NERVOUS SYSTEM ETIOLOGIES.***

  o ***Acute cerebrovascular accident.*** Typical features of cerebrovascular accident (CVA) include unilateral neurologic deficits. Signs and symptoms can be dynamic. See chapter 10.

o ***Acute intracranial hemorrhage.*** The patient suffering an acute intracranial hemorrhage may complain of a severe "thunderclap, worst headache of my life" type of pain, often accompanied by nausea and vomiting. This is a life-threatening illness that may rapidly progress. There may be few neurologic deficits initially.

o ***Traumatic brain injury.*** Although many traumatic brain injuries are apparent, some may be occult because the injury occurred several days earlier and is manifested by a gradual decline in mental status. See chapter 20.

o ***Seizure.*** Although there are many etiologies of seizures, the most common is epilepsy. Seizures may also occur as a component of alcohol withdrawal syndrome. EMS treatment consists of protecting the patient from injury, preventing or treating hypoxia, and observing the patient. Some patients may require benzodiazepines to halt a prolonged seizure or treat recurrent seizures or status epilepticus. See chapter 37.

o ***Tumors.*** Primary or metastatic brain tumors may cause an altered LOC with or without obvious focal neurologic findings. Symptoms may develop as the tumor compresses adjacent tissue or secondary to edema or bleeding of the tumor. Often the patient complains of new onset headaches.

• ***TOXICOLOGIC ETIOLOGIES.*** Select toxins are noted below. See chapter 34 for additional toxicology information.

o ***Ethanol and other alcohols.*** Ethanol is the most commonly abused alcohol that EMS personnel are called to treat. Typical clinical features include sedation, slurred speech, and ataxia. Patients can be agitated and uncooperative. Be alert for other occult illnesses or injuries when considering what appears to be alcohol intoxication.

o **_Opiates/narcotics._** The prototypical EMS opiate overdose is the IV heroin user. The patient has constricted pupils; slow, snoring respirations; and a depressed mental status. The goal of naloxone (Narcan) therapy is to improve the respiratory status of the patient. If there are atypical features, such as normal respirations, tachycardia, and hypertension, consider the presence of an additional drug.

o **_Carbon monoxide._** Carbon monoxide (CO), a colorless, tasteless gas, can cause an altered mental status. It is present in the environment when there is incomplete combustion. High-flow oxygen can significantly increase the elimination of CO from the blood. Patients with a serious illness may benefit from hyperbaric oxygen (HBO). See chapter 40 for information about CO poisoning.

o **_Drug abuse._** Chapter 34 provides a description of common toxidromes or toxicologic syndromes.

• **_INFECTIOUS ETIOLOGIES._**

o **_Meningitis._** Meningitis is an infection of the meninges. Patients present with a history of a headache, fever, and possibly nuchal rigidity (a stiff neck). The mental state may become altered as the disease progresses.

o **_Encephalitis._** Encephalitis is an inflammation of the brain that is typically caused by a viral infection. Encephalitis usually begins with a flulike illness characterized by mild headaches, fever, body aches, and poor appetite. The disease may progress to include an altered LOC, worsening headache, vomiting, possible nuchal rigidity, seizures, coma, and death.

o ***Sepsis.*** Sepsis is defined as a syndrome caused by an infection and associated with a systemic inflammatory response such as fever, hypothermia, altered mental status, tachycardia, tachypnea, hypotension, and poor capillary refill.

- **PULMONARY ETIOLOGIES.**

  o ***Hypoxia.*** Many pulmonary diseases can cause hypoxia. Often the addition of supplemental oxygen improves oxygenation.

  o ***Hypercapnia.*** Patients with hypercapnia typically develop mildly elevated carbon dioxide (CO_2) levels. If the CO_2 levels continue to increase, the patient may become sleepy, leading to a further decrease in ventilation. Thus the CO_2 can rapidly increase. Hypoxia occurs as well. This can be treated with ventilation.

  o ***Acute pulmonary embolism.*** Large pulmonary emboli can cause syncope. Hypoxia is often present, too. EMS treatment includes supplemental oxygen and IV fluid resuscitation, if needed. See chapter 11 and chapter 16.

- **METABOLIC ETIOLOGIES.**

  o ***Hypoglycemia.*** Hypoglycemia is one of the most common causes of altered mental status treated by paramedics. Generally these patients respond rapidly to oral or IV dextrose. See chapter 24 for more details.

  o ***Hyperglycemia.*** The history is one of a gradual onset. Patients often report malaise, polyuria, polydipsia and polyphagia. Hyperglycemia may be the initial presentation for a diabetic. See chapter 14.

  o ***Electrolyte disorders.*** Electrolyte disorders are usually not diagnosed by EMS providers because laboratory analysis of the blood is needed.

o **_Diabetic ketoacidosis and hyperosmolar hyperglycemic syndrome._** Diabetic ketoacidosis and hyperosmolar hyperglycemic syndrome share some of the features of hyperglycemia. EMS treatment involves IV fluid resuscitation. See chapter 14.

o **_Encephalopathy._** Encephalopathy is a progressive syndrome of brain dysfunction. Initially the patient may have a normal mental status but difficulty with memory and concentration. These symptoms may progress to confusion, impaired ability to perform mental tasks, disorientation, and coma. There are many causes, including hypertension, liver disease, and renal failure. EMS care is supportive.

o **_Uremia._** Uremia is a clinical syndrome of metabolic abnormalities associated with electrolyte, fluid, and hormonal imbalances that occur with renal failure. See chapter 4.

o **_Thyroid disorders._** Both hypothyroidism and hyperthyroidism can cause an alteration in mental status. See chapter 4.

• **_ENVIRONMENTAL ETIOLOGIES._**

o **_Heat-related emergencies._** Heat exhaustion and heatstroke are two heat-related emergencies that are associated with an alteration in mental status. See chapter 23.

o **_Hypothermia._** The mental status changes associated with hypothermia become apparent at about 93° F (34° C). See chapter 23.

o **_Near-drowning._** A combination of hypoxia and hypercapnia, such as that seen in near-drowning incidents, can lead to a change in mental status. See chapter 31.

• **_VASCULAR ETIOLOGIES._**

o **_Hypertensive encephalopathy._** Hypertensive encephalopathy is an acute, life-threatening alteration in

CNS function caused by severe hypertension. See chapter 22.

o ___Hypotension.___   The brain is sensitive to the poor perfusion that accompanies hypotension. See chapter 25.

KEY PHYSICAL EXAMINATION FINDINGS

- ✅ *Initial assessment.* Look for alterations in mental status, threats to the airway, respiratory compromise, and hemodynamic instability.

- ✅ *Vital signs.* Careful monitoring of the vital signs is needed. Many patients are tachycardic and hypertensive. Hypotension can occur. Hyperthermia may also be found.

- ✅ *HEENT.* Examine carefully and note signs of trauma or asymmetry. Examine pupils for responsiveness and equality.

- ✅ *Neck.* Assess for trauma. Assess for nuchal rigidity if this is a nontraumatic illness.

- ✅ *Lungs.* Listen to lung sounds for signs of pulmonary edema, bronchospasm, or pneumonia.

- ✅ *Abdomen.* Assess carefully for masses, tenderness, or peritoneal signs.

- ✅ *Extremities.* Assess for edema in the extremities. Check peripheral pulses to equality. Inspect for needle-track marks.

- ✅ *Neurologic examination.* An altered mental status is a sensitive indicator of cerebral perfusion. Severe withdrawal syndromes involve altered mental states. Assess cranial nerves and perform a motor and sensory examination. Unilateral deficits may be present in CVAs.

ELECTROCARDIOGRAM

Evaluate ECG results for signs of arrhythmias, cardiac ischemia, or injury.

SECTION 1

GLUCOMETER

Evaluate for hypoglycemia or hyperglycemia.

PULSE OXIMETER

Evaluate for hypoxia.

TREATMENT PLAN

- ***Patient assessment.*** Perform a rapid and systematic initial assessment, and institute treatment as life-threatening problems are discovered. Prompt transport to the appropriate ED is a key intervention. Frequent reassessment of patients with a suspected withdrawal syndrome is necessary because of the potential for worsening of their hemodynamic and neurologic status.

GENERAL TREATMENT GUIDELINES

- **Administer O$_2$ and provide ventilatory support** as needed.

- Place the patient in a **head-elevated position,** unless spinal immobilization is needed, or in the shock position, if shock is present.

- **Monitor the ECG and O$_2$ saturation. Perform blood glucose determination.**

- **Establish IV** access. Provide IV fluid resuscitation, if needed.

- **Treat hypoglycemia, if indicated.**

- **Treat seizures with a benzodiazepine.** Dosing may be repeated every 10 to 15 minutes, but all benzodiazepines can cause respiratory depression, hypotension, and decreased LOC:

  o **Diazepam** (Valium) 5 to 10 mg IV

  o **Lorazepam** (Ativan) 1 to 2 mg IV

or

o **Midazolam** (versed) 1 to 2 mg IV

- Frequently reassess the patient's airway and hemodynamic and neurologic status.

- **Transport to the appropriate ED.** Ensure patient comfort en route.

BIBLIOGRAPHY

Shockley, L. (2003). Withdrawal: Alcohol. In J. J. Schaider, S. R. Hayden, R. Wolfe, R. M. Barkin, & P. Rosen (Eds.), *Rosen & Barkin's 5-minute emergency medicine consult*, (2nd ed., pp. 1232–1233). Philadelphia: Lippincott Williams & Wilkins.

Shockley, L. (2003). Withdrawal: Drug. In J. J. Schaider, S. R. Hayden, R. Wolfe, R. M. Barkin, & P. Rosen (Eds.), *Rosen & Barkin's 5-minute emergency medicine consult* (2nd ed., pp. 1234–1235). Philadelphia: Lippincott Williams & Wilkins.

Wax, P. M. (2001). Withdrawal syndromes. In A. Harwood-Nus, A. B. Wolfson, C. H. Linden, S. M. Shepard, P. H. Stenklyft (Eds.), *The clinical practice of emergency medicine* (3rd ed., pp. 1628–1633). Philadelphia: Lippincott Williams & Wilkins.

NOTES

_____

_____

_____

_____

_____

_____

SECTION 1

CHAPTER 16

DYSPNEA

Walt Stoy, Ph.D., EMT-P
Thomas J. Rahilly, Ph.D.

PRESENTATION

Dyspnea is one of the most common medical complaints witnessed in the prehospital arena. Most patients describe it as a sensation of shortness of breath or a feeling of "air hunger" accompanied by labored breathing. Dyspnea may be caused by pulmonary or cardiac disease or by any mechanism that causes hypoxia. Dyspnea may be mild, manifesting as dyspnea on exertion, or severe, in which dyspnea occurs even at rest. This chapter focuses on dyspnea caused by mechanisms other than foreign body obstruction (see chapter 33) or croup and epiglottitis (see chapter 13).

IMMEDIATE CONCERNS

- **Is the patient's airway patent and stable?** Look and listen for indicators of airway obstruction. Check for equal bilateral chest movement and cyanosis in the patient's nail beds and mucous membranes. A patient experiencing difficulty breathing may show signs of labored respirations, such as the use of accessory muscles, tracheal tugging, or nasal flaring. Auscultation of the chest should always follow a visual inspection of the neck and chest.

- **What is the rate and depth of the respirations?** Most adults breathe at a resting rate of about 16 breaths per minute. Patients in respiratory distress usually have a rapid (greater than 25 breaths per minute) and deep pattern of breathing. The respiratory rate (RR) may be slow (less than nine breaths) and shallow if the respiratory drive has been depressed. Be alert for respiratory breathing patterns that may indicate central nervous system (CNS) impairment (Cheyne-Stokes respirations) and medical emergencies (Kussmaul's respirations).

● **Is the patient hypoxic?**   The question is easily answered by using pulse oximetry. If pulse oximetry is unavailable, clinical assessment must be used. The presence of either tachypnea or bradypnea, tachycardia, or cyanosis may suggest hypoxia. Restlessness, agitation, confusion, and occasionally combative behavior may also indicate hypoxia. The absence of cyanosis is not a reliable indicator of adequate oxygenation. Cyanosis occurs when 5 gm/100 cc of hemoglobin is unsaturated with oxygen. The normal adult has approximately 12 to 15 gm/100 cc of hemoglobin. A severely anemic patient may have significantly less hemoglobin. A patient with 6 gm/100 cc of hemoglobin, for example, will not be cyanotic if more than 1 gm/100 cc are oxygenated. These patients have a dramatically reduced oxygen-carrying capacity, approximately 40% to 50% of normal, and yet will not become cyanotic until they are carrying less than 9% of the oxygen of a normal healthy patient. Do not withhold oxygen from the hypoxic patient.

● **Does the patient produce abnormal breath sounds?** The breathing process is normally quiet. Listen to the chest for abnormal sounds that may indicate the nature of the problem. Absent breath sounds may indicate a pneumothorax or tension pneumothorax. If a tension pneumothorax is present, immediate needle decompression of the chest is indicated. Open pneumothoraces should be sealed immediately (on three sides) with an air occlusive dressing.

● **In what position was the patient found?**   Patients experiencing dyspnea are often found in a sitting or semi-sitting position. These patients do not tolerate lying flat and should be transported in a position that permits maximal comfort.

IMPORTANT HISTORY

❓ **Does the patient have a history of respiratory disease?**
Because many respiratory diseases are chronic in nature, there may be a history of the current problem. Persons who smoke tobacco products are especially prone to diseases of the respiratory system.

❓ **Was the onset sudden or gradual?**   Cases of dyspnea that have a sudden onset are usually more acute. Pulmonary embolism (PE), pneumothorax, bronchospasm, and acute pulmonary edema have a rapid onset.

❓ **What brought on this period of dyspnea?**   Was it the result of exertion or stress, or did the condition develop spontaneously?

❓ **Does the patient have any history of other medical problems?**   Because dyspnea is only a symptom of a particular disease, it is important to determine the underlying problem so that it may be treated. Respiratory and cardiovascular diseases are the most common causes of dyspnea, but other disease processes, such as diabetes and acquired immunodeficiency syndrome (AIDS), can result in breathing difficulty.

❓ **Is chest pain associated with the dyspnea?**   Cardiovascular problems often cause the patient to experience difficulty in breathing. Although not all chest pain indicates a cardiovascular event, it is a significant finding and may be the initial complaint.

❓ **Does the patient have evidence of infection?**   Cough (especially a productive cough), fever, and chills may indicate an infectious etiology such as pneumonia.

❓ **What medications is the patient currently taking?**
Knowing whether the patient takes medication and, if so, the type may help to identify the current cause of the dyspnea. Bronchodilator inhalers indicate an obstructive disease, such as chronic obstructive pulmonary disease (COPD) or asthma.

DIFFERENTIAL DIAGNOSIS

NOTE: Upper airway obstruction is covered in chapter 33, and croup and epiglottitis in chapter 13.

PULMONARY ETIOLOGIES

- **ACUTE ASTHMA.** Acute asthma is a reversible, episodic disease in which an obstruction results from one or more of the three "Ss": spasm, swelling, and secretions. Wheezes, most commonly heard during expiration, may also be heard on inspiration; however, if severe bronchospasm is present, there may be no wheezing. Status asthmaticus is a prolonged and life-threatening form of asthma that cannot be controlled with epinephrine.

- **ANAPHYLAXIS.** Wheezing may be a manifestation of anaphylaxis because histamine release and inflammation lead to narrowing of the airways. Usually, however, other clues are present to indicate an anaphylactic reaction, such as rash, edema, hypotension, and so forth.

- **ASPIRATION.** Persistent localized wheezing can suggest the diagnosis of foreign body aspiration, especially in individuals who may not protect their airways well. Foreign body aspiration, however, usually produces an obstruction of the upper airway and therefore is more likely to produce stridor (a continuous sound more prominent during inspiration than expiration) than frank wheezing. Aspiration is more likely to occur in young children and older debilitated patients who cannot protect their airway.

- **CHRONIC OBSTRUCTIVE PULMONARY DISEASE.** COPD is characterized by diffuse obstruction to airflow. The most common types are as follows:

  - o **Emphysema** is best described as distension beyond the bronchioles with destruction of alveolar septa. Patients with emphysema are usually thin as a result of weight loss and provide a history of dyspnea on exertion. Exhalation is prolonged and difficult, with the lungs still expanded after exhalation, resulting in a barrel-shaped appearance to the chest. Respirations are rapid, and breath sounds are distant and difficult to hear. Patients may appear short of breath and purse their lips during exhalation.

o **_Chronic bronchitis_** is characterized by inflammation, edema, and excessive mucus production in the bronchial tree. Patients with this condition use their neck and chest muscles to assist with breathing. They usually have a productive cough and a history of repetitive respiratory infections. On examination, they often cough, and rhonchi and wheezing can be heard on both inspiration and exhalation. They appear to struggle to get air into their lungs.

- **_PLEURAL EFFUSIONS._**   Pleural effusions, or collections of fluid, blood (hemothorax), or pus in the pleural space, may cause dyspnea by compressing the lungs. There are many etiologies, including congestive heart failure (CHF), pneumonia, cancer, tuberculosis, and cirrhosis.

- **_PNEUMONIA._**   Pneumonia causes lung inflammation and fluid- or pus-filled alveoli, leading to inadequate oxygenation of the blood. Pneumonia is most frequently caused by a bacterial or viral infection, although it may occur after aspiration of fluids, such as vomit, or inhalation of irritants, such as chemicals or smoke.

- **_PULMONARY EMBOLISM._**   Pulmonary embolism most often involves acute shortness of breath with tachycardia. Some patients also complain of a pleuritic type of chest pain that may be increased on inspiration. Common symptoms include chest pain in 88% of patients, dyspnea in 84% of patients, and cough in 53% of patients. Common physical findings include tachypnea (RR greater than 16) in 92% of patients, tachycardia (heart rate greater than 100 bpm) in 44% of patients, and temperature greater than 100.04° F in 43% of patients. Risk factors of pulmonary embolism include a history of atrial fibrillation, obesity, pregnancy, prolonged immobilization, posttrauma, oral contraceptive use, postsurgery, and cancer.

- **PNEUMOTHORAX.** A pneumothorax occurs when air enters the pleural sac surrounding the lungs. The pneumothorax can be caused by trauma or may occur spontaneously. Tension pneumothorax usually results from trauma. It may, however, result from a spontaneous pneumothorax. Physical exam findings of a simple pneumothorax include absent or diminished breath sounds, tracheal deviation, and hyperresonant percussion notes. Small pneumothoraces may not be detected by physical exam. The physical exam findings of a tension pneumothorax are similar to a simple pneumothorax, and also include JVD. The physical exam is an excellent tool for diagnosing a tension pneumothorax.

CARDIAC ETIOLOGIES

- **ACUTE MYOCARDIAL INFARCTION.** Some patients experiencing an acute myocardial infarction (AMI) may have a primary symptom of dyspnea and, after questioning, may also admit to chest pain.

- **ACUTE PULMONARY EDEMA.** Normally associated with CHF, acute pulmonary edema occurs when an excess of fluid builds up in the extravascular space in the lungs. Pulmonary edema usually results from a fluid overload in the pulmonary circulation due to an AMI-damaged left ventricle. Inadequate cardiac output may cause dyspnea in patients with symptomatic tachycardias or bradycardias. It can also be caused by drowning, aspiration pneumonia, and smoke or toxin inhalation.

- **PERICARDIAL TAMPONADE.** Persons suffering from pericardial tamponade often complain of difficulty breathing. It may result from penetrating or blunt trauma to the chest. It may develop over a time period from minutes to approximately 1 week. Muffled heart tones, together with JVD and narrowed pulse pressure, known as Beck's triad, may be found in pericardial tamponade. There are also several atraumatic etiologies (e.g., secondary to pericardial effusions resulting from renal disease, acute leukemias, lymphomas, breast cancer, lung cancer, and ovarian cancer).

NONCARDIAC AND NONPULMONARY ETIOLOGIES

- **HYPERVENTILATION.**   Usually brought on by psychological stress, hyperventilation typically occurs in young, anxious patients but may also be brought on by an overdose of aspirin or the need to compensate for metabolic acidosis. Hyperventilation is characterized by rapid, deep, or abnormal breathing. Although less common, organic causes of hyperventilation should not be excluded from the diagnosis.

- **ANEMIA.**   Anemia, or decreased red blood cell mass, results in a decreased oxygen-carrying capacity. Anemia may result from inadequate red blood cell production, blood loss, or premature destruction of red blood cells. The anemia may be chronic or acute, as in the case of hemorrhage.

- **CARBON MONOXIDE POISONING.**   Carbon monoxide poisoning may cause hypoxia and therefore dyspnea. Carbon monoxide has an affinity for hemoglobin 210 times greater than oxygen. Its half-life at room air is 4 to 6 hours. If 100% oxygen is given, the half-life is reduced to 60 to 90 minutes. The use of hyperbaric oxygen may decrease its half-life to 15 to 30 minutes.

KEY PHYSICAL EXAMINATION FINDINGS

- ✅ **Initial assessment.**   Look for signs of shock.

- ✅ **Vital signs.**   Assess for tachycardia and tachypnea, which usually accompany dyspnea. Hypotension may be present in patients who have experienced trauma, anaphylactic shock, or AMI. Fever may be present with pulmonary causes as well as with AMI.

✓ **Skin.** Look for peripheral cyanosis; patients experiencing dyspnea may be hypoxic.

✓ **Neck.** Assess the jugular veins for distension, indicating decompensated heart failure or pericardial tamponade.

✓ **Accessory muscles.** Observe the patient for use of the neck and chest wall muscles to assist with breathing, a sign that the work of breathing is too great for the diaphragm alone. Abdominal breathing is an even later sign that indicates the patient is beginning to tire. The energy required to breathe in this manner is great, and once fatigue sets in, the patient will no longer be able to compensate for the extra airway resistance.

✓ **Lungs.** Assess for evidence of abnormal breath sounds. Listen to the nature and character of the breath sounds. Beware, however, of being fooled into a sense of security by a previously noisy chest that has become quiet. Often this change is a sign of danger because, as the patient tires, the patient cannot generate enough airflow to create wheezes. Usually at this stage, the patient is rapidly deteriorating and steps should be taken immediately to prevent loss of the airway. Evidence of blunt trauma or penetrating trauma should raise suspicion of intrathoracic injury, including pericardial tamponade, tension pneumothorax, and hemothorax.

✓ **Heart.** Assess for muffled heart tones indicative of pericardial tamponade.

✓ **Abdomen.** Assess for evidence of diaphragmatic breathing that could indicate a problem with the CNS.

✓ **Extremities.** Check for peripheral pulses. They may be absent as perfusion decreases, which could indicate trauma as a cause of the dyspnea. Assess the fingers for clubbing and the nailbeds for cyanosis.

- ✪ ***Mental status.*** Look for signs of altered mental status, which is a sensitive indicator of inadequate cerebral perfusion and hypoxia.

- ✪ ***Neurologic examination.*** Evaluate for signs of head or spinal injury, which is quite common in the trauma victim.

ELECTROCARDIOGRAM

All patients with difficulty breathing should receive cardiac monitoring.

TREATMENT PLAN

The goal of the treatment plan is to relieve hypoxia and improve the oxygenation of the patient. Frequent reassessment of patients with dyspnea is necessary because of the potential for worsening of their respiratory status. Be prepared—the potential for respiratory arrest exists.

GENERAL TREATMENT GUIDELINES

- **Administer O$_2$ and provide ventilatory support** as needed. Monitor O$_2$ saturation with pulse oximetry if available. Ventilatory support includes relieving upper airway obstructions, suctioning, performing needle-chest decompression of the tension pneumothorax, and sealing an open pneumothorax with an air occlusive dressing or endotracheal intubation.

- **Continuous or bi-level positive airway pressure (CPAP or BiPAP).** CPAP or BiPAP may be employed to reduce the need for endotracheal intubation. The respiratory rate should be greater than 25/min with evidence of respiratory distress, such as respiratory accessory muscle use. Systolic BP must be greater than 100 mm Hg. The patient must be alert enough to protect his or her own airway. Typical starting pressures are 5 to 10 cm H$_2$O.

- Place patient in a comfortable position—usually the **sitting or semisitting position.**

- Establish **IV access with a saline lock.**

- Provide the specific treatment as indicated below for COPD, asthma, or CHF.

- **Transport to appropriate emergency department (ED).** Ensure patient comfort en route.

SPECIFIC TREATMENT GUIDELINES

Cardiac (chapter 11, chapter 44, chapter 6), croup and epiglottitis (chapter 13), and traumatic (chapter 28) causes of dyspnea should be treated according to the recommendations established for these purposes.

PULMONARY ETIOLOGIES: CHRONIC OBSTRUCTIVE PULMONARY DISEASE, ASTHMA, STATUS ASTHMATICUS

- **Measure peak expiratory flow rate.** The peak expiratory flow rate (PEFR) provides the only objective measurement of the degree of airway obstruction and can be used to follow the patient's progress. PEFR depends on the patient's technique and efforts; therefore the patient must be coached in its use and encouraged to give his or her best effort.

- **Provide aerosolized albuterol, 2.5 mg in 3 ml 0.9% NaCl via nebulizer** (pediatric dose: younger than 12 years, one half of the adult dose [1.25 mg], older than 12 years, use full adult dose). Dose may be repeated every 6 hours; however, in cases of severe bronchospasm, it may be given as frequently as back to back. More frequent dosing may result in greater incidence of side effects.

- NOTE: You may also consider metaproterenol (Alupent) isoproternol Bronkosol, or;

- **Administer epinephrine 0.3 to 0.5 mg of a 1:1000 solution SC** (pediatric dose: 0.01 mg/kg SC, not to exceed 0.5 mg) if the patient is hemodynamically stable, or;

- **Provide aerosolized ipratropium bromide (Atrovent) 1 unit dose (2.5 ml (500 µg) of a 0.2% solution).** [Pediatric dosing: age < 12 years: 1/2 unit dose (1.25 ml (250 µg) of a 0.2% solution); age >12 years: 1/2 to 1 unit dose (1.25 ml (250 µg) to 2.5 ml (500 µg) of a 0.2% solution.] May be repeated in 4 to 6 hours.

* **Administer Terbutaline 0.25 mg SC. May be repeated once in 15 to 30 minutes if improvement is insufficient.** Maximum total dose 0.5 mg in a 4 hour period. [Pediatric dosing: age > 6 years: 5–10 µg/kg SC. May be repeated once in 15 to 50 minutes if improvement is insufficient. Maximum single dose 0.4 mg.]

* **Administer methylprednisolone (Solumedrol) 2mg/kg IV.** Not to exceed 125 mg IV. [Pediatric dosing is the same as the adult.]

CARDIAC ETIOLOGIES—CHF

* **Administer nitroglycerin, 1/150 grain (0.4 mg) SL** (for systolic BP greater than 90 mm Hg). Dose may be repeated every 5 minutes as needed. High-dose nitroglycerin may be used for CHF associated with hypertension. If SBP is greater than 160, use 3 metered doses SL every 3 to 5 minutes.

* **Administer morphine sulfate, 1 to 3 mg IV** (for systolic blood pressure greater than 90 mm Hg). Dose may be repeated every 5 minutes as necessary.

* **Administer Lasix (furosemide) 40 mg to 80 mg IV** (pediatric dose: 1.0 to 3.0 mg/kg IV). Higher doses may be necessary if the patient is on chronic diuretic therapy at home.

* **Administer enalaprilat (Vasotec) 0.625 to 1.25 mg IV.**

HYPERVENTILATION

Treatment is aimed at restoring the patient's P_{CO_2} to a normal state. This may be accomplished by either calming the patient or having the patient rebreathe his or her own carbon dioxide. Use caution with the rebreathing method because the carbon dioxide and oxygen mixture cannot be precisely monitored.

BIBLIOGRAPHY

Mahler, D. A. (2003). Evaluation of dyspnea in the elderly. *Clinical Geriatric Medicine, 19*, 19–33.

Mitchell, E. (2003). Dyspnea. In J. J. Schaider, S. R. Hayden, R. Wolfe, R. M. Barkin, & P. Rosen (Eds.), *Rosen & Barkin's 5-minute emergency medicine consult* (2nd ed., pp. 344–345). Philadelphia: Lippincott Williams & Wilkins.

NOTES

CHAPTER 17

FEVER

Owen T. Traynor, M.D.

PRESENTATION

Most patients with fever will not ask for EMS assistance. The fever is typically an associated symptom. Patients at the extremes of age, infants and the elderly, or those who are immunosuppressed are more likely to present for evaluation of a fever. These patients are also more likely to have atypical presentations. Although an infection is commonly sought as the cause of a fever, other causes include medications, neoplasms, and inflammatory disorders, such as rheumatoid arthritis and sarcoidosis. This chapter focuses on infectious etiologies. Many patients with a fever do not have a serious illness. The paramedic must be vigilant to recognize those who are at risk. Environmental exposures leading to an elevated temperature are discussed in chapter 23.

IMMEDIATE CONCERNS

❶ **Is the crew safe?** Most infectious diseases do not pose a significant risk to healthcare workers. Some diseases are communicable, however. Tuberculosis (TB), bacterial meningitis, human immunodeficiency virus (HIV), hepatitis, severe acute respiratory syndrome (SARS), and chicken pox are some of the diseases that are communicable from person to person. You can significantly reduce the danger of transmission by being aware of the modes of transmission and following standard body substance isolation (BSI) procedures, including wearing disposable gowns, gloves, eye protection, and respiratory protection (N-95 masks for TB and SARS). EMS agencies should have an up-to-date infection control policy. Local hospitals and the Centers for Disease Control (CDC) may serve as useful resources.

● **Is the airway safe?** Most patients with a fever have intact airway protection reflexes. Infection in the mouth, pharynx, epiglottis, or neck may compromise the airway as a result of inflammation and swelling. It may be difficult and possibly dangerous to manipulate these airways. Patients with a decreased level of consciousness may also be at risk of aspiration.

● **Is there evidence of respiratory distress?** Pulmonary infections, such as pneumonia and bronchitis, may cause fever. The fever also increases the respiratory rate. Patients with significant pulmonary or cardiac disease may decompensate with the stress of a febrile illness. Supplemental oxygen may be beneficial.

● **Is there evidence of poor perfusion or shock?** Sepsis, an infectious process associated with a systemic inflammatory response, can cause tachycardia, tachypnea, and hypotension. IV fluid resuscitation may be needed.

● **Is there an altered mental status?** Consider meningitis as a cause of an altered mental status when the patient has fever, headache, and altered mental status. Septic patients frequently have an altered mental state. The patient may be at risk for aspiration.

IMPORTANT HISTORY

❷ **Is there a respiratory source of infection?** Common infections include sinusitis, pneumonia, and bronchitis. Young pediatric patients may also present with croup. Ask about runny nose, nasal congestion, cough, shortness of breath, and sputum production.

❷ **Is there an intraabdominal source of infection?** Ask about abdominal pain, nausea, vomiting, and diarrhea. Some intraabdominal processes (e.g., appendicitis, cholecystitis, and perforated ulcers) may require surgery as well as antibiotics.

❓ **Is there a urinary source of infection?**   Common symptoms of a urinary tract infection include dysuria, urinary frequency, and urgency. Pain may be suprapubic or, in the case of pyelonephritis, in the flank or back.

❓ **Is there evidence of a skin infection?**   Search for cellulitis, a skin infection characterized by redness, swelling, and pain. An abscess is a painful, red, swollen collection of pus.

❓ **Does the patient have any indwelling catheters or prostheses?**   Catheters and prostheses can become infected. Inspect the surrounding tissue for redness, pain, and discharge. The devices may be infected even without external evidence of infection.

❓ **Is the patient an IV drug user?**   In addition to HIV and hepatitis infections, patients who use intravenous drugs are at increased risk of endocarditis and osteomyelitis. Endocarditis is an infection of the endothelium (inner surface of the heart). Vegetations, bacteria-containing thrombi, form on the heart valves. The heart valves may become diseased and require surgical replacement. Septic emboli may travel to remote areas of the body. Osteomyelitis is a bone infection that may require weeks of IV antibiotics and surgical debridement.

❓ **Is the patient immunosuppressed?**   Patients with diabetes, AIDS, leukemias, and lymphomas and patients receiving chemotherapy, steroids, or other immunosuppression drugs may be at higher risk of infection. In addition, they may not be able to mount a significant fever. Atypical presentations of disease are more likely in this group.

❓ **Has there been an exposure to an infected or ill person?** A known exposure may simplify the diagnosis.

❷ **Has there been recent travel to an area identified with an infectious disease outbreak?** Air travel has made it possible for patients to acquire unusual disease exposures.

❷ **Has there been an occupational exposure to an infectious agent?** Healthcare workers and laboratory workers have a potential for occupational exposures. Less obvious occupations may also entail exposure. Recall postal workers, newsroom staff, and other government employees who were exposed to anthrax in October and November 2001.

❷ **Are there associated symptoms?** The associated symptoms may indicate the severity of the illness or point toward the source of the fever.

DIFFERENTIAL DIAGNOSIS

INFECTIOUS ETIOLOGIES

* **_CNS INFECTIONS._** Headache, altered mental status, and possible focal neurologic deficits may be found.

    o **_MENINGITIS._** Meningitis is typically a viral or bacterial infection of the meninges. Patients present with a history of a headache, fever, and possibly nuchal rigidity (a stiff neck). The mental state may become altered as the disease progresses. Meningococcal meningitis, caused by *Neisseria meningitidis* bacteria, is associated with a petechial (small red or purple spots) or purpuric (larger red or purple spots) rash. It can be rapidly fatal, even if treated with IV antibiotics. Infants and the elderly may have less typical presentations.

    o **_ENCEPHALITIS._** Encephalitis is an inflammation of the brain that is typically caused by a viral infection, although nonviral etiologies are possible, too. The mortality rate is approximately 10%. West Nile virus encephalitis has recently increased in incidence in North America. Encephalitis usually begins with a flulike illness, often with a history of mild headaches, fever, body aches, and poor appetite. The disease may progress to include an altered level of consciousness (LOC), worsening headache, vomiting, possible nuchal rigidity, seizures, coma, and death. The diagnosis may be made in the ED after an extensive evaluation.

- **EAR, NOSE, AND THROAT INFECTIONS.**

  o **_Sinusitis._**   Patients with sinusitis report headache or facial pain, nasal congestion, purulent (pus) nasal discharge, cough, and fever. A viral (most common etiology) or bacterial infection causes inflammation of the mucous membranes in the sinuses. The patient's pain is usually least when his or her head is upright. Physical exam reveals tenderness over the affected sinuses. The neurologic exam is normal.

  o **_Otitis media._**   Otitis media is an infection of the middle ear. Although more common in pediatric patients, it does occur in adults. Patients typically report ear pain and a sensation that the ear is clogged. Some patients complain of vertigo and tinnitus (ringing in the ears). Young pediatric patients may exhibit poor feeding, fever, irritability, and a runny nose. No EMS intervention is necessary.

  o **_Pharyngitis._**   Although not a common reason for an EMS call, pharyngitis is a common reason to visit the ED. Patients report a sore throat, painful swallowing, decreased oral intake, fevers, and "swollen glands" (cervical lymphadenopathy). A viral infection is the most common cause. The most common reason for antibiotics is for a group A beta hemolytic streptococcus (GABHS) infection. GABHS has been associated with acute rheumatic fever, a complication that can damage heart valves. GABHS accounts for 15%

to 30% of childhood pharyngitis infections and only 5% to 10% of adult cases. Mononucleosis is another important etiology of pharyngitis in children and adolescents. Consider a possible ruptured spleen in a patient with recent sore throat and hypotension following mild abdominal trauma.

o ***Epiglottitis.*** Epiglottitis involves an inflammation of the epiglottis and surrounding tissues that can compromise the upper airway. This was primarily a disease of children until widespread immunization against the most common organism, *Hemophilus influenza*, dramatically reduced its incidence. The incidence in adults is increasing, but it is not clear if there is more disease or just improved diagnostic accuracy. Patients present with fever, sore throat, drooling and a "hot-potato voice." The voice is generally muffled or hoarse. Adults and children appear ill. Pediatric patients usually have a greater degree of respiratory distress owing to the smaller-caliber airway. Airway management can be difficult in either group. It is best to minimize airway manipulations until more help is available, for example, in the OR should a surgical airway be needed. Patients are treated with antibiotics. The use of steroids is controversial. Some pediatric patients have been temporarily treated with racemic epinephrine, with care taken not to agitate the patient. EMS care involves keeping the patient calm and administering oxygen. Positive pressure ventilation with a bag-valve-mask device is usually possible.

- ***RESPIRATORY INFECTIONS.***

  o ***Pneumonia.*** Typical complaints of patients with pneumonia include cough, sputum production, fever, chills, shortness of breath, pleuritic chest pain, fatigue, and poor appetite. The vital signs are abnormal, and tachycardia and tachypnea are common. Some patients are hypoxic. The physical examination may reveal crackles, rhonchi, or wheezing. There may be dullness to percussion. The patient may be using respiratory accessory muscles. Pediatric patients may have retractions, grunting respirations, and nasal flaring. Some patients are dehydrated and hypotensive. Supplemental oxygen and possibly nebulized bronchodilators and IV fluids may be needed. Intubation may be required for those with severe respiratory distress.

o **_Bronchitis._** Bronchitis is a milder and generally self-limiting disease that is caused primarily by a viral infection. It is characterized by an initially dry cough that becomes productive, wheezing, fever, chest pain related to cough, and malaise. EMS treatment involves supplemental oxygen and possibly nebulized bronchodilators.

o **_Severe acute respiratory syndrome._** SARS was first diagnosed in Asia in November 1992. It is caused by the SARS-associated coronavirus (SARS-CoV). Early clinical features include fever, chills, myalgias, headache, diarrhea, sore throat, and runny nose. Later the patient will develop a fever greater than 100.4 F (> 38 C) and coughing and shortness of breath. The clinical features match many respiratory infections. The case definition includes criteria regarding possible or likely exposure. In addition, there are radiographic and laboratory criteria. Please see the CDC's SARS webpage at http://www.cdc.gov/ncidod/sars/index.htm for the most up-to-date information.

• **_CARDIAC INFECTIONS._**

o **_Endocarditis._** Endocarditis is an infection of the lining of the heart or heart valves. Vegetations (an abnormal growth of thrombi and bacteria) form and may embolize to distant locations. Patients may present with fever, malaise, night sweats, and weight loss.

When there has been embolization, patients may have a stroke or a cold or pulseless extremity. If there has been significant damage to the heart valves, the patient may present with congestive heart failure or shock. Heart murmurs may be present. Some skin findings may help with the diagnosis. Splinter hemorrhages may be evident under the nails. Osler nodes are tender, erythematous nodules that appear on the tips of the fingers and toes. Janeway lesions are nontender red macules or nodules on the palms and soles. Patients at risk for endocarditis include IV drug users; those with poor dental hygiene, prosthetic valves, indwelling catheters, and congenital heart disorders; and those with diseased heart valves. EMS care is supportive.

o ***Pericarditis.*** Pericarditis is commonly caused by inflammation or infection of the pericardial sac. The most common variety is without a known cause. Viruses, bacteria, fungi, neoplasms, uremia, and trauma can all cause pericarditis. A pericardial effusion and tamponade can occur. Patients may complain of fever, pleuritic retrosternal, or precordial chest discomfort that improves when they sit forward or worsens in a supine position. Patients also report mild dyspnea. The physical findings may include hypotension, a narrowed pulse pressure, a cardiac friction rub, muffled heart sounds, and evidence of right and left heart failure. At times the clinical picture can be difficult to distinguish from an AMI. The 12-lead ECG may reveal diffuse ST-segment elevations early in the disease, followed by a return to baseline. PR-segments become depressed later in the disease. Eventually all changes resolve. No Q waves will form. In addition, there are no reciprocal changes as in the AMI. EMS care involves oxygen and monitoring. Hypotensive patients should be treated with aggressive fluid resuscitation.

• **ABDOMINAL INFECTIONS.** See chapters 1 and 2.

  o **Hepatitis.**   Hepatitis is an inflammatory disease of the liver. Most cases are viral. In viral hepatitis the early symptoms can be mild but include a flulike illness with fever, malaise, nausea, and vomiting. Many patients report a poor appetite. Later symptoms can include right upper quadrant (RUQ) tenderness, jaundice, dark-colored urine, and clay-colored stools. The incubation period can be 2 to several weeks.

  o **Cholecystitis.**   Cholecystitis, or inflammation of the gallbladder, is associated with right upper or epigastric crampy pain. Fever is common. The pain occurs when prolonged bile stasis caused by a stone in the duct leads to increased intraluminal pressure and eventually to inflammation and edema. These patients typically have a Murphy's sign, an inspiratory arrest on palpation of the RUQ caused by an increase in pain as the gallbladder bumps into the examiner's hand.

  o **Cholangitis.**   Cholangitis is a bacterial infection of the biliary tract associated with fever and chills, RUQ pain, and jaundice. Obstruction of the biliary tree causes bacterial infection and possible sepsis. These patients have RUQ tenderness and often peritoneal signs, such as rebound tenderness, rigidity, and guarding.

  o **Appendicitis.** The classic presentation of appendicitis involves periumbilical abdominal pain followed by anorexia and mild fever. The pain eventually moves to the RLQ. Many patients report vomiting and either diarrhea or constipation. The location of the pain is quite variable, with many people reporting back or flank pain, testicular pain, suprapubic pain, and even RUQ or LLQ pain. Patients with appendicitis prefer not to move. The exam reveals tenderness, guarding, and rebound tenderness.

  o **Diverticulitis.**   Patients with diverticulitis complain of persistent, vague abdominal pain in the lower abdomen. Over time, the pain worsens and localizes to the LLQ. Fever, nausea, and poor appetite are common. Patients may report constipation or diarrhea. The exam reveals LLQ tenderness and possibly a mass (inflamed colon or abscess).

o **_Peritonitis._** Inflammation of the peritoneal lining, or peritonitis, can come from many sources, including perforation of a hollow organ, bacterial infection of ascites, and those intraabdominal processes listed above. Fever, tenderness, rebound tenderness, guarding, and a rigid abdomen may be present. Shock can occur.

• **_SKIN AND CONNECTIVE TISSUE INFECTIONS._**

o **_Cellulitis._** Cellulitis is a superficial infection of the skin. The patient reports a painful, erythematous, edematous rash that spreads. Lymphangitis (a red streak) and lymphadenopathy (painful lymph nodes) are common. EMS care is required when the patient is septic.

o **_Abscess._** An abscess is a pocket of pus that has been contained or walled off by inflamed tissue. The physical exam reveals a painful, erythematous, area of swelling beneath the skin. It may be surrounded by cellulitis. There is often lymphadenopathy and, at times, lymphangitis. Although this is a local infection, it may be accompanied by systemic symptoms such as fever, malaise, altered mental status, and hypotension. EMS care is limited to unstable patients.

o **_Osteomyelitis._** Osteomyelitis is an infection of the bone with destruction caused by the body's inflammatory response. Patients complain of a localized deep pain. It can be described as dull or throbbing. The infected site may be warm, erythematous, and tender. Usually the patient is unwilling to use the affected limb. The infection can come from a local wound or via the blood from a remote infection.

Patients with cancer, IV drug users, and patients with diabetes are at higher risk for this disease. Osteomyelitis can occur in children as well. There is no acute EMS intervention. A prolonged course (weeks) of IV antibiotics and surgical debridement may be necessary.

- **URINARY INFECTIONS.** See chapter 1.

  o **Cystitis.**   Cystitis is defined as a urinary tract infection involving the bladder. Patients complain of dysuria, urinary frequency, and urgency. Fever and suprapubic pain may be present. The physical exam reveals suprapubic tenderness.

  o **Pyelonephritis.**   Pyelonephritis is an infection of the upper urinary tract. Patients typically report the same urinary symptoms as in cystitis. Patients also complain of back pain, flank pain, or abdominal pain. The pain can be unilateral or bilateral. Fever and chills, nausea and vomiting, and malaise are common. The physical exam reveals costovertebral angle tenderness or suprapubic tenderness.

- **GYNECOLOGIC INFECTIONS.** See chapter 2.

  o **Pelvic inflammatory disease.**   Pelvic inflammatory disease (PID) is an acute infection of the uterus, fallopian tubes, ovaries, and adjacent tissues. If untreated it may lead to a tuboovarian abscess. It often develops during or after menses. Patients report fever, bilateral lower abdominal pain, vaginal discharge or bleeding, nausea, and vomiting. The patient can develop inflammation of the capsule of the liver, or Fitz-Hugh-Curtis syndrome. These patients have RUQ pleuritic pain and tenderness.

  o **Tuboovarian abscess.**   Tuboovarian abscess is a complication of PID. The abscess can often develop when treatment fails to resolve PID. The patient may have a palpable, tender abdominal mass. Peritonitis and sepsis may develop if the abscess ruptures.

- **SYSTEMIC INFECTIONS.**

  o **HIV infection and AIDS.** Primary HIV infection appears as a typical viral illness with mild fever, body aches, and malaise. Patients are at increased risk of opportunistic infections. See chapter 21.

  o **Sepsis.** Sepsis is defined as an infectious process associated with a systemic inflammatory response. Typical features include fever, hypothermia, tachycardia, tachypnea, hypotension, poor perfusion, and altered mental status. EMS treatment focuses on improving oxygenation and providing IV fluid resuscitation if needed.

NONINFECTIOUS ETIOLOGIES

- **CENTRAL NERVOUS SYSTEM LESIONS.** The core temperature is set by the hypothalamus.

- **MEDICATIONS.** Almost any medication can cause a fever.

- **SYSTEMIC INFLAMMATORY DISORDERS.** Sickle cell disease, rheumatoid arthritis, systemic lupus erythematosus, polymyalgia rheumatica, sarcoidosis, and vasculitis are a few of the inflammatory disorders that are associated with fever.

- **NEOPLASMS.** Leukemias, lymphomas, and metastatic tumors are associated with fever.

- **ENDOCRINE DISORDERS.** Hyperthyroidism and pheochromocytomas may cause fevers.

KEY PHYSICAL EXAMINATION FINDINGS

✓ **Initial assessment.** Look for alterations in mental status, threats to the airway, respiratory compromise, and hemodynamic instability.

SECTION 1

- ✅ **Vital signs.**   Careful monitoring of the vital signs is needed. Check temperature, if possible.

- ✅ **HEENT.**   Examine carefully and note signs of swelling, redness, or unusual warmth. Examine pupils for responsiveness and equality. Look for pharyngeal exudate, erythema, or tonsillar enlargement. Evaluate for dental abscess if the patient complains of toothache. Palpate over the frontal and maxillary sinuses for tenderness.

- ✅ **Neck.**   Assess for nuchal rigidity, cervical adenopathy, jugular venous distension, and stridor.

- ✅ **Lungs.**   Listen to lung sounds for signs of pulmonary edema, bronchospasm, or pneumonia. Percuss for areas of consolidation (dull percussion notes).

- ✅ **Heart.**   Assess for pericardial friction rub.

- ✅ **Abdomen.**   Assess carefully for masses, tenderness, ascites, or peritoneal signs.

- ✅ **Extremities.**   Assess for edema in the extremities. Check peripheral pulses to equality. Inspect for needle-track marks. Look for regional lymphadenopathy (tender lymph nodes)

- ✅ **Skin.**   Assess for rashes, swelling, lymphangitis, wounds, and abscesses.

- ✅ **Neurologic examination.**   An altered mental status can be a sign of a CNS infection or sepsis.

ELECTROCARDIOGRAM

Evaluate ECG results for signs of arrhythmias, pericarditis, cardiac ischemia, or injury.

GLUCOMETER

Evaluate for hypoglycemia or hyperglycemia.

PULSE OXIMETER

Evaluate for hypoxia.

TREATMENT PLAN

- ***Patient assessment.*** Perform a rapid and systematic initial assessment, and institute treatment as life-threatening problems are discovered. Prompt transport of seriously ill or unstable patients to the appropriate ED is a key intervention. Frequent reassessment of patients with an altered mental status, hemodynamic instability, or sepsis is necessary because of the potential for worsening of their condition.

GENERAL TREATMENT GUIDELINES

- Institute **BSI precautions** as appropriate.

- **Administer O₂ and provide ventilatory support** as needed.

- Place the patient in a **head-elevated position**, unless spinal immobilization is needed, or in the shock position if shock is present.

- **Monitor the ECG and O₂** saturation of all unstable patients and those at risk of becoming unstable.

- **Establish IV** access if there is evidence of a potentially serious infection or if IV fluid resuscitation is warranted.

- **Perform blood glucose determination** in patients with diabetes, unstable or potentially unstable patients, and those with an altered mental status. Treat hypoglycemia as in chapter 24. Treat hyperglycemia as per chapter 14.

- Do not overbundle patients, especially pediatric patients.

- Consider the following interventions:

   o IV fluid resuscitation with 0.9% NaCl or lactated Ringer's solution.

o Patients who fail to respond to IV fluid resuscitation should be treated with vasopressors as in chapter 38.

o Acetaminophen (Tylenol) 325 to 1000 mg PO (pediatric dose 15 mg/kg PO) if no doses in last 4 hours.

- Frequently reassess the patient's airway and hemodynamic and neurologic status.

- **Transport to the appropriate ED**. Ensure patient comfort enroute.

BIBLIOGRAPHY

Ciccone, T. J. J. (2003). Fever, adult. In J. J. Schaider, S. R. Hayden, R. Wolfe, R. M. Barkin, & P. Rosen (Eds.), *Rosen & Barkin's 5-minute emergency medicine consult* (2nd ed., pp. 408–409). Philadelphia: Lippincott Williams & Wilkins.

Hawkins, R. R. L. & D. F. Danzl (2004). Infectious disease emergencies. In C. K. Stone & R. L. Humphries (Eds.), *Current emergency diagnosis and treatment* (5th ed., pp. 824–866). New York: McGraw-Hill.

Mick, N., D. A. Peak & A. S. Ulrich (2003). Fever, pediatric. In J. J. Schaider, S. R. Hayden, R. Wolfe, R. M. Barkin, & P. Rosen (Eds.), *Rosen & Barkin's 5-minute emergency medicine consult* (2nd ed., pp. 410–411). Philadelphia: Lippincott Williams & Wilkins.

Thomas, H. A. & J. H. Brian (2001). Fever and night sweats. In A. Harwood-Nuss, A. B. Wolfson, C. H. Linden, S. M. Shepard, & P. H. Stenklyft (Eds.), *The clinical practice of emergency medicine* (3rd ed., pp. 21–27). Philadelphia: Lippincott Williams & Wilkins.

NOTES

_____

_____

_____

CHAPTER 18

GASTROINTESTINAL BLEEDING

Owen T. Traynor, M.D.

PRESENTATION

Patients with gastrointestinal (GI) bleeding may present in several ways: with shock, syncope, hematemesis (bright-red blood) or coffee-ground emesis, melena (the passage of black, tarry stool indicating blood in the GI tract), or hematochezia (bright-red blood around the rectum).

IMMEDIATE CONCERNS

❶ **What is the patient's hemodynamic status?** If the patient is hemodynamically unstable, immediate resuscitation is warranted, including oxygen administration, establishment of large-bore IV access, and IV fluid administration.

IMPORTANT HISTORY

❷ **Has there been hematemesis, melena, or hematochezia?** Vomiting blood or coffee-ground matter suggests upper GI bleeding. Melena suggests acute blood loss in the upper GI tract whereas hematochezia indicates likely bleeding in the distal colon or rectum. However, there are exceptions to these guidelines: Massive upper GI bleeding may involve hematochezia. Vomiting and retching before vomiting bright-red blood may indicate a Mallory-Weiss tear of the esophagus.

❷ **Is there a history of GI bleeding?** If the history is positive, determine the nature of previous bleeding. Although bleeding may recur from the same location, it is not uncommon for bleeding to occur from another site. Be sure to ask about a history of diseases associated with GI bleeding, such as peptic ulcer disease, esophageal varices, diverticular disease, colon cancer, polyps, inflammatory bowel disease, and hemorrhoids or other anal disease.

❷ Is the patient taking any medication? Anticoagulants, steroids, and nonsteroidal anti-inflammatory agents (NSAIDs), including aspirin, are associated with GI bleeding. Patients who have a history of peptic ulcer disease or gastritis may take proton pump inhibitors (PPIs) or H_2 blockers.

❷ Is there a history of alcohol abuse? Alcohol abuse can cause gastritis and esophageal varices. Patients with cirrhosis have an increased incidence of duodenal ulcers.

DIFFERENTIAL DIAGNOSIS

UPPER GI BLEEDING

- **PEPTIC ULCER DISEASE.** The most common cause of upper GI bleeding is peptic ulcer, which accounts for up to 50% of all cases.

- **GASTRITIS AND ESOPHAGITIS.** Gastritis and esophagitis account for up to 20% of upper GI bleeds. Alcohol use, aspirin use, and hiatal hernia are predisposing factors.

- **MALLORY-WEISS SYNDROME.** Mallory-Weiss syndrome is characterized by upper GI bleeding caused by a longitudinal tear in the mucosal lining of the esophagus. The classic presentation is one of repeated retching followed by hematemesis. It is associated with recent alcohol intake and causes up to 15% of upper GI bleeds.

- **ESOPHAGEAL VARICES.** Varices result from portal hypertension; in the United States, the condition is most commonly caused by alcoholic liver disease. Varices account for up to 15% of all upper GI bleeds. Varices are prone to rebleed and carry the highest mortality rate of upper GI bleeds. Many patients with esophageal varices never bleed. However, patients with documented varices and GI bleeding may bleed from a site other than the varices.

- **OTHER SOURCES.** Cancer causes approximately 1% to 2% of upper GI bleeding—look for a history of weight loss. Sources of bleeding from the ears, nose, and throat (ENT) should be investigated sources because they can masquerade as GI bleeding.

LOWER GI BLEEDING

- **UPPER GI BLEEDING.** The most common cause of apparent lower GI bleeding is actually upper GI bleeding.

- **DIVERTICULAR DISEASE.** The most common cause of massive lower GI bleeding is diverticular disease. Diverticulosis is the presence of small outpouchings in the wall of the colon. These may become infected and erode into blood vessels in the wall of the colon, causing painless bleeding. The typical patient is over 50 years of age.

- **HEMORRHOIDS.** Hemorrhoids cause most lower GI bleeding; however, they usually do not cause life-threatening hemorrhage.

- **OTHER SOURCES.** Vascular malformations of the colon may cause bleeding in the elderly. Cancer and polyps usually do not cause significant bleeding in the lower GI tract. Patients with cancer often present with weight loss, a change in bowel habits, or both. Inflammatory bowel diseases, such as ulcerative colitis and Crohn's disease, are an infrequent cause of significant bleeding.

KEY PHYSICAL EXAMINATION FINDINGS

- ✅ **Initial assessment.** Look for signs of shock.
- ✅ **Vital signs.** Include orthostatic vital signs.
- ✅ **HEENT.** Look for ENT source of bleeding.
- ✅ **Abdomen.** Hyperactive bowel sounds may indicate blood in the upper GI tract. Check for masses, tenderness, and ascites.

TREATMENT PLAN

- *Patient Assessment.* Frequent reassessment is necessary because of the potential for massive hemorrhage and shock. Cardiac monitoring is necessary for patients with blood loss and a documented heart disease or risk of heart disease. Because these patients may vomit, be prepared to protect the airway.

HEMODYNAMICALLY UNSTABLE PATIENT

- **Administer O_2 and provide ventilatory support** as needed.

- **Treat for shock** (see chapter 38).

- **Establish large-bore IV access** and begin fluid resuscitation with 0.9% NaCl or LR.

- **Transport expeditiously to appropriate emergency department (ED).** Do not needlessly delay patient transport—expedite transport.

HEMODYNAMICALLY STABLE PATIENT

- **Establish large-bore IV access.**

- **Transport to appropriate ED.** Ensure patient comfort en route.

BIBLIOGRAPHY

Johnson, D. E. (2003). Gastrointestinal bleeding. In J. J. Schaider, S. R. Hayden, R. Wolfe, R. M. Barkin, & P. Rosen (Eds.), *Rosen & Barkin's 5-minute emergency medicine consult* (2nd ed., pp. 450–451). Philadelphia: Lippincott Williams & Wilkins.

Pianka, J. D. (2001). Management principles of gastrointestinal bleeding. *Primary Care, 28,* 557–575.

CHAPTER 19

HEADACHE

Jonathan S. Rubens, M.D., FACEP

PRESENTATION

Headache is a common entity, known to most adult patients at some time in their lives. Consequently, the fact that a patient has summoned a paramedic because of a chief complaint of headache should immediately send a signal that in the patient's perception, at least, this headache is somehow different or more severe than prior headaches. Associated symptoms of visual, motor, or sensory disturbances; nausea and vomiting; or fever are often a part of the patient's complaint.

IMMEDIATE CONCERNS

❗ **Is the patient able to protect the airway?** Most headache patients have no trouble protecting their airway; however, those with serious intracranial pathology may require assistance.

❗ **Has there been recent head trauma?** The patient with headache may have an injury that requires a neurosurgeon. Cervical spine immobilization may be necessary.

❗ **Is there an altered mental status?** Headaches associated with an altered mental status may indicate intracranial hemorrhage, cerebral edema, tumor, or infection.

❗ **Has the patient had a seizure?** Although headache following a seizure is common, some serious causes of headache, such as intracranial hemorrhage, may also cause seizures.

❶ **Are there focal neurologic deficits?** The presence of an abnormal neurologic exam suggests the possibility of intracranial mass, blood, or CVA.

IMPORTANT HISTORY

❷ **Is the patient febrile?** The presence of fever suggests an infectious etiology. Although nonlife-threatening illnesses may cause headaches and fever, the paramedic should consider the possibility of meningitis as the etiology.

❷ **Did the headache have a sudden or gradual onset?** Onset is one of the most important parameters to establish. A severe headache of acute onset with associated symptoms suggests a serious illness, such as hemorrhage. Knowledge of preceding events (i.e., trauma, exercise, exertion) can be helpful.

❷ **What is the nature of the pain?** A throbbing, pulsatile headache is usually of vascular etiology and generally due to vasodilation, hypertension, or fever. The shock-like, transient pain in the distribution of the fifth cranial nerve (the face) is characteristic of trigeminal neuralgia, whereas the deep, boring, intense, unilateral pain of cluster headaches helps to differentiate them.

❷ **Is this a new headache?** Many patients have a history of headaches. Often the headache has a characteristic typical location, typical quality, and common features. Headaches that are either new or different from the patient's typical headache require careful evaluation.

❷ **Are there associated symptoms?** The associated symptoms may help suggest a diagnosis. Ask specifically about photophobia, lacrimation, rhinorrhea, ptosis, neck pain or stiffness, visual disturbances, fever, syncope, and seizures. In addition, ask about a history of eye pain, clouding of the cornea, nasal congestion, and facial and jaw pain.

DIFFERENTIAL DIAGNOSIS

LIFE-THREATENING ETIOLOGIES

- **SUBARACHNOID HEMORRHAGE.** Subarachnoid hemorrhage is caused by the rupture or leakage from a cerebral aneurysm or bleeding from an arteriovenous malformation (abnormal tangle of blood vessels). The patient complains of the sudden onset of "the worst headache of my life." It may be associated with a transient loss of consciousness or syncope. Nausea and vomiting are common associated symptoms. Patients may also report neck or back pain. Up to 50% of patients will initially have a nonfocal neurologic exam. The most common location of the headache is occipital or nuchal.

- **EPIDURAL HEMATOMA.** The classic presentation for epidural hematoma involves a loss of consciousness following acute head trauma, with an intervening lucid interval before the patient loses consciousness again. The more common presentation is one of an altered mental status after head trauma. See chapter 20 for additional details.

- **SUBDURAL HEMATOMA.** Subdural hematomas also occur following head trauma; however, the trauma may be remote, especially in the elderly and in alcoholics. Altered mental status, seizures, nausea, and vomiting may be found, as well as unilateral weakness or paralysis. See chapter 20 for additional details.

- **BRAIN TUMOR.** Primary or metastatic brain tumors may cause an altered LOC with or without obvious focal neurologic findings. Symptoms may develop as the tumor compresses adjacent tissue or secondary to edema or bleeding of the tumor. Often the patient complains of new onset headaches. The classic presentation includes morning headaches that change with position and are associated with nausea and vomiting.

- **MENINGITIS.**   Meningitis is typically a viral or bacterial infection of the meninges. Patients present with a history of a headache, fever, and possibly nuchal rigidity (a stiff neck). The mental state may become altered as the disease progresses. Meningococcal meningitis, caused by *Neisseria meningitidis* bacteria, is associated with a petechial (small red or purple spots) or purpuric (larger red or purple spots) rash. It can be rapidly fatal, even if treated with IV antibiotics. Infants and the elderly may have less typical presentations.

IMPORTANT HEADACHE SYNDROMES

- **MIGRAINE HEADACHES.**   Migraine is a common cause of headaches. Patients generally begin experiencing migraines in their teens or twenties. Migraines are more common in women and seem to run in families. They can be temporally related to menstruation and exacerbated by ingestion of chocolate, cheeses, nuts, alcohol, sulfites, and monosodium glutamate (MSG). The common migraine is a recurrent headache that is typically unilateral and pulsating or throbbing in nature. It worsens with physical activity and is associated with photophobia and phonophobia (i.e., light and noise make it worse), nausea, and vomiting. The classic migraine shares the features of the common migraine with the addition of a prodromal aura. The aura can involve any of the senses but commonly involves a sense of wavy lines or flashing lights before the eyes. Migrainous infarction, previously called a "complex migraine," is a migraine headache with focal neurologic findings including hemiparesthesia, hemiparesis, aphasia, or other speech difficulties. Its aura may last more than 7 days.

- **TENSION HEADACHES.**   Tension headache is the most common headache syndrome. Commonly bilateral, nonpulsatile, and not associated with vomiting, tension headaches are three times more common in women than men, with a typical onset between the ages of 30 and 50. Muscle spasm or tension in the neck is often present. There are no abnormal neurologic findings.

- **CLUSTER HEADACHES.** Cluster headache is an uncommon cause of severe unilateral headache. It is found in men more often than women. The pain is typically around or above the eye or in the temple. It is associated with ptosis, lacrimation, constricted pupil, conjunctival injection, nasal congestion, and rhinorrhea. All of these features are found on the same side as the headache. Each attack lasts up to 3 or 4 hours and occurs several times per day. The attacks can occur daily for weeks, followed by a pain-free interval of months to years. High-flow supplemental oxygen resolves 75% of these headaches.

IMPORTANT EXTRACRANIAL ETIOLOGIES

- **TEMPOROMANDIBULAR JOINT SYNDROME.** The pain associated with temporomandibular joint (TMJ) syndrome is in the region of the TMJ. It often worsens with movement. The patient may report clicking and locking of the jaw.

- **TRIGEMINAL NEURALGIA.** Trigeminal neuralgia involves severe, stabbing pain in the distribution of the mandibular or maxillary division of the trigeminal nerve. The pain is usually unilateral and recurs over seconds to minutes. Trigger zones on the face appear to bring about the pain. Onset is usually after the fourth decade of life. Women are affected more often than men. The physical examination detects no abnormalities of the trigeminal nerve function. There may be pain-free periods that last minutes to weeks, but remission is rare without treatment.

- **EAR INFECTIONS, SINUSITIS, AND DENTAL DISEASE.** Facial pain is often associated with infections of the ear, sinus passages, and teeth. A careful history and physical examination can usually identify the cause.

- **OPHTHALMIC CAUSES.** Patients with acute narrow-angle glaucoma may present with severe eye or forehead pain, headache, nausea, and vomiting. The pain is usually associated with blurred vision, visual halos, and a hazy cornea. Iritis and other corneal injuries are associated with eye pain, headaches, a red eye, photophobia, and lacrimation.

- **HYPERTENSION.**   Headache is not a common feature of chronic hypertension. It can be found as a component of a hypertensive crisis, however. See chapter 22.

- **TOXIC ETIOLOGIES.**   Although many toxic exposures may result in a headache, it is a particular feature of carbon monoxide poisoning. Additional symptoms include dizziness, ataxia, altered mental status, syncope, nausea, and vomiting. A toxic etiology should be considered in any patient with potential exposure. See chapter 40.

KEY PHYSICAL EXAMINATION FINDINGS

✅ **Initial Assessment.**   Look for alterations in mental status, threats to the airway, respiratory compromise, and hemodynamic instability.

✅ **Vital Signs.**   Monitor blood pressure and respiratory pattern and rate. Diastolic blood pressure elevations greater than 130 mm Hg associated with mental status changes or other focal neurologic findings is a true neurologic emergency. In cases of cerebral edema and increased intracranial pressure, Cushing's reflex, increased blood pressure associated with a decrease in pulse rate may be found. Changes in respiratory pattern or rate may suggest a toxic etiology of the headache.

✅ **HEENT.**   Assess for evidence of traumatic injury. Assess pupillary response and extraocular movements. Assess the eye for redness or corneal haziness. Palpate over the frontal and maxillary sinuses. Palpate the TMJ for instability and clicks while the patient opens and closes the mouth. Inspect the mouth for a dental cause of the pain.

- ✓ **Neck.** Assess for nuchal rigidity, which may be found in cases of meningeal irritation.

- ✓ **Neurologic examination.** An altered mental status is a sensitive indicator of cerebral perfusion. Assess cranial nerves, and perform a motor and sensory examination. Unilateral deficits may be present in CVAs.

TREATMENT PLAN

SECTION 1

- **Patient assessment.** Perform continued evaluation of vital signs and mental status. Changes in any of these parameters may require immediate intervention during transport.

- **Patient assessment.** Perform a rapid and systematic initial assessment, and institute treatment as life-threatening problems are discovered. Prompt transport to the appropriate emergency department (ED) is a key intervention if a life-threatening headache is suspected. Frequent reassessment of patients with a potentially serious headache is necessary because of the potential for worsening of their neurologic status.

GENERAL TREATMENT GUIDELINES

- **Administer O$_2$ and provide ventilatory support** as needed.

- Place the patient in a **head-elevated position**, unless spinal immobilization is needed, or in the shock position, if shock is present.

- **Perform blood glucose determination** if the patient is a diabetic.

- **Establish IV** access if a serious etiology is suspected.

- **Transport to the appropriate ED.** Ensure patient comfort en route.

DIAGNOSIS-SPECIFIC TREATMENT GUIDELINES

- Acute CVA—see chapter 10.

- Acute intracranial hemorrhage—see chapter 10.

- Seizures—see chapter 37.

- Carbon monoxide poisoning—see chapter 40.

- Hypertensive encephalopathy—see chapter 22.

- Traumatic head injuries—see chapter 20.

BIBLIOGRAPHY

Gallagher, E. J. & A. J. Birnbaum (2001). Headache. In A. Harwood-Nuss, A. B. Wolfson, C. H. Linden, S. M. Shepard, & P. H. Stenklyft (Eds.), *The clinical practice of emergency medicine* (3rd ed., pp. 969–978). Philadelphia: Lippincott Williams & Wilkins.

Mehrotra, A. (2003). Headache. In J. J. Schaider, S. R. Hayden, R. Wolfe, R. M. Barkin, & P. Rosen (Eds.), *Rosen & Barkin's 5-minute emergency medicine consult* (2nd ed., pp. 480–481). Philadelphia: Lippincott Williams & Wilkins.

Stone, C. K. & N. J. Antonacci (2004). Headache. In C. K. Stone & R. L. Humphries (Eds.), *Current emergency diagnosis and treatment* (5th ed., pp. 379–390). New York: McGraw-Hill.

NOTES

_____

_____

_____

_____

_____

CHAPTER 20

HEAD INJURY

Russell Bradley, M.D.
Owen T. Traynor, M.D.

PRESENTATION

Patients with a traumatic head injury vary in presentation, from nearly asymptomatic with mild and transient headache after a concussion, to comatose or dead after a major head injury. The presentation of CNS injury is generally related to the level along the CNS at which the injury takes place. With trauma, injuries may occur at multiple sites, and a paramedic must take this fact into account when assessing the patient. Key in assessing multiple presentations of CNS injury is to identify a cause and mechanism of injury, such as a direct blow to the head or body by some object; a penetrating injury from bullets, knives, or other sharp objects; or an indirect cause of injury, such as a transmitted force from a blow to the body, as in a motor vehicle accident (MVA), explosion, or fall. This information will prove vital in the subsequent treatment and care of the patient. Because a CNS injury can have significant morbidity and mortality, the prehospital emergency medical services (EMS) provider must have a high index of suspicion and treat suspected cases of CNS injury on the basis of mechanism of injury, history, and physical findings.

IMMEDIATE CONCERNS

❶ **Is there a mechanism of injury that could cause CNS injury?** Direct trauma to the head, spine, and back can obviously injure the CNS. The mechanism of injury is often apparent. However, sometimes a history of trauma must be actively sought. For example, alcoholic patients with subacute subdural hematomas may have fallen and hit their head several days before becoming unconscious. Family members may not have taken notice of the fall because the patient falls frequently. Again, the paramedic must have a high index of suspicion. Although significant force is usually necessary to cause CNS injury, consider the elderly to be at higher risk owing to the more brittle nature of their bones. A cervical fracture may result from a fall to the ground while standing. The paramedic should use spinal immobilization liberally and be aware that signs or symptoms of spinal cord damage may not be apparent. Vertebral spine injury can remain silent until something causes a change in the status of the injured area (i.e., a fracture becomes displaced when the patient moves). Once again, any signs, symptoms, or relevant mechanism of injury warrant appropriate cervical and spinal column immobilization.

❶ **Is there evidence of a primary brain injury?**   Primary brain injuries result from direct trauma to the brain. They are characterized by alterations in mental status and abnormal neurologic exams.

❶ **Is there evidence of a secondary brain injury?**   Secondary brain injuries are insults that occur following the primary injury. These include hypoxia, hypotension, seizures, and infection. Paramedics can intervene here to reduce the amount of injury. High-flow oxygen, airway management, and IV fluid resuscitation should be initiated as needed.

❶ **Is the patient's airway patent and stable?**   Patients with a CNS injury may be unable to protect their airway. Often, associated facial injuries cause both bleeding and swelling, leading to airway compromise. All airway interventions must be performed without endangering the cervical spine. Endotracheal intubation may be required.

❶ **Is the patient hemodynamically stable?**   Hemodynamic instability in the context of a CNS injury usually means that there are other "hidden" injuries—look for evidence of internal trauma (intrathoracic, intraabdominal, intrapelvic, and so forth). Treat the patient for shock while protecting the spine. Expedite transport to the closest appropriate ED.

● **Does the patient have an altered mental status?** The patient's mental status is the most sensitive indicator of brain function. The range of alteration of consciousness extends from the transient and mild (e.g., seeing stars, momentary amnesia, restlessness, vomiting, and headache), to the profound (focal neurologic deficits, stroke, paralysis, seizures, coma, shock, respiratory arrest, and death). It is prudent to assume that any patient with altered consciousness has also suffered damage to the cervical spine and spinal cord, and subsequent immobilization of the neck and spine must be used.

● **Did you inspect or gain information at the scene?** Some information, if not recorded by the paramedic, will not be available at the ED. For example: In an MVA, telltale signs such as a cracked or "spidered" windshield, deformed steering column, the presence or absence of seatbelt use, and the location of automobile damage (i.e., front, back, or side) can all help in determining the mechanism of injury. If the patient has fallen, it is important to note from how high and onto what type of surface. A fall that produces obvious gluteal, feet, or ankle injury might also cause compressive spinal fractures. Note the position in which the patient was found: Extremity flexion and extension (known as decorticate and decerebrate posturing, respectively) can indicate a certain level of brain injury.

● **Are there distracting injuries, or is the patient's ability to feel pain impaired?** Often, the paramedic must rely on a patient's self-reporting of symptoms to discover injury. If there are other significant painful injuries, the patient may not accurately report the pain of a skull or vertebral fracture. A patient who has been drinking alcohol or using pain medications or substances of abuse may be impaired and not report pain. These patients should be immobilized and treated as if they have an injury.

IMPORTANT HISTORY

❶ **Is the patient's neurologic injury improving or worsening?** The treatment on arrival at the ED may depend on the severity and progression of the injury. This requires serial neurologic assessment. The Glasgow Coma Scale (GCS) should be noted initially and monitored during transport. A loss in the GCS of two or more points is an alarming sign: expedite transport. Know the signs of increasing intracranial pressure (ICP) that might indicate impending herniation: hypertension associated with bradycardia and an altered mental state. The development of a fixed and dilated pupil, implying third cranial nerve compression and possible herniation, should also spur quickened transportation. A simple way to look at CNS injuries is that they are of three types: those that are improving, those that are stable, and those that are worsening. Those that are worsening may require a more aggressive neurosurgical approach.

❷ **Has there been a loss of consciousness?** If the patient lost consciousness, for how long? Loss of consciousness requires significant force transmitted to the brain. Patients may not be reliable historians regarding loss of consciousness. A change in mental status for the better might have already occurred, and this information will be important in terms of future management in hospital. The patient might have lost consciousness before the event, thus precipitating the accident. Causes might include myocardial infarction (MI), seizure, cerebrovascular accident (CVA), syncope, or intoxication. A lucid interval may precede deterioration in an acute epidural hemorrhage. All trauma patients who have suffered loss of consciousness require immobilization of the spine and transport to the hospital.

❓ **Is there any history of vomiting?** Children frequently vomit with any degree of head injury, but in the adult vomiting can be a sign of deterioration. A history of vomiting might suggest a possible cause for a blocked airway or possible aspiration.

❓ **Are there any comorbid medical problems or injuries?** The patient's loss of consciousness may have actually been caused by hypoglycemia, cardiac arrhythmia, MI, alcohol or drug abuse, hypoxia, blood loss, or seizure. There is no substitute for an accurate medical history— even in the face of an "obvious" injury. Often treatment and history may be obtained simultaneously.

SECTION 1

DIFFERENTIAL DIAGNOSIS

SKULL FRACTURES

Skull fractures may be divided into two major groups: open fractures and closed fractures. In open fracture, a communication exists between the brain substance through the fracture to the outside of the skull. The dura, a layer of tissue around the brain that contains the cerebrospinal fluid (CSF), is disrupted in an open fracture. The dura is not disrupted in a closed fracture. Skull fractures may also be classified as depressed or nondepressed. A depressed skull fracture means that there is a step-off between the fractured piece of bone and the surrounding skull. Although skull fractures do not always cause brain injury, there is a greater risk of underlying brain injury when they are present. The mechanism of injury can be secondary to penetration or crushing of the brain substance by a piece of bone. It can also be caused by the fracture disrupting cerebral vessels, leading to bleeding into or around the brain parenchyma (tissue). A basal skull fracture is another type of fracture wherein the fracture occurs through the bones at the base of the skull. Physical examination findings that suggest a basal skull fracture include Battle's sign, an ecchymosis found over the mastoid process that develops several hours after the trauma; raccoon eyes, a bilateral periorbital ecchymosis found without trauma to the eyes; and CSF leak from the nose or ears.

DIFFUSE BRAIN INJURIES

- **CONCUSSION.**   Concussion may be defined as a temporary loss of neurologic function. It may involve loss of consciousness. The duration of unconsciousness ranges from seconds or minutes to several hours. It typically occurs as a result of a blow to the head. The movement of the brain within the skull may cause a transient impairment of the reticular activating system (RAS), which regulates consciousness. Although recovery is normally complete, some patients experience headache, anxiety, memory difficulties, insomnia, and dizziness for weeks to months after the injury. More often than not, by the time the patient has been brought to the ED, return of consciousness has occurred. Concussion can be mild, moderate, or severe and potentially accompanies more critical brain injury.

- **DIFFUSE AXONAL INJURY.**   Diffuse axonal injury can be described as a very severe concussion. It is characterized by prolonged coma and often requires long-term care. The pathology is described as microscopic injury scattered throughout the brain. This entity is often termed closed head injury (CHI) or brainstem injury, and its overall mortality rate is 33%.

FOCAL BRAIN INJURIES

- **CONTUSION.**   Contusion can be thought of as a bruise to the brain. Contusions can be small, large, single, or multiple. They usually occur directly under the site of impact or on the side of the head opposite to the injury. The latter type is caused by rebound of the brain and is known as a coup or contrecoup injury. A contusion might not exhibit any neurologic findings, but if the sensory or motor cortex is injured, focal deficits will result. Edema and hemorrhage can cause swelling, leading to increased intracranial pressure, and possible herniation or brainstem compression, both of which can cause immediate death.

INTRACRANIAL HEMORRHAGE

- ***ACUTE EPIDURAL HEMATOMA.*** In the majority of cases, acute epidural hematoma results from an arterial injury in the dural covering of the brain causing bleeding between the skull and the dura. Bleeding can also occur from a disruption of venous vessels. Epidural hematomas are usually associated with a fracture over the middle meningeal artery (i.e., a fracture of the temporal or parietal bones of the skull). This can be a rapidly fatal process. Because the skull is a confined space, an increase in the quantity of material—in this case, blood where it should not be—compresses the brain and can cause herniation. In the classic description of an epidural hematoma, there is an initial LOC, followed by a lucid (but not necessarily symptom-free) interval, progressing to another LOC. Although this is the classic description, it is not the most common presentation. There might be either no LOC or prolonged unconsciousness with this injury. A fixed and dilated pupil on the side of the head injury is a hallmark of this injury. Immediate surgical intervention is the cure.

- ***ACUTE SUBDURAL HEMATOMA.*** In acute subdural hematoma, the blood comes from bridging veins that span the gap between the brain tissue and the dura. The accumulation of blood is, therefore, between the dura and the brain. Acute subdural hematoma is much more common than epidural hematoma; in fact, 30% of severe head injuries are subdural hematomas. Acceleration-deceleration forces are frequently the cause of injury. There is often quite extensive contusion, as well as injury caused by the increasing volume of blood compressing brain tissue. Acute subdural hematomas usually become symptomatic within 24 hours of injury, but subacute and chronic forms of this hemorrhage do exist. These forms take longer to show up after injury. Acute subdural hematomas require surgical intervention, and, even with surgery, the mortality rate is 30%. Elderly and alcoholic patientss are particularly susceptible to this type of injury because these patients' brains have undergone some atrophy and the bridging veins must therefore span a wider gap.

- ***SUBARACHNOID HEMORRHAGE.*** Subarachnoid hemorrhage (SAH) occurs from bleeding vessels in the arachnoid space. Patients usually present with a severe headache, stiff neck, photophobia, or some combination of these features. Patients may report that this is the worst headache of their life. SAH may occur in the absence of trauma secondary to a rupture of a cerebral aneurysm.

- ***BRAIN HEMORRHAGES AND LACERATIONS.*** Brain hemorrhages and lacerations can result from penetrating injuries and depressed skull fractures. If a major artery or venous sinus within the brain tissue is injured, the hemorrhage can be significant and life-threatening. If an object is impaled in the head or spine, it must be left in place until removal is performed by a neurosurgeon. Bullet wounds inflict injury greater than suggested by the bullet tract, secondary to the large amount of force dissipated into surrounding tissue. A bullet does not have to penetrate the skull to cause intracranial injury because of these transmitted forces.

KEY PHYSICAL EXAMINATION FINDINGS

- ✅ ***Initial assessment.*** Look for compromised airway, difficult breathing, and signs of shock or acute hemorrhage. Consider the mechanism of injury and institute spinal precautions when indicated. If the patient is in shock, look for a hidden injury. Closed head injuries should not cause hypovolemia in adults.

- ✅ ***Vital signs.*** Be alert for signs of increased intracranial pressure: hypertension, bradycardia, and altered mental status.

⊘ **HEENT.** Look for raccoon eyes; Battle's sign; and CSF or blood drainage from the nose or ears, a sign of basal skull fracture. Palpate skull for depression. Check facial bone instability. Check pupil size, symmetry, and reactivity to light. A specific measurement of size can provide precise information. Check for facial symmetry and document deviation. Look for ecchymosis that might suggest underlying fracture. Facial fracture might be associated with airway compromise and cervical spine injury. Palpate cervical spine.

⊘ **Extremities.** Assess for any gross motor or sensory deficits.

⊘ **Neurologic examination.** Assess the level of consciousness, record GCS, and perform assessment of motor and sensory status.

TREATMENT PLAN

- **Patient assessment.** Perform a rapid and systematic primary survey initially, and institute treatment as life-threatening problems are discovered. Prompt transport to the appropriate ED is a key intervention. A secondary survey should be performed once the primary survey and all primary survey interventions have been accomplished. Frequent reassessment of the patient with a CNS injury is necessary because of the potential for a rapidly worsening neurologic status. Be prepared—potential for cardiac arrest exists.

- **Communications.** Consult with the medical control physician for guidance and institution of appropriate orders. Such consultation may prove valuable in the care of the patient with a CNS injury.

- Administer O_2 and **provide ventilatory support,** including endotracheal intubation, as indicated. Protect the cervical spine if indicted. **If GCS is at or below 8, the patient should be intubated.** Modest hyperventilation may be used when there is evidence of increased intracranial pressure and herniation. Excessive hyperventilation may worsen the injury by decreasing blood flow in watershed areas. The goal is a target $pCO_2 = 30$.

- If no mechanism of injury suggests cervical spine injury, place patient in the **Semi-Fowler or Fowler position.** The **coma position** is also useful to **reduce the aspiration risk** in patients with a compromised gag reflex or depressed consciousness.

- If there is a mechanism of injury that suggests the possibility of cervical spine injury, the patient requires spinal immobilization.

- Establish **IV access.**

- **Treat for shock.** See chapter 38.

- If the patient has an altered mental status, consider the administration of the following agents:

    o **Naloxone** (Narcan), 0.4 to 2.0 mg IV bolus. Dose may be repeated in 2 to 3 minutes.

    o **Dextrose 50%, 25 g IV if the patient is hypoglycemic** or if hypoglycemia is suspected in a patient with diabetes.

- Treat symptomatic arrhythmias. See chapters 6 and 44 for specific options.

- Treat nonlife-threatening injuries as appropriate (e.g., control bleeding, splint fractures).

- Transport to appropriate ED. Ensure patient comfort en route. Do not needlessly delay patient transport—expedite transport.

BIBLIOGRAPHY

Borczuk, P. & S. H. Thomas (2001). Head injuries. In A. Harwood-Nuss, A. B. Wolfson, C. H. Linden, S. M. Shepard, & P. H. Stenklyft (Eds.), *The clinical practice of emergency medi-*

cine (3rd ed., pp. 460–464). Philadelphia: Lippincott Williams & Wilkins.

Marik, P. E., J. Varon, & T. Trask (2002, August). Management of head trauma. *Chest, 122,* 699–711.

Shepard, S. (n.d.). Head injury: The eMedicine web page. Retrieved March 11, 2004, at http://www.emedicine.com/med/topic2820.htm.

NOTES

CHAPTER 21

HUMAN IMMUNODEFICIENCY VIRUS AND ACQUIRED IMMUNODEFICIENCY SYNDROME

Andrew W. Stern, M.P.A., M.A., NREMT-P

PRESENTATION

The presentation of patients infected with human immunodeficiency virus (HIV) or those who have acquired immunodeficiency syndrome (AIDS) may vary from asymptomatic to critically ill. Late in the disease the patient may have pneumonia, wasting, mental illness, and other complications resulting from opportunistic infections. With the availability of effective antiretroviral therapy (ART), increasing numbers of people with HIV infection or AIDS are living normal and healthy lives. For this reason, it is important to stress that universal precautions are necessary when providing care to any individual, regardless of whether he or she appears otherwise healthy.

IMMEDIATE CONCERNS

❶ **What is the patient's respiratory status?** More than 80% of patients with AIDS will develop pulmonary disease. The etiologies include infections and malignancies. *Pneumocystis carinii* pneumonia (PCP) occurs in 70% of patients with AIDS. Tuberculosis (TB) may also be found in these immunocompromised patients. In addition to the routine care of a patient in respiratory distress, paramedics may need to take precautions regarding the transmission of TB.

❶ **What is the patient's mental status?** CNS disease occurs in 90% of patients with AIDS. The symptoms may be mild, ranging from headache or focal neurologic findings to life-threatening, with altered mental status, coma, and seizures. Infection is the most common cause.

❶ **Is the patient hemodynamically stable?** Patients with AIDS may present in shock caused by sepsis and dehydration.

IMPORTANT HISTORY

❷ **What is the patient's CD-4 count?** Many patients who have HIV know their CD-4 counts. HIV selectively attacks the CD-4 lymphocytes (helper T lymphocytes). The helper T lymphocytes play a pivotal role in activating and coordinating an immune response. HIV infects these cells, converting them to virus-producing factories. When the CD-4 count drops below 500 cells/µL, the patient will begin to have infections that occur in normal hosts but in more severe forms. Opportunistic infections and malignancies begin to occur at 200 cells/µL. This CD-4 level is one of the defining criteria for AIDS. Average survival is 24 months at this level. Median survival of 12 to 18 months occurs at a CD-4 count of 50 cells/µL. Severe life-threatening infections can be seen at this level.

❷ **Is the patient having constitutional symptoms and fever?** Constitutional symptoms such as malaise, weakness, and weight loss are common. Fever is also a common symptom. Fever caused by HIV alone typically occurs in the afternoon or evening. It usually responds to antipyretics. A search for systemic infection or malignancy should be undertaken if patients with HIV present with a change in their usual fever pattern or a febrile illness.

❷ **Is the patient complaining of a respiratory illness?** As previously mentioned, respiratory complaints are common. Typical complaints include cough, hemoptysis, shortness of breath, and chest pain. Specifically diagnosing the cause in the prehospital environment is usually impossible. A productive cough with fever suggests a bacterial infection. Nonproductive coughs suggest PCP, viral or fungal pneumonias, and neoplasm. Hemoptysis may be found with TB and pneumococcal pneumonia.

❷ **Is the patient reporting any GI symptoms?** Approximately 50% of patients with AIDS report GI symptoms such as abdominal pain, diarrhea, and bleeding. Prehospital treatment of these patients is similar to the treatment of immunocompetent patients.

❷ **Is the patient taking medications?** Patients with HIV and AIDS may be taking many medications, including antiretroviral drugs, PCP prophylaxis and treatment, antiviral drugs, antibacterial drugs, antifungal agents, toxoplasmosis therapies, steroids, and analgesics.

❷ **Is there a history of other preexisting medical conditions?** Patients who become infected with HIV may also have a history of other preexisting medical problems.

DIFFERENTIAL DIAGNOSIS

A small list of the diseases associated with HIV infection and AIDS are presented here. Patients with HIV are subject to all of the other illnesses and injuries that plague immunocompetent patients. These illnesses and injuries are not discussed here.

- *PRIMARY HIV INFECTION.* In the weeks following infection with HIV, the patient presents with an acute viral syndrome—fever, malaise, sore throat, myalgias, and lymphadenopathy. This period lasts approximately 2 weeks. A typical patient is symptom-free for up to 10 years. Viral RNA is high during the initial flulike illness. There is usually a transient significant drop in CD-4 counts during this period. Seroconversion, defined as the presence of anti-HIV antibodies, averages 2 months, but longer periods (up to 11 months) have been reported.

  o *OPPORTUNISTIC INFECTIONS.* Opportunistic infections are often related to the CD-4 counts.

- **CD-4 < 500 cells/µL:**

  o ***ORAL CANDIDIASIS.*** Oral candidiasis is an infection of the mouth caused by the fungus *Candida*. The most common symptoms are discomfort and burning of the mouth. Patients also report a bad taste in the mouth. Physical exam will reveal a white or yellow plaque in the mouth. The infection can also extend down into the esophagus. It is treated with antifungals such as ketoconazole, fluconazole, itraconazole, and amphotericin B.

  o ***PNEUMOCOCCAL DISEASE.*** Pneumococcal disease is caused by the bacteria *Streptococcus pneumoniae*. It can cause pneumonia but can also spread to the blood, middle ear and CNS. Common symptoms of pneumococcal pneumonia include fever, cough, dyspnea, tachypnea, and chest pains. Pneumococcal disease is treated with antibiotics.

  o ***HAIRY LEUKOPLAKIA.*** Hairy leukoplakia is a nonpainful white plaque found along the sides of the tongue. It is associated with the Epstein-Barr virus (EBV). It is decreasing in incidence because of the use of protease inhibitors. It is usually not treated.

  o **IMMUNE THROMBOCYTOPENIC PURPURA.** Immune thrombocytopenic purpura (ITP) results in the destruction of platelets by an autoantibody. The patient may report easy bruising or bleeding. The risk of bleeding increases as the platelet count declines. ITP may be treated by splenectomy or with IV immunoglobulins.

- **CD-4 < 200 cells/µL:**

  o **PNEUMOCYSTIS CARINII *PNEUMONIA.*** The organism that causes PCP is a parasite that has features of a protozoa and a fungus. The clinical features include cough, fever, shortness of breath, and hypoxia. PCP is treated with Bactrim. Patients are often placed on prophylaxis when their CD-4 counts are low.

o **CRYPTOCOCCAL INFECTION.** The cryptococcus fungus can cause CNS infection. The clinical presentation can be subtle with symptoms such as headache, dizziness, or depression, or severe, with signs of meningitis, cranial nerve palsies, and seizures. The diagnosis is made by finding the organism in the cerebrospinal fluid. The treatment involves antifungal agents.

o **TUBERCULOSIS.** *Mycobacterium* tuberculosis usually infects the lungs but may be carried i n the blood to any tissue. Bacteria is found in the sputum and may be aerosolized when the patient coughs. TB is transmissible. The classic presentation of pulmonary TB includes cough, hemoptysis, fever, night sweats, and weight loss. The incidence of TB infections that are resistant to antibiotics is increasing. AIDS patients with TB will be empirically treated with 4 agents.

o **CRYPTOSPORIDIOSIS.** Cryptosporidiosis is a diarrheal illness caused by the microscopic parasite *Cryptosporidium parvum.* This parasite lives in the colon of humans and other animals. It is spread via the fecal-to-oral route. It has a hardy outer shell that enables it to survive long periods outside of the body and to resist chlorination. Common symptoms include nausea, diarrhea with watery stools, abdominal cramps, and fever. Therapy is usually supportive.

o **TOXOPLASMOSIS.** *Toxoplasma gondii* is the causative agent in toxoplasmosis, the most common CNS infection of patients with AIDS. This parasite is found in animal feces and soil. One stage of its life cycle occurs in the intestines of cats. Up to 50% of the U.S. population have been infected, but the infection is latent. The parasite reactivates as the CD-4 counts decline. Although toxoplasmosis may occur in various tissues in the body, most infections occur in the brain. CNS toxoplasmosis can cause fever, headache, personality changes, altered mental status, blindness, seizures, coma, and death. Combination therapy with pyrimethamine and sulfadiazine is standard treatment.

o **HISTOPLASMOSIS.** Histoplasmosis infection is caused by breathing in spores of the fungus *Histoplasma capsulatum*. The organism is found in soil contaminated by certain bird droppings. People with healthy immune systems do not typically have symptoms with the initial infection. Histoplasmosis usually involves the lungs. It can also infect the GI tract, skin, and CNS. Immunosuppressed patients are at risk of a progressive disseminated infection. The most common symptoms of disseminated histoplasmosis are fever, weight loss, skin lesions, dyspnea, anemia, and enlarged lymph nodes. CNS and eye inflammation can occur also. Treatment is with antifungal agents.

- **CD-4 < 50 cells/µL:**

  o **CNS LYMPHOMA.** CNS lymphoma is a type of cancer that occurs when abnormal white blood cells proliferate in the lymphocyte cell line. The cancer can occur in the lymph nodes or at other sites, such as the brain, spinal cord, bone marrow, and GI tract. The most common AIDS-related lymphoma is non-Hodgkin's lymphoma. This lymphoma involved antibody-producing lymphocytes and frequently produces tumors outside of the lymph nodes. Early symptoms include fever and weight loss. Enlarged asymmetric lymph nodes are common. Other symptoms are identified according to the location of the tumor. CNS lymphomas can cause headaches, altered mental status, personality changes, focal neurologic deficits, and seizures. Lymphomas are treated with chemotherapy.

  o **MYCOBACTERIUM AVIUM COMPLEX.** *Mycobacterium avium* complex (MAC) is caused by two bacteria, *Mycobacterium avium* and *Mycobacterium intracellulare*. The bacteria, commonly found in soil, water, and bird droppings, do not typically cause symptoms in healthy people. Those with immune suppression cannot contain the small numbers of bacteria that are usually found in the GI tract and lungs of many people. The bacterium can then make its way to the blood and therefore can spread to distant tissues. Common symptoms include fever, night sweats, weight loss, and diarrhea. Disseminated illness can cause brain, bone, and skin infections. A multiple antibiotic regimen is used to treat this infection.

o **CYTOMEGALOVIRUS.** Cytomegalovirus (CMV) is a member of the herpes virus family. It is primarily a sexually transmitted disease but may be transmitted via blood and bodily fluids and close personal contact. Initial infection causes fever and body aches. Many people are asymptomatic during the initial infection. Approximately 50% of adults are infected with this common disease. Nearly 90% of people infected with HIV show signs of CMV infection at autopsy. It is the primary cause of death in 10% of people infected with HIV. This virus can affect many areas of the body, but in AIDS patients its most common site is the eye. CMV retinitis can lead to blindness. CMV colitis, an inflammatory disease of the colon, causes diarrhea, fever, and weight loss. CNS infection can also occur. Antiviral therapy is used to treat CMV infection.

KEY PHYSICAL EXAMINATION FINDINGS

- ✓ **Initial assessment.** Look for respiratory distress and signs of shock.

- ✓ **Vital signs.** Assess for tachycardia and tachypnea. Hypotension may be present.

- ✓ **HEENT.** Look for dry mucus membranes in the dehydrated patient. Oral candidiasis may also be present.

- ✓ **Neck.** Lymphadenopathy may be present.

- ✓ **Lungs.** Evaluate for abnormal breath sounds, which may indicate possible pneumonia.

- ✓ ***Abdomen.*** Evaluate for tenderness, rigidity, and masses.

- ✓ ***Neuro.*** Evaluate mental status. Perform cranial nerve exam. Look for motor weakness and sensory deficits.

TREATMENT PLAN

- **Administer O$_2$ and provide ventilatory support** as needed.

- **Treat for shock as needed**. Establish **large-bore IV with 0.9% normal saline or lactated Ringer's, if needed.**

- **Provide psychological support.**

- **Transport to appropriate ED.** Ensure patient comfort en route.

BIBLIOGRAPHY

Centers for Disease Control and Prevention. (n.d.). The division of HIV/AIDS prevention. Retrieved March 3, 2004, at http://www.cdc.gov/hiv/dhap.htm.

National Institutes of Health. (n.d.). The AIDSinfo page. Retrieved March 4, 2004, at http://aidsinfo.nih.gov/.

Rothman, R. E., C. A. Marco, & G. D. Kelen (2001). Human immunodeficiency virus infection and related disorders. In A. Harwood-Nuss, A. B. Wolfson, C. H. Linden, S. M. Shepard, & P. H. Stenklyft (Eds.), *The clinical practice of emergency medicine* (3rd ed., pp. 926–935). Philadelphia: Lippincott Williams & Wilkins.

NOTES

_____

_____

_____

_____

SECTION 1

CHAPTER 22

HYPERTENSIVE EMERGENCIES

Heidi S. Betler, NREMT-P

PRESENTATION

Hypertension affects nearly 60 million Americans. Because of diagnosis and treatment of this disease, only 1% of these patients will ever experience a hypertensive emergency. Patients experiencing this type of emergency must be managed properly to prevent devastating injury to the central nervous system (CNS), heart, blood vessels, and kidneys. Most hypertensive emergencies occur in patients with a history of hypertension. A hypertensive emergency is defined as elevated blood pressure accompanied by diastolic pressure greater than 120 to 130 mm Hg with the presence of end-organ damage.

IMMEDIATE CONCERNS

❶ **Is there evidence of central nervous system involvement?** Patients with hypertensive encephalopathy may present with severe headache, nausea, vomiting, alterations in mental status, seizures, and visual disturbances. The symptoms may progress rapidly and lead to death. Hypertensive encephalopathy mostly occurs in middle-aged individuals who have a long-standing history of hypertension. The objective in management of these patients is controlled lowering of the blood pressure over minutes to hours. It may be difficult to determine whether a CNS event, such as a hemorrhagic stroke, led to elevated intracranial pressure and hypertension or whether the elevated blood pressure led to the CNS injury.

❶ **Is there evidence of cardiovascular injury?** Patients with a cardiovascular hypertensive emergency may present with chest pain, shortness of breath, myocardial ischemia, or acute pulmonary edema. The paramedic should also be aware that patients with hypertension are predisposed to aortic aneurysm and aortic dissection.

❶ Is the patient pregnant? Preeclampsia occurs in pregnant women with hypertension, causing swelling of the extremities and face, headache, and possibly confusion. These patients are at increased risk of seizure. Once the patient has a seizure, the diagnosis becomes eclampsia. Uterine blood flow is decreased in patients with preeclampsia, increasing fetal risk. The objective during prehospital management is reduction of blood pressure and prevention of seizures.

IMPORTANT HISTORY

❷ Does the patient have a history of hypertension? Most patients presenting with hypertensive emergencies have a history of hypertension. Approximately 32% of adults in the U.S. suffer from hypertension. Hypertension has been called a "silent killer" because there are few symptoms until the blood pressure is dangerously high and end-organ damage has occurred.

❷ Does the patient have a history of any end-organ illness? A history of kidney disease, cardiac disease, or stroke suggests a poorly controlled hypertension.

❷ Is the patient taking any medications? Medications prescribed to patients with hypertension are many and varied. Some of these may include alpha and beta blockers, calcium channel blockers, ACE inhibitors, angiotension II receptor antagonists, and diuretics. Determine whether the patient has been taking medications as prescribed. Rapid discontinuation of sympathetic agents may cause severe rebound hypertension and precipitate end-organ injury. Psychiatric patients taking monoamine oxidase inhibitors (MAOIs), such as phenelzine (Nardil), tranylcypromin (Parnate) and isocarboxazid (Marplan), may become hypertensive if they take tyramine-containing foods (aged cheeses or wines) or sympathomimetic agents. Also inquire about the use of recreational (illicit) drugs, specifically sympathomimetic drugs (i.e., cocaine, amphetamines). Include in the history a listing of any herbal medications that the patient may have taken as well.

DIFFERENTIAL DIAGNOSIS

- **HYPERTENSIVE ENCEPHALOPATHY.** Hypertensive encephalopathy is an acute life-threatening alteration in CNS function caused by hypertension. Common findings include headache, vision changes, altered mental status, or neurologic deficits. The onset is gradual, over hours to days. Cerebral blood flow remains constant over a wide range of mean arterial blood pressures (MAP). At very high blood pressures, the cerebral blood flow increases as well. As cerebral blood flow continues to increase, the blood-brain barrier becomes damaged, allowing cerebral edema to develop, which results in decreased blood flow in the brain. Although a paramedic may be tempted to reduce the arterial blood pressure to normal levels, this may be dangerous. Over time, hypertensive patients have adapted to elevated mean arterial pressures, achieving normal cerebral blood flow at higher blood pressures. Acutely lowering their MAP below 120 mm Hg may cause inadequate cerebral perfusion. Safe reduction in MAP is best accomplished gradually with medications that can be titrated.

- **PRIMARY CNS INJURY.** CNS injuries that cause elevated intracranial pressure may cause herniation and brainstem injury. Hypertension and bradycardia, known as a Cushing's response, may occur. The hypertension may be needed to perfuse the brain subjected to elevated intracranial pressures. Less aggressive blood pressure reduction is undertaken for fear of further decreasing cerebral blood flow and extending the injury. Distinguishing between hypertensive encephalopathy and primary CNS injuries can be difficult. Acute subarachnoid hemorrhage is an important primary CNS injury to recognize. Patients present with a sudden headache, often described as the "worst headache" of their life. These patients will require neurosurgical evaluation.

- **MYOCARDIAL ISCHEMIA.** The excessive afterload caused by the hypertensive emergency of myocardial ischemia increases the workload of the heart and its oxygen demand. These patients present with symptoms typical of ischemic chest pain, ECG changes, and possibly acute pulmonary edema. Treatment involves aspirin, oxygen, nitrates, and possibly morphine and diuretics.

- **AORTIC DISSECTION.** Aortic dissections are false passages created in the media of the thoracic aorta. These can be caused by long-standing hypertension, which damages the endothelium of the aorta. The false passages can grow and actually dissect the aorta. If the dissection involves the arch of the aorta, the arch vessels, including the carotid arteries, can become occluded, causing neurologic deficits similar to those associated with cerebrovascular accident (CVA), as well as back pain. If the dissection involves the root of the aorta, coronary arteries may become occluded, causin g an acute myocardial infarction (AMI). Dissections that extend distally can lead to differential blood blow in the arteries of the arms and legs. Differences in blood pressure greater than 10 mm Hg are cause for concern. Patients with a thoracic aortic dissection are usually hypertensive initially but may become hypotensive if the dissection leaks. The goal of therapy in the hypertensive aortic dissection patient is to reduce the blood pressure and the force of the pulse wave. Nitroprusside and beta blockers are typically used. Patients with hypotensive dissection should receive fluid resuscitation and be transported expeditiously.

- **PREECLAMPSIA AND ECLAMPSIA.** Preeclampsia and eclampsia are known as the toxemias of pregnancy. There are many common findings, including hypertension (systolic blood pressure > 140/90), peripheral edema, proteinuria, renal failure, hyperreflexia, altered mental status, and seizures. Intense vasoconstriction is believed to be the cause of the disease. In severe preeclampsia there is also epigastric and right upper quadrant abdominal pain caused by liver injury. The diagnosis becomes eclampsia when a seizure occurs. The goal of therapy is blood pressure reduction and seizure prevention. Despite the peripheral edema, these patients may be intravascularly hypovolemic. The vasodilator of choice has historically been hydralazine. IV fluid administration is beneficial. Magnesium sulfate is used to prevent seizures.

NOTE: Nitroprusside is contraindicated in the pregnant patient.

KEY PHYSICAL EXAMINATION FINDINGS

- ✓ **Initial assessment.** Look for alterations in mental status, respiratory compromise, and hemodynamic instability.

- ✓ **Vital signs.** Careful monitoring of the blood pressure is needed. Be sure to record pressures in both arms of patients presenting with chest or back pain.

- ✓ **HEENT.** Examine carefully and note signs of facial swelling or asymmetry. Examine pupils for responsiveness and equality.

- ✓ **Lungs.** Listen to lung sounds for signs of pulmonary edema.

- ✓ **Heart.** Assess heart tones and apical pulse. Heart tones may be muffled, and apical pulse may be very prominent.

- ✓ **Abdomen.** Assess carefully for pulsatile masses, which may indicate the presence of an abdominal aortic aneurysm.

- ✓ **Extremities.** Assess for edema in the extremities. Check peripheral pulses to equality.

ELECROCARDIOGRAM

Evaluate for signs of cardiac ischemia or injury.

TREATMENT PLAN

- **Patient assessment.** Perform a rapid and systematic initial assessment, and institute treatment as life-threatening problems are discovered. Prompt transport to the appropriate ED is a key intervention. Frequent reassessment of patients with a hypertensive emergency is necessary because of the potential for worsening of their cardiovascular and neurologic status. Be prepared—potential for cardiac arrest exists. Patients experiencing a hypertensive emergency must be managed carefully because lowering the blood pressure too quickly may result in end-organ damage. Early contact with medical command is recommended.

HYPERTENSIVE ENCEPHALOPATHY

- **Administer O$_2$ and provide ventilatory support** as needed.

- Place the patient in a **head-elevated position**, unless spinal immobilization is needed.

- **Monitor the ECG and O$_2$ saturation**.

- **Establish large-bore IV** access.

- Consider the following interventions:

    o **Nitroprusside infusion** (50 mg/500 mL D5W). Start at 0.5 µg/kg/min, titrating to a systolic blood pressure decrease of 30 to 40 mm Hg and a diastolic blood pressure decrease of 10 to 20 mm Hg. Nitroprusside is the drug of choice because of its short duration of action and the excellent control of blood pressure reduction afforded by its infusion. Monitor BP continuously. If the patient's BP falls precipitously, discontinue the infusion and consider a 250 mL fluid bolus. NOTE: If the patient has a history of coronary artery disease or is demonstrating evidence of cardiac ischemia, consider pretreatment with nitroglycerin before starting nitroprusside.

- o **Nitroglycerin, 0.4 mg SL** every 3 to 5 minutes, or

- o **Nitroglycerin infusion** (25 mg/250 mL D5W) starting at 10 µg/min and titrating by 5 µg/min every 5 to 20 minutes until there is a SBP decrease of 30 to 40 mm Hg and a DBP decrease of 10 to 20 mm Hg.

- o **Labetolol, 20 mg IV** over 2 minutes. Repeat at 20 to 80 mg IV every 10 minutes to a maximum total dose of 300 mg. Therapeutic goal: SBP decrease of 30 to 40 mm Hg and a DBP decrease of 10 to 20 mm Hg. Hold for patients whose heart rate drops below 60.

- Frequently reassess the patient's hemodynamic and neurologic status.

- **Transport to the appropriate ED**. Ensure patient comfort en route.

THORACIC AORTIC DISSECTION

- **Administer O_2 and provide ventilatory support** as needed.

- Place the patient in a position of comfort, unless spinal immobilization is needed.

- **Monitor the ECG and O_2 saturation.**

- **Establish large-bore IV** access.

- Consider the following interventions:

- o **Propranolol, 1.0 mg IV.** Repeat 1.0 mg dose as needed to a maximum total of 0.1 mg/kg. Stop the administration for patients whose heart rate drops below 60.

- o **Nitroprusside infusion** (50 mg/500 mL D5W). Start at 0.5µg/kg/min, titrating to a systolic blood pressure between 90 and 120 mm Hg.

- o **Nitroglycerin, 0.4 mg SL** every 3 to 5 minutes, or

o **Nitroglycerin infusion** (25 mg/250 mL D5W) starting at 10 µg/min and titrating by 5 µg/min every 5 to 20 minutes until the chest pain is relieved, the SBP is below 100 mm Hg, or the patient demonstrates evidence of poor perfusion.

o **Normal saline (NS) or lactated Ringer's (LR) IV** fluid bolus if the patient is hypotensive.

- **Transport to the appropriate ED.** Ensure patient comfort en route.

CHEST PAIN, CARDIAC ISCHEMIA, AND PULMONARY EDEMA

- **Administer O$_2$ and provide ventilatory support** as needed.

- Place the patient in a position of comfort, unless spinal immobilization is needed.

- **Monitor the ECG and O$_2$ saturation. Obtain a 12-lead ECG,** if available.

- **Establish IV** access

- Consider the following interventions:

o **Aspirin, 160 to 325 mg PO**. Have the patients chew the tablets.

o **Nitroglycerin, 0.4 mg SL** every 3 to 5 minutes, as needed. Hold for systolic blood pressures below 100 mm Hg.

o **Morphine sulfate, 1 to 5 mg IV.** May be repeated every 5 minutes, as needed.

- **Treat symptomatic arrhythmias** per AHA ACLS guidelines. See chapters 6 and 44.

- **Treat cardiogenic shock** as described in chapter 38.

- If pulmonary edema is present, consider the following interventions:

  o **High-dose nitroglycerin, 0.4 to 1.2 mg SL** every 3 to 5 minutes. Titrate to respiratory distress and SBP greater than 100 mm Hg.

  o **Furosemide (Lasix), 40 mg IV.** Higher doses may be given if the patient is already taking furosemide.

  o **Morphine sulfate, 1 to 5 mg IV.** May be repeated every 5 minutes, as needed.

- **Transport to the appropriate ED.** Ensure patient comfort en route.

PREECLAMPSIA AND ECLAMPSIA

- **Administer O_2 and provide ventilatory support** as needed.

- Place the patient in the **left lateral recumbent position**.

- **Monitor the ECG, O_2 saturation, and fetal heart rate,** if available.

- **Establish IV** access.

- Consider the following interventions:

  o **Hydralazine, 5 mg IV** over 3 minutes. Repeat 5 mg IV every 5 minutes until DBP is between 90 to 100 mm Hg. Maximum total dose is 20 mg.

  o **Labetolol, 10 mg IV** over 2 minutes. May be repeated every 10 minutes at 10 to 80 mg. The maximum total dose is 300 mg.

  o **Magnesium sulfate 2 to 4 g IV** over 5 to 10 minutes if a seizure occurs. May also be given for seizure prophylaxis. After the loading dose, run as an infusion at 2 g/hour. Magnesium causes CNS depression. Watch for decreased respiratory rate and decreased deep tendon reflexes. If CNS depression occurs or there are additional seizures or evidence of fetal distress, contact medical command for guidance. The magnesium may need to be discontinued.

- **Transport to the appropriate ED.** Ensure patient comfort en route.

BIBLIOGRAPHY

Bledsoe, B. E., R. S. Porter, & R. A. Cherry (2001). *Paramedic emergency care principles and practice* (Vol. 3). Upper Saddle River, NJ: Prentice-Hall.

Brown, D. F. & C. Courban (2003). Hypertensive emergencies. In J. J. Schaider, S. R. Hayden, R. Wolfe, R. M. Barkin, & P. Rosen (Eds.), *Rosen & Barkin's 5-minute emergency medicine consult* (2nd ed., pp. 560–561). Philadelphia: Lippincott Williams & Wilkins.

Sapiro, E. M. Preeclampsia/eclampsia. (2003). In J. J. Schaider, S. R. Hayden, R. Wolfe, R. M. Barkin, & P. Rosen (Eds.), *Rosen & Barkin's 5-minute emergency medicine consult* (2nd ed., pp. 892–893). Philadelphia: Lippincott Williams & Wilkins.

SECTION 1

NOTES

_____
_____
_____
_____
_____
_____
_____
_____

CHAPTER 23

HYPERTHERMIA

Mark Scheatzle, M.D.

PRESENTATION

Hyperthermia, or heat illness, is common during the hot and humid season. Patients with heat exhaustion are hemodynamically stable, with a normal mental status. Typically, they are nauseated and fatigued, with a temperature of 102° F or less. Unlike patients with heat exhaustion, patients with heatstroke have an abnormal mental status (e.g., bizarre behavior, seizure, coma, confusion) and often hemodynamic instability.

IMMEDIATE CONCERNS

❶ **What is the patient's temperature?** The patient with heatstroke has a temperature above 104° F (usually greater than 106°). Hyperthermia is a medical emergency that necessitates immediate cooling and transport to the nearest appropriate ED. The patient may also be hemodynamically unstable, requiring aggressive resuscitation with airway control, oxygen, large-bore IV access, and IV fluids.

IMPORTANT HISTORY

❷ **What are the circumstances of the event?** Pertinent information includes duration of onset, general health of the patient, and degree of activity at onset. Heatstroke is commonly separated into classic heatstroke and exertional heatstroke. Classic heatstroke occurs in infants, the elderly, and the chronically ill, who tend to become severely dehydrated over several days. Their skin is hot and dry on presentation. Exertional heatstroke occurs in the young, unacclimatized athlete who is not dehydrated. These patients will thus sweat profusely.

❓ Is the patient taking any medications? Medications, both over the counter and prescription, can have a profound impact on a patient's ability to tolerate heat. For example, drugs with anticholinergic properties, tricyclic antidepressants, and cold medications decrease the body's ability to dissipate heat through sweating. Cocaine, amphetamines, and salicylate intoxication increase the body's heat production, as do overdoses of synthetic thyroid hormone. In addition, patients recently administered neuroleptics, most commonly haloperidol (Haldol), are susceptible to neuroleptic malignant syndrome (NMS). NMS causes the basal metabolic rate to greatly increase, leading to severe hyperthermia.

SECTION 1

DIFFERENTIAL DIAGNOSIS

- ***FEVER.*** Fever is an entity separate from hyperthermia, with a different pathopysiology and treatment. Fever is best distinguished from hyperthermia by history, although the distinction is not always clear. Look for evidence of infection: respiratory symptoms; abdominal complaints, such as diarrhea and pain; urinary tract symptoms, such as burning on urination, foul-smelling urine, increased urinary frequency, and hesitancy; and evidence of meningitis, such as stiff neck, photophobia, and an altered mental status.

- ***SEVERE DEHYDRATION.*** Severe dehydration is a common cause of hyperthermia. Total body volume depletion leads to vasoconstriction, causing a decrease in the body's ability to dissipate heat through sweating.

- ***MEDICATIONS.*** Hyperthermia may occur secondary to medication use.

- ***HYPERTHYROIDISM OR THYROID STORM.*** Thyroid storm most commonly occurs in patients with nondiagnosed or undertreated hyperthyroidism. However, it may occur with overdose of exogenous thyroid hormone. Symptoms are identical to those found in patients with hyperthermia. Physical findings may be subtle and include the presence of a goiter (thyroid nodule in the neck) or exopthalmus (i.e., prominent, bulging eyes).

- **NEUROLEPTIC MALIGNANT SYNDROME.** NMS is a rare complication of neuroleptic medications. It can occur during early therapy or years later. It is characterized by fever, an altered mental status, and muscular rigidity. Patients are often profoundly diaphoretic. Medicines associated with NMS include phenothiazines (Thorazine, Prolixin, Trilafon, Compazine, Mellaril), butyrophenones (droperidol, haloperidol), and thiothixene.

- **DELIRIUM TREMENS.** Delirium tremens (DTs) typically occur 3 or 4 days after cessation of excessive alcohol intake. Symptoms can be identical to heatstroke, with a significant tremor or seizure activity. History and a careful physical examination provide the best clues in diagnosing DTs.

- **HEAT CRAMPS**. Heat cramp is a relatively benign condition characterized by painful muscle cramps, usually in the acclimatized patient working in a hot, humid environment. The cramps may begin during or after several hours of exertion and are caused by inadequate fluid or electrolyte replacement.

- **HEAT EXHAUSTION.** Heat exhaustion usually occurs in an unacclimatized person who has worked under hot, humid conditions. There are two varieties of heat exhaustion: water-depletion type and salt-depletion type. The water-depletion type is characterized by thirst, dizziness, fever, confusion, and poor motor coordination. The salt-depletion type is characterized by weakness, headache, muscle cramps, nausea, and vomiting. Patients are usually without thirst or fever. Patients experiencing both varieties of heat exhaustion present with diaphoretic skin, tachycardia, and possibly hypotension. Although two varieties of heat exhaustion exist, most patients present with a combination of the two. Heat exhaustion may progress to heatstroke if untreated.

- **HEATSTROKE.** The typical patient experiencing heatstroke is either very young or elderly. Heatstroke can have a gradual onset over several days or occur suddenly. When the onset is gradual, the patient may be markedly dehydrated. When heatstroke develops acutely, it is usually in the younger, unacclimatized patient working under significant heat stress for several hours. Patients with heatstroke are tachycardic, tachypneic, hypotensive, and febrile (temperature above 104° F) and have an altered mental status. They are usually still able to sweat. All organ systems are damaged by the elevated temperature, with the damage related to both the magnitude of the fever and the duration of the elevation. If the temperature is not rapidly reduced, death may occur. The cause of death is usually caused by disseminated intravascular coagulation (a severe clotting abnormality characterized by the widespread formation of microthrombi and by difficult-to-control bleeding), acute renal failure, acute liver failure, or acute respiratory distress syndrome.

- **CENTRAL NERVOUS SYSTEM LESIONS.** Cerebrovascular accidents (CVAs) or tumors, which damage the hypothalamic thermoregulatory center, can cause marked temperature elevations accompanied by neurologic deficits.

KEY PHYSICAL EXAMINATION FINDINGS

❓ **Initial assessment.**   Look for signs of shock.

❓ **Vital signs.**   Monitor vital signs, particularly temperature, because they indicate the severity of the disease.

❓ **Skin condition.**   Inspect for redness and flushing or profuse sweating.

❷ *Mental status.* Assess for neurologic deficit or decrease in mental status. Hyperthermia with these features indicates heatstroke.

TREATMENT PLAN

- *Patient assessment.* Frequent reassessment is necessary because the patient's temperature may continue to increase despite cooling efforts. The patient's mental status may deteriorate, requiring aggressive airway management. In addition, these patients are prone to vomit, seize, or develop hypotension.

GENERAL TREATMENT GUIDELINES

- Remove patient from the heat stress and place in a cool environment.

- **Administer O$_2$ and provide ventilatory support** as needed.

SPECIFIC TREATMENT GUIDELINES

HEATSTROKE

- Follow general guidelines.

- Continuously monitor the patient's temperature.

- **Institute rapid cooling.** The patient must be placed in a cool environment, and his or her clothes should be removed. There are several effective methods for decreasing temperature. The most effective is spraying the patient with a mist of room-temperature water while constantly fanning. Sponging the patient with water while fanning is also effective. Do not sponge the patient with alcohol. Ice packs may be placed at the patient's groin, axial, and neck; however, this method is not as effective as the previously mentioned ones.

- **Establish large-bore IV** and begin fluid resuscitation with 0.9% NaCL or lactated Ringer's solution if the patient is hypotensive.

- **If patient is seizing, give diazepam (Valium), 5 to 10 mg IV bolus.** Dose may be repeated every 10 to 15 minutes (pediatric dose: 0.2 to 0.5 mg/kg by slow IV bolus, maximum dose: age younger than 5 years, 5 mg; age older than 5 years, 10 mg).

- **Transport expeditiously to appropriate ED.** Do not needlessly delay transport—expedite transport. Continue cooling efforts en route.

HEAT EXHAUSTION

- **Establish large-bore IV** and begin fluid resuscitation with 0.9% NaCL or lactated Ringer's solution if the patient is hypotensive.

- Transport expeditiously to appropriate ED because progression to heatstroke can occur.

BIBLIOGRAPHY

Walker, J. S. & D. E. Hogan (2004). Heat emergencies. In J. E. Tintinelli, G. D. Kelen, & J. S. Stapczynski (Eds.), *Emergency medicine: A comprehensive study guide* (6th ed., pp. 1183–1190). New York: McGraw-Hill.

Doucette, M. (2003). Hyperthermia. In P. Rosen, R. M. Barkin, S. R. Hayden, J. J. Schnider, & R. Wolfe (Eds.), *The 5-minute emergency medicine consult* (pp. 562–563). Philadelphia: Lippincott Williams & Wilkins.

Simon, H. B. (1993). Hyperthermia. *New England Journal of Medicine, 329,* 483–487.

CHAPTER 24

HYPOGLYCEMIA

Steve Shurgot, EMT-P

PRESENTATION

Hypoglycemia is the most common endocrine emergency treated by EMS professionals. Many of the signs and symptoms of hypoglycemia, such as altered mental status, headache, seizures, and strokelike motor weakness, reflect the brain's sensitivity to low blood sugar. Other signs and symptoms—diaphoresis, tachycardia, palpitations, and hypertension—reflect the release of stress hormones and epinephrine designed to increase blood sugar. In adults and children, hypoglycemia is uncommon and is usually a side effect of diabetes treatment. However, it can result from other disease, medications, hormone or enzyme deficiencies, and tumors. Young children and infants have small glycogen stores and may become hypoglycemic in the face of poor oral intake.

IMMEDIATE CONCERNS

❶ **What is the patient's mental status?** Consider hypoglycemia in all patients who present with an altered mental status or abnormal behavior. If the patient is not alert, first assess the patient's ABCs. Look for treatable etiologies early, such as hypoglycemia, hypoxia, opiate overdose, and shock.

IMPORTANT HISTORY

❷ **Does the patient have a history of diabetes?** Most of the hypoglycemic patients treated by EMS providers have a history of diabetes. Excess insulin administration relative to dietary intake is the most common reason for hypoglycemia.

❓ **Is the patient taking any medications?** Insulin and oral hypoglycemic agents are the most common medications implicated in causing hypoglycemia. Patients who use oral agents are at increased risk of recurrent hypoglycemia because of the long duration of action of these agents.

❓ **When did the patient last eat?** Skipping meals or eating later than usual is a common reason for hypoglycemia in diabetic patients.

❓ **Does the patient have an infection or fever?** Sepsis is a common nondiabetic cause of hypoglycemia, especially in infants and the elderly.

❓ **Has the patient been exercising?** Exertion decreases insulin requirements. The diabetic must balance dietary intake with exertion and insulin administration. A change in exertion levels without concomitant changes in diet or insulin dosing can lead to hypoglycemia.

❓ **Has the patient been drinking alcohol?** Alcohol consumption in diabetic patients may cause hypoglycemia secondary to inhibition of glucose release by the liver between meals. In addition, alcoholic patients may have hypoglycemia caused by liver disease or starvation.

DIFFERENTIAL DIAGNOSIS

• *POSTPRANDIAL HYPOGLYCEMIA.* Hypoglycemia after eating a meal occurs in patients who are "prediabetics" and patients who have recently undergone gastric surgery.

• *FASTING OR STARVATION STATES.* Fasting or starvation states occur primarily with patients with diabetes who continue their medications while fasting. Hypoglycemia has been reported in patients who are not diabetic who have received insulin or oral hypoglycemic agents as part of Munchausen's syndrome, suicide, or attempted homicide.

- **INSULINOMAS.** Insulin-secreting tumors are a rare cause of hypoglycemia.

- **ORGAN FAILURE.** Liver failure is the most common type of organ failure to cause hypoglycemia. Other causes include adrenal failure, renal failure, and hypothyroidism.

- **PEDIATRICS.** Neonates and infants are at high risk because they need frequent feedings and have small glucose stores.

KEY PHYSICAL EXAMINATION FINDINGS

- **Initial assessment.** Look for alterations in mental status, respiratory compromise, and hemodynamic instability.

- **Vital signs.** Assess for tachycardia, fever, or hypotension.

- **HEENT.** Examine carefully and note signs of trauma. Examine pupils for responsiveness and equality.

- **Skin.** Assess for edema in the extremities. Check peripheral pulses to equality.

- **Neurologic examination.** Assess for decreased level of consciousness, postictal states, and acute CVA.

GLUCOMETER

Evaluate for evidence of hypoglycemia.

TREATMENT PLAN

- **Patient assessment.** Perform a rapid and systematic initial assessment, and institute treatment as life-threatening problems are discovered. Prompt transport to the appropriate ED is a key intervention. Frequent reassessment of patients with an altered mental status is necessary because of the potential for worsening of their neurologic status and airway compromise.

- **Administer O$_2$ and provide ventilatory support** as needed.

- **Monitor the ECG and O$_2$ saturation.**

- Place the patient in the **Fowler or semi-Fowler position.** The coma position is also helpful to reduce aspiration risk in patients with a decreased mental status or compromised gag reflex.

- If hypoglycemia is suspected or the patient has an altered mental status, perform blood glucose testing on peripheral blood. If the patient is hypoglycemic, administer dextrose.

- Consider the following interventions:

  o **Oral glucose** solution administration in awake patient with an intact gag reflex. If this is not safe, establish IV access.

  o **Dextrose 50%, 25 g IV** (pediatric dose, D25 [dilute D50 1:1 with NS or sterile water] 1 to 2 mL/kg IV, infant dose, D10 [dilute D50 1:4 with NS or sterile water] 2 to 4 mL/kg IV). May be repeated if there is insufficient improvement.

  o If there is no immediate IV access, give **glucagon 1 mg IM** (pediatric dose 0.1 mg/kg IM, maximum 1 mg). May repeat in 10 to 30 minutes, if needed. As the patient's mental status improves, you may administer an oral glucose solution.

  o If there is no response to the above interventions, follow the treatment recommendations in chapter 4.

- Frequently reassess the patient.

- **Transport to the appropriate ED.** Ensure patient comfort en route. Some hypoglycemic patients may refuse transport to the ED following treatment. There may be potential for further episodes of hypoglycemia, especially when the patient is taking oral hypoglycemic agents. If the patient's decision-making capacity is intact and he or she is aware of the risks of not seeking further care immediately, the patient's wishes must be followed. Establish a backup plan that will include prompt consumption of a meal, presence of another responsible adult, frequent measurement of the patient's blood sugar, and early follow-up with the patient's family doctor.

BIBLIOGRAPHY

Harrigan, R. A., M. S. Nathan, & P. Beattie (2001). Oral agents for the treatment of type 2 diabetes mellitus: Pharmacology, toxicity, and treatment. *Annals of Emergency Medicine, 38,* 68–78.

Ervin, M. & S. Friedman (2003). Hypoglycemia. In J. J. Schaider, S. R. Hayden, R. Wolfe, R. M. Barkin, & P. Rosen (Eds.), *Rosen & Barkin's 5-minute emergency medicine consult* (2nd ed., pp. 574–575). Philadelphia: Lippincott Williams & Wilkins.

NOTES

_____

_____

_____

_____

_____

_____

_____

_____

_____

_____

_____

_____

CHAPTER 25

HYPOTENSION

Myles Greenberg, M.D.

PRESENTATION

Patients with low blood pressure may present any-where along the clinical spectrum, from completely asymp-tomatic to exhibiting profound shock. Usually, hypotension is discovered during the evaluation.

IMMEDIATE CONCERNS

❶ **Is the patient hemodynamically stable?** Stability is defined by both symptoms and signs. The primary sign of hemodynamic instability is poor mentation (e.g., confusion, agitations, or decreased level of conscious-ness). Signs include cyanosis, poor capillary refill, sys-tolic blood pressure less than 90 mm Hg in both arms, new dysrhythmias, urine output less than 0.5 ml/kg per hour, and tachycardia without another explanation. Any patient who is unstable warrants immediate resuscita-tion. The type of resuscitation depends on the etiology of the hypotension. All patients, however, should receive oxygen administration, ventilatory assistance if neces-sary, and large-bore IV access.

❶ **Is there any immediately obvious source of the patient's low blood pressure?** Respiratory arrest or hypoventilation should be treated with all necessary measures, including endotracheal intubation if indicated. External hemorrhage should be controlled, including the use of pneumatic antishock garment (PASG) for lower extremity open fractures. Obvious evidence of a hypovo-lemic cause for hypotension, such as gastrointestinal (GI) bleeding or trauma, is justification for immediate, large-volume fluid resuscitation. An unstable cardiac rhythm should prompt the initiation of ACLS protocols.

● **Does the patient have a ruptured abdominal aortic aneurysm?** Patients who have a history of an abdominal aortic aneurysm (AAA) are at risk for rupture. The typical patient is elderly, with a history of atherosclerosis and hypertension. The classic triad of hypotension, pains and a pulsatile mass is found in only half of these patients. The risk of rupture increases with the size of the aneurysm. Unexplained hypotension in an elderly patient with or without a history of AAA warrants the consideration of this diagnosis. Early transport to a facility that can repair the AAA is essential if the patient is to survive.

● **Is there evidence of uncontrollable bleeding?** Some evidence suggests that patients with uncontrollable hemorrhage might benefit from being treated without the traditional IV fluid resuscitation. This concept is presently controversial, but its premise is that IV fluids may actually increase the rate of bleeding. Proposed mechanisms for the increased bleeding include hydraulic acceleration of bleeding caused by elevated blood pressure, dislodgment of soft clots, and dilution of clotting factors. Proponents of this theory suggest withholding preoperative IV fluids in patients with uncontrollable bleeding.

IMPORTANT HISTORY

❓ **Does the patient have a history of blood loss or dehydration?** Search for hypovolemia by asking about recent trauma or bleeding; recent GI bleeding, hematemesis, melena, or hematochezia; previous history of GI bleeding; history of a bleeding disorder; recent history of poor oral intake; and a recent history of severe diarrhea or vomiting.

❓ **Are there any symptoms of cardiac ischemia?** Coronary disease is the primary killer in the United States. Hypotension may occur as a result of ineffective cardiac performance caused by pump failure or dysrhythmias.

❓ **Has the patient been febrile or had other symptoms of an infectious process?** Is the patient immunocompromised or elderly? Hypotension may be the presenting sign of sepsis in certain populations. The elderly, nursing home residents, and HIV positive patients are particularly susceptible to fulminant infections.

❓ **Is the patient taking any medications that may predispose the patient to hypotension or bleeding?** A wide variety of medications, particularly antihypertensives, can cause hypotension. Look for any new medications or recently increased doses. A patient on anticoagulant therapy may be bleeding. Patients with poorly controlled diabetes who are on insulin may present with hypotension.

❓ **Is there evidence of allergic reaction?** A patient in anaphylactic shock needs prompt attention to the ABCs as well as specific therapy with epinephrine, antihistamines, IV fluids, and possibly steroids.

DIFFERENTIAL DIAGNOSIS

SHOCK

For more detailed information on shock, refer to chapter 38.

- ***HYPOVOLEMIC SHOCK.*** Hypovolemic shock is caused by loss of blood volume secondary to bleeding or dehydration. The most common causes are trauma, GI bleeding, intractable vomiting or diarrhea, and diabetic ketoacidosis. Hypovolemic shock is by far the most common type of shock among young patients.

- ***CARDIOGENIC SHOCK.*** Cardiogenic shock is caused by loss of myocardial pumping ability. Myocardial ischemia or infarction causes this loss of pumping action directly or indirectly through the inducement of nonlife-sustaining dysrhythmias. This form of shock occurs in older patients, particularly those who have a history of previous cardiac disease or a history of diabetes, hypertension, smoking, hypercholesterolemia, or obesity. Other common causes of pump failure include cardiomyopathies, valvular disease, and prosthetic valve dysfunction.

- **SEPTIC SHOCK.** Septic shock is caused by loss of vascular integrity and subsequent loss of intravascular volume owing to bacterial toxins. Septic shock occurs only in the setting of acute infection and is much more common in elderly, debilitated, or immunocompromised individuals.

- **NEUROGENIC SHOCK.** Neurogenic shock is caused by loss of vascular tone resulting from the loss of sympathetic nervous tone. It can occur after high spinal (cervical) trauma, but this is fairly uncommon.

- **ANAPHYLACTIC SHOCK.** Anaphylactic shock is caused by systemic release of potent vasoactive substances, particularly histamine, resulting in airway compromise, vascular collapse, and extensive skin reactions. This response can be caused by any substance to which the patient has developed an allergy; often foods and bee stings are the culprits. Patients can also develop allergic reactions that cause hypotension but do not result in shock. See chapter 3.

OTHER CAUSES OF HYPOTENSION

All of the processes listed previously under shock can occur in less severe form, causing hypotension without the shock syndrome. Other causes of low blood pressure include the following:

- **DYSRHYTHMIAS**. Bradycardias or tachycardias often cause low blood pressure without progressing to frank shock. Common etiologies are second- and third-degree heart block, sinus bradycardia, pacemaker failures, sinus tachycardia, atrial fibrillation or flutter, paroxysmal supraventricular tachycardia (PSVTs), and ventricular tachycardia.

- **HYPOVOLEMIA WITHOUT SHOCK.** A multitude of conditions can cause hypovolemia with hypotension. Bleeding, GI losses (vomiting or diarrhea), renal losses, infection (insensible losses), and adrenal insufficiency are examples.

- **PULMONARY EMBOLISM.** Pulmonary embolism should be suspected in any patient who is tachycardic and tachypneic and has any predisposing factors, such as inactivity, recent surgery, malignancy, and old age.

- **TENSION PNEUMOTHORAX.** Tension pneumothorax should be considered in patients who have recently experienced trauma and patients with advanced chronic obstructive pulmonary disease or asthma.

- **MEDICATIONS.** As mentioned previously, many medications can be the cause of a lower-than-normal blood pressure. Antihypertensives that have recently been started or increased in dosage can cause either orthostatic hypotension or resting hypotension.

- **VASOVAGAL RESPONSE.** Commonly known as fainting, the vasovagal response is caused by stressful situations. The vasovagal response consists of bradycardia and hypotension that often result in syncope. The episode usually resolves quickly after the patient is placed in the supine position.

- **PHYSIOLOGIC MECHANISMS.** Some patients, particularly young women and pregnant women, may normally have a low blood pressure. If the patient is asymptomatic and nonorthostatic, a low pressure may be normal.

KEY PHYSICAL EXAMINATION FINDINGS

✓ **Initial assessment.** Monitor ABCs. If the patient has ventilatory or circulatory compromise, this issue must be addressed first.

⊘ **Vital signs.** Monitor heart rate and rhythm, BP in both arms, temperature, and respiratory effort. All these steps are essential to diagnosing the etiology of the patient's low BP.

⊘ **Focused physical exam.** Look for evidence of bleeding or trauma.

⊘ **Neck.** Examine for cervical fractures, which can cause neurogenic shock.

⊘ **Abdomen.** Look for peritoneal signs (e.g., extreme tenderness, guarding, rebound) as a source of bleeding or infection.

⊘ **Extremities.** Assess for long bone fractures, which may be a cause of hypovolemia.

⊘ **Neurologic examinations.** Assess for depressed level of consciousness, which may indicate shock.

⊘ **Skin.** Inspect for hives, pallor, cool temperature, and delayed capillary refill—an indication of allergic reaction.

TREATMENT PLAN

• **Patient assessment.** Constantly evaluate any hypotensive patient for deterioration to a shock state. All patients should receive cardiac monitoring and frequent reassessments of mental status, which are the best indictors of adequate perfusion. If a specific etiology of the patient's shock is known, institute specific shock therapy as outlined in chapter 38. General guidelines for the care of patients with nontraumatic hypotension are as follows:

PATIENTS WHO ARE HEMODYNAMICALLY UNSTABLE WITHOUT TRAUMA

• **Administer O$_2$ and provide ventilatory support** as needed. This includes needle-chest decompression of the tension pneumothorax.

- Place patient in the **shock position** (supine with legs elevated).

- **Establish large-bore IV access** and begin fluid resuscitation with 0.9% NaCl or lactated Ringer's solution. [Controversial therapy note: Some experts recommend withholding IV fluid resuscitation in the context of penetrating trauma with uncontrollable hemorrhage unless the patient is in extremis.] If transportation is delayed or if there is inadequate response to 2 to 3 liters of crystalloid infusion, consider infusing colloid solutions, such as plasmanate or hespan. If there has been inadequate response to ongoing fluid resuscitation, consider using vasopressors such as dopamine 2 to 20 µg/kg per minute IV infusion (pediatric dosing: start at 1.0 µg/kg per minute), titrated to systolic blood pressure greater than 90 mm Hg. Vasopressors are a temporary last-ditch effort to be used only after fluid resuscitation is inadequate. Remember, the patient is not bleeding dopamine.

- **Expeditiously transport to appropriate ED.** Do not needlessly delay patient transport—expedite transport.

PATIENTS WHO ARE HEMODYNAMICALLY STABLE WITHOUT TRAUMA

- **Establish large-bore IV** access with a 0.9% NaCl or lactated Ringer's solution.

- **Transport to appropriate ED.** Ensure patient comfort en route.

PATIENT WITH HYPOTENSION SECONDARY TO DYSRHYTHMIA

- Treat the patient with shock secondary to a tachycardia or a bradycardia according to guidelines in chapters 6 and 44.

BIBLIOGRAPHY

Imperato, J. & C. L. Rosen (2003). Abdominal aortic aneurysm. In J. J. Schaider, S. R. Hayden, R. Wolfe, R. M. Barkin, & P. Rosen (Eds.), *Rosen & Barkin's 5-minute emergency medicine consult* (2nd ed., pp. 2–3). Philadelphia: Lippincott Williams & Wilkins.

Shapiro, N. (2003). Shock. In J. J. Schaider, S. R. Hayden, R. Wolfe, R. M. Barkin, & P. Rosen (Eds.), *Rosen & Barkin's 5-minute emergency medicine consult* (2nd ed., pp. 1016–1019). Philadelphia: Lippincott Williams & Wilkins.

NOTES

_____

_____

_____

_____

_____

_____

_____

_____

_____

_____

_____

_____

_____

_____

_____

_____

_____

CHAPTER 26

HYPOTHERMIA

Thomas J. Rahilly, Ph.D.

PRESENTATION

Patients experiencing generalized cooling of the body (hypothermia) mostly present in two specific manners. The first is a situation wherein a person has suffered from direct exposure to a very cold (less than 30° F) environment. The other is a more common finding: The body has been exposed to a more passive cooling condition, one in which the patient has been subjected to relatively warmer temperatures (30° F to 50° F) but for longer periods of time. The very old or very young are especially at risk in this situation because their ability to generate and conserve heat is less than adequate for their environment. Substance abusers who use central nervous system (NS) depressants are at increased risk of hypothermia because of a decreased ability to respond appropriately to a cold environment.

IMMEDIATE CONCERNS

❶ **What is the patient's hemodynamic status?** Ordinarily this question is not difficult to answer. In the presence of hypothermia, however, it may be more difficult to assess the status of the patient because the body may have instituted several mechanisms in an attempt to counteract the drop in body temperature. For patients with hypothermia, standard resuscitative measures may be inappropriate and even contraindicated. Your immediate concern should be to stop the cooling process by insulating the body from the cold environment. Warmed, humidified oxygen should be administered. If positive pressure ventilation is needed, ventilate using a bag-valve-mask device at a rate of 5 to 10 breaths per minute. NOTE: Rough handling of a hypothermic patient may precipitate cardiac arrest. Initial measures should be directed at preventing ventricular fibrillation because the hypothermic myocardium is extremely susceptible to lethal arrhythmias.

IMPORTANT HISTORY

❓ **To what environment has the patient been subjected in the past 24 hours?** Hypothermia is most common in patients who have been exposed to temperatures of 30° F to 50° F for several days in an indoor environment. It is not difficult to recognize accidental hypothermia caused by exposure to the extreme temperatures of the outdoors. However, patients who present with an altered mental status and depressed vital signs may be suffering from hypothermia. It is important to note and record the environmental conditions in which the patient is found.

❓ **Is there a history of a chronic illness?** Patients suffering from a chronic illness may have lost the ability to respond to extremes in temperature as a result of damage to their thermoregulatory functions. Sepsis has been known to cause a change in the hypothalamic temperature set point, which can bring about hypothermia. Hypothermia should be suspected in any individual with a chronic disease found in an environment that is below 50° F.

❓ **Is there evidence of a serious infection?** In one study, 41% of the hypothermic patients admitted to the hospital had a serious infection. Pneumonia and urinary tract infections are major causes of these infections. Be sure to examine the respiratory system thoroughly. Ask patients if they experience any abnormal urination patterns or pain while urinating.

❓ **Is the patient taking any medication?** Certain medications, such as barbiturates and phenothiazines, can disrupt the thermoregulation of body temperature. Any substance that depresses the CNS can impair the ability of the body to respond to the cold. Insulin, thyroid medication, and steroids can do the same.

❼ **Is there a history of substance abuse?** Alcohol is most often associated with hypothermia because it causes vasodilation in addition to depressing the CNS. Alcoholics are frequently thiamine-depleted.

DIFFERENTIAL DIAGNOSIS

It is often difficult for the paramedic to diagnose hypothermia because the thermometers used in the prehospital environment are not capable of measuring a temperature below 94° F.

* **SEPSIS.** Because of the large number (41%) of cases of sepsis causing hypothermia, sepsis must be given adequate consideration.

* **ENVIRONMENTAL EXPOSURE.** Was the patient found outdoors or in a nonheated or poorly heated building? Remember that alcohol may also be a factor.

* **HYPOGLYCEMIA.** Patients suffering from hypothermia may have hypoglycemia as either the cause of the problem or as a result of shivering muscles depleting glycogen stores.

* **CNS DYSFUNCTION.** Hypothermia brought about by insult to the CNS may be caused by the ingestion of a depressant, by a CVA, head injury, or damage to the spinal cord. Assessment of the patient's neurologic functions is essential.

KEY PHYSICAL EXAMINATION FINDINGS

✔ **INITIAL ASSESSMENT.** Monitor ABCs.

✔ **VITAL SIGNS.** There are two grades of hypothermia: moderate and severe. The preferred method of determining whether the patient is suffering from moderate or severe hypothermia is by obtaining a body core temperature with a rectal thermometer capable of measuring lower-than-normal body temperatures.

MODERATE HYPOTHERMIA (90° TO 95° F)

During this stage the body attempts to compensate for the loss of heat through physiologic adjustments, such as shivering. The patient is alert and responsive. The heart rate is elevated, and the blood pressure is normal.

SEVERE HYPOTHERMIA (LESS THAN 90° F)

As the body temperature falls below 90° F, decreased myocardial and cerebral blood flow cause depressed metabolic function, including oxygen use and CO_2 production. Shivering stops while the heart rate slows and the blood pressure falls. Cardiac dysrhythmias appear as the myocardium becomes extremely irritable. Atrial fibrillation or flutter, atrioventricular block, premature ventricular contractions, and asystole may appear at any time. A classic electrocardiographic sign of hypothermia is the Osborne (J) wave, a slow positive deflection at the end of the QRS complex. Ventricular fibrillation may be caused by any actions that stimulate the heart, including rough handling of the patient. The pulmonary function will decline and may progress from an initial tachypnea to a declining respiratory rate and tidal volume. Expect the cough and gag reflex to disappear and aspiration pneumonia to result if the airway is not secured.

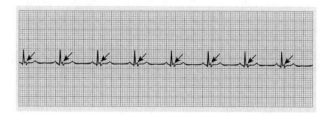

INSPECTION AND PALPATION. Assess for muscle rigidity and papillary reaction to light. Muscle rigidity may be present as the core temperature decreases. Pupillary reaction to light stimulus is lost in severe hypothermia.

NEUROLOGIC EXAMINATION. The patient's level of consciousness will gradually decline to a coma state. During this decline the patient will have difficulty making rational decisions and may actually exhibit behavior that will exacerbate their condition, such as removing clothing.

TREATMENT PLAN

- **Maintain body temperature and prevent further heat loss.** Gently remove any wet clothing, and cover the patient with blankets to insulate the patient against heat loss. Avoid measures that will cause rapid rewarming.

- **Secure the airway.** Endotracheal intubation is indicated in the same circumstances as with a normothermic patient; however, it should be performed as gently as possible to avoid causing ventricular fibrillation. **Oxygenate with warm, humidified oxygen** if available.

- **Treat shock or hemodynamic instability.** Because many patients with hypothermia are hypovolemic owing to extravascular plasma fluid shifts, a fluid challenge using 0.9% NaCl may improve tissue perfusion.

- **Monitor cardiac electrical activity.** Early tachycardia followed by bradycardia is common. Potentially lethal cardiac dysrhythmias are likely to arise in patients with hypothermia. Most of these dysrhythmias will self-correct after rewarming. Dysrhythmias are usually refractory to conventional treatment modalities, such as drug therapy, pacing, and defibrillation. CPR should be performed on patients in cardiac arrest. The medical control physician will determine whether aggressive field resuscitation is warranted before rewarmng.

NOTE: Hypothermic patients are not dead until they are warm and dead.

- **Transport to appropriate ED.** Field-specific therapy is relatively limited for the patient with hypothermia. Continue to monitor the patient, maintain body warmth, and transport as gently as possible. Passive rewarming may cause "afterdrop," a condition in which the body core temperature actually decreases as a result of peripheral vasodilation and subsequent return of cooler blood to the central circulation.

BIBLIOGRAPHY

Haist, S. A. & J. B. Robbins (Eds.) (2002). *Internal medicine on call* (3rd ed., pp. 229–233). Columbus, OH: McGraw-Hill/Appleton & Lange.

Tintinalli, J. E., L. R. Krome, & E. Ruiz (Eds.) (2003). *Emergency medicine: A comprehensive study guide* (6th ed., pp. 1231–1235). New York: McGraw-Hill.

NOTES

CHAPTER 27

DOMESTIC VIOLENCE AND INTIMATE PARTNER VIOLENCE

Debra Lejeune, M.Ed., NREMT-P

PRESENTATION

Domestic violence is defined as actual or threatened physical, emotional, or sexual abuse by a partner involved in an intimate relationship (i.e., current or former spouse, boyfriend, or girlfriend). The term *intimate partner violence* (IPV) began to appear in the medical literature in the late 1990s. It is replacing the term *domestic violence* because it highlights the relationship between the abuser and the victim, and separates IPV from other forms of abuse, such as elder abuse or child abuse.

Although *IPV* may be the term that is currently found in literature on this subject (especially by federal agencies), most EMS providers are more familiar with, and more apt to use, the term *domestic violence*; therefore *domestic violence* is the term that will be used for this discussion. Although most research has focused on women who have been abused by men, the term *violence* has been chosen to reflect the awareness that any person—man or woman—may be abused by his or her partner. The relevance of the research on women abused by men to the abuse that may occur in gay or lesbian relationships or abuse of men by women is not yet known. The EMS provider must be aware of the potential for violence under these circumstances as well.

Just how bad is the problem of violence? It is hard to know the exact magnitude of the problem because many incidents go unreported. Statistics from a survey conducted by the National Institute of Justice and the Centers for Disease Control and Prevention indicate that 22.1% of surveyed women and 7.4 % of surveyed men have been physically assaulted by an intimate partner. Approximately 1.5 million women and 800,000 men are assaulted by their intimate partners in the United States every year.

The consequences of domestic violence are not limited to physical injuries; the victim often experiences psychological trauma, such as increased depression, stress, and feelings of helplessness. Children who witness domestic violence are also at increased risk of being abused, experiencing psychological trauma, and perpetrating physical violence. Domestic violence is clearly of epidemic proportion.

The patient who is a victim of violence may present to the paramedic with any type of injury. The paramedic may not be aware initially that violence is the cause of the injury.

IMMEDIATE CONCERNS

- ❶ **Is the scene safe?** Domestic violence provides a potentially dangerous situation for prehospital care providers. Aggressive individuals are often jealous and overly possessive of the battered partner and will not allow the patient to be separated from them. If the aggressive person is still at the scene, wait for law enforcement assistance.

- ❶ **Does the patient have any serious injuries?** Serious injuries should be treated immediately. Minor injuries should be treated in the safety of the ambulance. Try to separate the patient from the aggressor before beginning treatment.

- ❶ **Are there other potential victims in the house?** An abusive partner may experience rage or helplessness and turn on another weaker victim. If the patient is being transported to the hospital, all potential victims of violence, such as children, should be transported as well.

IMPORTANT HISTORY

❓ **How was this injury obtained?** Abuse victims often take responsibility for their injury to protect the abuser. Suspect abuse in the following situations:

o The injury is not consistent with the patient's account of how the injury was obtained.

o The patient has injuries in various stages of healing.

o The partner appears overly concerned, will not be separated from the patient, and answers questions directed toward the patient.

o The patient has injuries to the head, face, back, chest or breasts, or buttocks.

❓ **Are there risk factors that place a person at increased risk for domestic violence?** Abuse can happen in any type of intimate relationship, in any socioeconomic situation, and in any age group. However, the following factors place a person at greater risk for domestic violence:

o Single, separated, or divorced (or planning a separation or divorce) women

o Women who are 17 to 28 years old

o Pregnant women

o Women who abuse alcohol or drugs

o Partners of substance abusers

o Women whose partners are excessively jealous or possessive

❓ **How should the victim of suspected domestic violence be interviewed?** Maintain a nonjudgmental and supportive attitude. In addition, interview the patient and partner separately. The interview goal is not only to discover the presence of domestic violence but also to assess the safety of the patient. The following questions should be asked in the EMS provider's own words.

o Are you in a relationship in which you have been physically hurt or threatened by your partner?

o Are you in a relationship in which you have been treated badly? In what way?

o Has your partner ever forced you to have sex when you did not want to?

o Has your partner ever threatened or abused your children?

o Do you ever feel afraid of your partner?

o You have mentioned that your partner uses drugs or alcohol. How does your partner act when drinking or using drugs? Is your partner ever verbally or physically abusive?

o Do you have guns in the home? Has your partner ever threatened to use them when angry?

DIFFERENTIAL DIAGNOSIS

Remember, the victim of domestic violence is likely to present with a wide variety of injuries and may conceal the way they occurred. Have a high index of suspicion when the reported mechanism of injury does not seem believable, when there has been a delay in seeking care, when there are multiple injuries in various stages of healing, and when there are repeated or chronic injuries.

KEY PHYSICAL EXAMINATION FINDINGS

Assess the patient as you would any trauma patient. Remember, the patient may downplay the extent or severity of injury to protect the partner, so a thorough assessment is vital.

- ☑ ***Initial assessment.*** Look for signs of head injury or shock. Assess the home environment, and look for other potential victims.

- ☑ ***HEENT.*** Look for contusions, abrasions, and minor lacerations.

- ☑ ***Neck.*** Look for contusions and other soft tissue injury.

- ☑ ***Chest.*** Suspect abuse when injury to the chest, and particularly to the breasts, is present.

- ☑ ***Skin.*** Suspect abuse when burns or bruises of various stages of healing and in unlikely areas for accidental injuries are present.

- ☑ ***Abdomen.*** Look for abdominal tenderness, distension, or hypoactive bowel sounds. External signs of injury are often absent. Be suspicious of injuries to a pregnant woman.

- ☑ ***Orthopedic examination.*** Assess for extremity pain, deformity fractures, and strains.

- ☑ ***Neurologic examination.*** Be alert for seizures, coma, or change in mental status because any of these conditions is suggestive of head injury.

TREATMENT PLAN

- Rapidly **evaluate hemodynamic instability and mental status.**

- **Assess both patient and home environment. Consider other victims** in the home and evidence suggestive of abuse or neglect.

- **Even if the patient's injuries do not require transport, consider transport to remove the patient from the violent situation so that counseling and shelter options may be discussed.**

- Separate patient from partner when possible to allow the patient to speak freely.

SECTION 1

- Provide information for shelters in your area or the telephone number for **National Domestic Violence Hotline: (800) 333-SAFE.**

- Always report your suspicions to the medical control physician or the staff at the receiving ED.

GENERAL TREATMENT GUIDELINES FOR PATIENT WHO IS HEMODYNAMICALLY STABLE

- **Administer O_2 and provide ventilatory support** as needed. Protect cervical spine as indicated.

- Place patient in the **shock position** (supine with legs elevated) or use **PASG, if indicated.** The use of PASG is currently controversial; follow local protocol.

- Establish **large-bore IV access** and begin **fluid resuscitation with 0.9% NaCl or lactated Ringer's solution.**

- **Rapid transport to appropriate ED.** Do not needlessly delay patient transport—expedite transport.

- **Treat nonlife-threatening injuries** as appropriate (e.g., control bleeding, splint fractures).

- **Transport to appropriate ED.** Ensure patient comfort en route.

- ***Collect supporting documentation.*** Clear statements of history, using quotes when possible, and accurate descriptions of injuries in laymen's terms are invaluable in court.

BIBLIOGRAPHY

Centers for Disease Control and Prevention. (n.d.). Full report of the prevalence, incidence, and consequences of violence against women. Retrieved on October 30, 2003, at http://www.ncjrs.org/txtfiles1/nij/183781.txt.

Cole, T. B. (2000). Is domestic violence screening helpful? *Journal of the American Medical Association, 284,* 551–553.

Sanders, M. J. (2001). *Mosby's paramedic textbook* (Rev. 2nd ed.). St. Louis, MO: Mosby.

CHAPTER 28

THE MAJOR TRAUMA PATIENT

Owen T. Traynor, M.D.

PRESENTATION

Major trauma involves a significant mechanism of injury or an altered level of consciousness after the trauma. There is a trimodal distribution of deaths following major trauma: immediate, early, and late. Half of all trauma deaths are classified as immediate. These patients have unsalvageable injuries, usually major brain injuries or cardiovascular injuries. The early deaths occur from 15 minutes to 6 hours after the injury. These patients often have major torso or head injuries. Modern trauma systems, including its prehospital component, are capable of treating injuries that lead to early deaths. The late deaths peak at days to weeks following the injury. Multisystem organ failure and sepsis are the major causes of late deaths.

IMMEDIATE CONCERNS

❶ **Is the scene safe?** Performing a scene size-up is an important initial step. Be alert for signs of danger. Ensure the scene is safe before entering the environment.

❶ **Does the patient have an altered mental status?** Use the AVPU mnemonic to quickly assess the patient's initial mental status. Multitrauma patients may have several significant reasons for an altered mental status, including head injury and shock.

❶ **Is the airway endangered?** Perform basic and advanced airway management as needed. Protect the cervical spine as needed.

- ❗ **Is the patient's breathing adequate?**   The multitrauma victim may have inadequate breathing caused by chest injuries, including pneumothorax, tension pneumothorax, flail chest, and pulmonary contusion, or secondary to shock. Treat open pneumothoraces with occlusive dressings, decompress tension pneumothoraces, stabilize flail segments, and supply supplemental oxygen to all with inadequate breathing.

- ❗ **Is the circulation adequate?**   Begin CPR as needed. Control major bleeding. Treat for shock if present.

- ❗ **Is the patient a "top priority" patient?**   These patients may benefit from expeditious transport to a trauma center.

IMPORTANT QUESTIONS

- ❓ **What was the mechanism of injury?**   The mechanism of injury (MOI) suggests the amount and manner of energy transfer that may have occurred during the incident. In general, the greater the energy transfer to the patient, the greater the potential for significant injury. The MOI helps the paramedic understand the possible injuries that may be present.

- ❓ **Does the patient report pain?**   The patient can direct the paramedic to areas of injuries that might not be obvious.

- ❓ **Is there evidence of uncontrollable bleeding?**   Some evidence suggests that patients with uncontrollable hemorrhage might benefit from being treated without the traditional IV fluid resuscitation. This concept is presently controversial, but its premise is that IV fluids may actually increase the rate of bleeding. Proposed mechanisms for the increased bleeding include hydraulic acceleration of bleeding caused by elevated blood pressure, dislodgment of soft clots, and dilution of clotting factors. Proponents of this theory suggest withholding preoperative IV fluids in patients with uncontrollable bleeding.

❷ **What is the patient's past medical history?** Patients with a significant past medical history may not be able to tolerate the major trauma as well as healthy patients. Their ability to compensate for the injuries will be decreased. Be prepared for potential worsening of their hemodynamic status.

❷ **Is the patient taking any medication?** Beta blockers will eliminate or decrease the tachycardia typically found with significant blood loss. Patients who are using anticoagulants, such as warfarin (Coumadin), or the low-molecular-weight heparins, enoxaparin (Lovenox), ardeparin (Normiflo), dalteparin (Fragmin), and danaparoid (Orgaran), are at increased risk of hemorrhage.

❷ **Is the patient pregnant?** Trauma during pregnancy may cause abruptio placentae, ruptured fetal membranes, or direct fetal trauma, in addition to the injury to the patient. In addition, assessment may become difficult because of the normal physiologic changes of pregnancy.

DIFFERENTIAL DIAGNOSIS

HEAD INJURIES

• ***TRAUMATIC BRAIN INJURY.*** Traumatic brain injury (TBI) may be classified as mild, moderate, or severe depending on the neurologic dysfunction at the time of the initial assessment. Mild TBI characteristics include a Glasgow Coma Scale (GCS) score of 13 to 15 and possibly a brief loss of consciousness. The mortality rate is less than 1%. The prognosis is excellent. Moderate TBI characteristics include a GCS of 9 to 12. This patient is typically confused and may have focal neurologic findings. The mortality rate is less than 5%. The prognosis is good. Severe TBI characteristics include a GCS at or below 8. These patients are unable to follow commands. Mortality rate is greater than 30%. The prognosis is poor. Many survivors will have significant disability.

- **PRIMARY AND SECONDARY BRAIN INJURIES.**   Brain injuries can be classified as primary and secondary injuries. The primary brain injury results from direct trauma to the brain. Secondary brain injuries are insults that occur after the primary injury. These include hypoxia, hypotension, seizures, and infection. Paramedics can intervene here to reduce the amount of secondary injury. High-flow oxygen, airway management, and IV fluid resuscitation should be initiated as needed.

- **SPECIFIC BRAIN INJURIES.**   See chapter 20.

SPINE INJURIES

- **SPINAL CORD AND SPINAL COLUMN INJURIES.**   Spinal cord and spinal column injuries are injuries of the musculoskeletal portion of the neck and back, including fractures, dislocations, and subluxations, as well as injuries to the cervical ligaments, muscles, and tendons. These injuries can exist without spinal cord injury. Some spinal column injuries may be unstable. The conscious patient typically reports neck or back pain and possibly stiffness. Posterior midline bony tenderness suggests the possible presence of an injury that would benefit from immobilization. Patients who have experienced major trauma are likely to have other distracting injuries and may not be able to report injuries with any accuracy.

- **SPINAL CORD INJURIES.**   Although spinal cord injuries (SCIs) may be associated with vertebral fractures or disruption of the spinal ligaments, they may also occur in the absence of bony or ligamentous injury (e.g., where there is a hematoma or vascular compromise). Complete or partial cord syndromes are possible. Complete spinal cord lesions create a total loss of motor and sensation distal to the site of injury. The partial cord syndromes include a central cord syndrome, anterior cord syndrome, and a lateral, or Brown-Sequard, syndrome. See chapter 41 for more details.

CHEST INJURIES

- **"THE LETHAL SIX."** The following injuries are immediately life-threatening.

  o **AIRWAY OBSTRUCTION.** The tongue, bleeding, vomitus, dentures, and teeth can block the airway. Expanding neck hematomas can produce compression of the trachea. Tracheal tears or transection and laryngeal trauma can obstruct the airway as well. Physical exam findings may include snoring respirations, debris in the mouth and pharynx, cyanosis, stridor, hoarseness, neck hematomas, subcutaneous emphysema, and respiratory distress. Protect the cervical spine and use advanced airway devices as needed.

  o **TENSION PNEUMOTHORAX.** Elevated intrathoracic pressure caused by air leaking into the pleural space can compress the great vessels, impair venous return, decrease cardiac output, and impair ventilation of the opposite lung. Tension pneumothorax can follow a penetrating chest injury, blunt trauma with lung parenchyma injury, mechanical ventilation with high airway pressures, and spontaneous pneumothorax. Physical exam findings include respiratory distress, hypotension, unilateral absence of breath sounds with a hyperresonant percussion note, and tracheal deviation away from the affected lung (a late sign). Perform a needle thoracostomy (needle-chest decompression).

  o **PERICARDIAL TAMPONADE**. The pericardial sac cannot acutely distend. Less than 100 ml of bleeding into the sac can cause tamponade. Tamponade can be caused by penetrating and blunt trauma. The classic signs—jugular venous distension, muffled heart sounds, and hypotension—are found in about a third of patients. Shock or ongoing hypotension without blood loss should suggest pericardial tamponade as a possible cause. EMS treatment includes prompt recognition, IV fluid resuscitation, and possibly pericardiocentesis. Pericardiocentesis should be performed by those skilled in its use and authorized by medical command.

o **OPEN PNEUMOTHORAX.** Usually easy to recognize and treat, the sucking chest wound, or open pneumothorax, can cause severe respiratory distress. Use an air occlusive dressing. Frequently reassess for the development of a tension pneumothorax.

o **MASSIVE HEMOTHORAX.** The massive hemothorax is primarily caused by penetrating trauma with injury to the large vessels in the chest, including the intercostal and internal mammary vessels. Physical exam reveals findings consistent with hypovolemia, unilateral decreased or absent breath sounds with a dull percussion note. EMS treatment is to treat for shock.

o **FLAIL CHEST.** High-energy blunt chest trauma can cause the multiple rib fractures and formation of the flail segment. The chest wall injury is not as serious as the underlying pulmonary contusion. Hemothoraces and pneumothoraces are possible as well. High-flow oxygen, possible intubation, and stabilization of the flail segment are EMS interventions.

ABDOMINAL INJURIES

• **BLUNT ABDOMINAL TRAUMA.** Motor vehicle collisions account for 75% of blunt abdominal trauma injuries. The injuries result from compression forces, which cause a crush injury; a shearing force, which causes tears of organs or their vascular attachments; or a sudden rise in intraabdominal pressure, which causes rupture of hollow organs. Clinical findings include abdominal pain and tenderness, peritonitis, and shock.

- **PENETRATING ABDOMINAL TRAUMA.** The common causes of penetrating abdominal trauma are gunshot wounds and stab wounds. The clinical findings are similar to those associated with blunt abdominal trauma.

EXTREMITY INJURIES

- **SOFT-TISSUE INJURIES.** Soft-tissue injuries include lacerations, abrasions, contusions, and penetrating wounds. Although not usually life-threatening, they may be dramatic. EMS treatment typically involves treating immediate life threats first and, if time permits, lower priority injuries later.

- **FRACTURES, SPRAINS, AND STRAINS.** Once the life-threatening injuries are treated, splinting fractures, sprains, and strains is possible. See chapter 29 for more details.

SHOCK

- **HYPOVOLEMIC SHOCK.** The patient who has experienced multiple trauma will likely be in hypovolemic shock caused by acute blood loss. Attend to the problems identified during the initial assessment. Expedite transport to a trauma center. Establish IV access and fluid resuscitation if indicated. See chapter 38 for more details.

- **OBSTRUCTIVE SHOCK.** Tension pneumothorax and pericardial tamponade are two examples of obstructive shock. See previous discussions for more details.

THE PREGNANT PATIENT

- **NORMAL PHYSIOLOGIC CHANGES.** The systolic and diastolic blood pressures decrease by 10 mm Hg by the middle of the second trimester. The resting heart rate typically increases by 10 to 15 beats. The maternal blood volume can increase by 40% to 50% during the pregnancy. Uterine blood flow increases to 17% of the cardiac output. Although tidal volume increases, there is a decrease in residual volume capacity (the volume of gas in the lungs at the end of a maximal exhalation) and functional residual capacity (the volume of gas in the lungs at the end of a normal breath). The functional residual capacity serves as an oxygen reservoir. Thus pregnant trauma patients may suffer oxygen desaturation more readily. The gravid uterus expands from the pelvis and displaces intraabdominal organs, thereby altering injury patterns.

- **MECHANISMS OF INJURY.** Motor vehicle collisions are the leading nonobstetric cause of maternal and fetal death. Placental abruption is the leading cause of fetal death when the mother survives. Pelvic fractures are the most common maternal injury associated with fetal death. The most common fetal injury is skull fracture with intracranial bleeding. Gunshot wounds are more common than stab wounds. These are often associated with intimate partner violence. The risk of uterine injury increases during the second and third trimester as the uterus enlarges. Upper abdominal penetrating injuries are associated with significant gastrointestinal injury and bleeding.

- **ABRUPTIO PLACENTAE.** Abruptio placentae is the separation of the placenta from the uterine wall. It may occur spontaneously or after trauma. It typically occurs after the twentieth week of pregnancy. The patients report vaginal bleeding, uterine cramps, and abdominal pain. Hypotension may occur secondary to blood loss. It is possible that the patient may develop disseminated intramuscular coagulation.

- **UTERINE RUPTURE.** Uterine rupture is an uncommon emergency, occurring with abdominal trauma or labor. In the context of trauma, the most common MOI is ejection from the vehicle. The patient reports severe abdominal pain and vaginal bleeding. Shock may occur. Treatment for shock is recommended. Risk factors include prior uterine surgeries and prolonged or obstructed labor.

- **PRETERM LABOR.** Preterm labor, which occurs in up to 10% of all pregnancies, is defined as labor of significant intensity and duration to cause changes in the cervix before 37 weeks of gestation. It is a common sequela of maternal trauma. Treatment includes magnesium sulfate or beta agonists such as terbutaline.

- *MANAGEMENT PRINCIPLES.*   The initial treatment priorities remain the same as for all patients. Treatment of the mother provides the best treatment for the fetus. See chapter 32 for more details.

- *PERIMORTEM CESAREAN DELIVERY.*   Fetal survival is time dependent aftrer maternal cardiac arrest. The best survival is when a cesarean delivery is performed within 4 or 5 minutes after the maternal arrest. A perimortem cesarean delivery should be performed only by those clinicians who are skilled in its use and authorized by medical command. It is indicated when there is maternal cardiac arrest and the fetus is of sufficient gestational age to survive outside the uterus (older than 23 to 28 weeks of gestation).

KEY PHYSICAL EXAMINATION FINDINGS

- ✓ *Initial assessment.*   Look for compromised airway, difficult breathing, and signs of shock or acute hemorrhage. Consider the mechanism of injury and institute spinal precautions when indicated. Treat for shock if indicated.

- ✓ *Vital signs.*   Obtain and reassess vital signs often.

- ✓ *Rapid trauma assessment.*   After the initial assessment, perform a rapid trauma assessment to discover other life-threatening injuries. Use the DCAP-BTLS (**D**eformities, **C**ontusions, **A**brasions, **P**enetrations, **B**urns, **T**enderness, **L**acerations, **S**welling.) mnemonic to recall the signs of injury.

- ✓ *HEENT.*   Look for signs of head injury. If force was sufficient to cause head trauma, also suspect SCI.

- ✓ *Neck.*   Stabilize the cervical spine as needed. Assess neck veins. Flat neck veins are expected in hypovolemic shock. Jugular venous distension may indicate tension pneumothorax or pericardial tamponade. Assess for expanding hematomas and laryngeal injury.

✔ ***Chest.***   Assess for chest wounds, hemothorax, pneumothorax, and flail segment. Assess for respiratory distress. Assess for muffled heart sounds.

✔ ***Abdomen/pelvis.***   Assess for wounds, tenderness, rigidity, guarding, and masses.

✔ ***Extremities.***   Assess for any wounds, soft-tissue injuries, and deformities.

✔ ***Posterior body.***   Carefully palpate the spine for wounds, pain, tenderness, and deformity.

✔ ***Neurologic examination.***   Assess the level of consciousness, record GCS score, and perform assessment of motor and sensory status.

ELECTROCARDIOGRAM

Continuous ECG monitoring, if time permits, provides continuous evaluation of the heart rate and discovery of possible arrhythmias.

PULSE OXIMETER

Pulse oximetry can provide real-time assessment of the patient's oxygenation.

BLOOD GLUCOSE DETERMINATION

Blood glucose determination should be used when hypoglycemia may be present.

TREATMENT PLAN

• **Patient assessment.**   Perform a rapid and systematic initial assessment, and institute treatment as life-threatening problems are discovered. Prompt transport to the appropriate ED, preferably to a trauma center, is a key intervention. A rapid trauma assessment should be performed once the initial assessment and all attendant interventions have been accomplished. Frequent reassessment of the patient with multiple trauma is necessary owing to the potential for rapid deterioration.

- Administer **O₂** and **provide ventilatory support,** including endotracheal intubation, as indicated. Protect the cervical spine. **If GCS is at or below 8, the patient should be intubated**.

- If there is a mechanism of injury that suggests the possibility of SCI, the patient requires spinal immobilization.

- Establish **large-bore IV access** with 0.9% NaCl or LR. Consider IV fluid resuscitation if there is hypovolemic shock. [Controversial therapy note: Some EMS experts recommend withholding IV fluid resuscitation in the context of penetrating trauma with uncontrollable hemorrhage unless the patient is in extremis.]

- **Treat for shock.** See chapter 38.

- If the patient has an altered mental status, treat for head injury. See chapter 20.

- If spinal cord injury is present, see chapter 41.

- Treat nonlife-threatening injuries as time permits (e.g., control bleeding, splint fractures).

- Transport to appropriate trauma center. Ensure patient comfort en route. Do not needlessly delay patient transport—expedite transport.

- Frequently reassess the patient. The potential for worsening exists after multiple trauma.

BIBLIOGRAPHY

Martin, J. & M. McClurg (2004). The multiply injured patient. In C. K. Stone & R. L. Humphries (Eds.), *Current emergency diagnosis and treatment* (5th ed., pp. 208–221). New York: McGraw-Hill.

Peitzman, A. B., M. Rhodes, C. W. Schwab, D. M. Yealy, & T. C. Fabian (Eds.) (2002). *The trauma manual* (2nd ed.). Philadelphia: Lippincott Williams & Wilkins.

NOTES

_____

_____

_____

_____

_____

_____

_____

_____

_____

_____

_____

_____

_____

_____

_____

_____

_____

_____

_____

_____

_____

CHAPTER 29

MUSCULOSKELETAL TRAUMA

Owen T. Traynor, M.D.

PRESENTATION

Musculoskeletal and soft tissue injuries are generally nonlife-threatening; however, they can be associated with other life-threatening injuries. In addition, they can jeopardize the limbs if not properly managed. Their often obvious and dramatic nature may distract you from treating the immediate life-threatening injuries. A stepwise, systematic approach to patient assessment will keep you from transporting a well-splinted, but dead, patient. Early proper management of patients with musculoskeletal and soft-tissue injuries can significantly reduce morbidity and mortality.

IMMEDIATE CONCERNS

❶ **Are there any life-threatening injuries present?** A rapid and thorough initial assessment should be performed on all patients before treatment of obvious nonlife-threatening injuries. Prompt intervention in cases of life-threatening airway, respiratory, and circulatory emergencies should be carried out as the problems are discovered. Patients who have life-threatening injuries should be expeditiously transported to the appropriate ED, with care continued throughout transport. A rapid trauma assessment and treatment of the high-priority injuries may be carried out en route to the ED if time and patient condition permits. Patients who are not immediate-transport patients should receive a focused history and physical exam. Their injuries should then be ranked according to priority and treated before transport.

IMPORTANT HISTORY

❓ **What is the mechanism of injury?**   Often the patient's injuries can be predicted according to the mechanism of injury. Essentially, injury results from the absorption of kinetic energy by the patient's body. A knowledge of the kinetics of the injury can help you search for occult injury. For example, a fall on an outstretched hand can result in injury from the fingers up through the shoulder and neck.

❓ **What is the age of the patient?**   Certain injuries are more common at various ages: Greenstick fractures are common in pediatric patients, whereas dislocations are rare. Elderly patients have higher incidences of fractures even without significant mechanisms of injury.

❓ **What is the patient's chief complaint?**   Under most circumstances, the patient's chief complaint will lead you to the site of the injury. Exceptions to this rule are when the patient has an altered mental status, is under anesthesia or the influence of alcohol or other substances, and when there are other significant distracting injuries. The pain of a fractured femur is likely to distract the patient from the pain of a fractured metacarpal bone.

❓ **What is the patient's past medical history?**   The patient's medical history may provide important information about the nature of a patient's injury or predisposition to injury. Patients who have osteoporosis (an atrophy or reduction in bone mass), bone cancer or bony metastases, multiple myeloma, or a history of chronic steroid use are at higher risk of fractures. In fact, a fracture, particularly compression fractures of the spine, may occur in the absence of significant trauma.

DIFFERENTIAL DIAGNOSIS

In this section, common or significant musculoskeletal injuries of the upper and lower extremities are reviewed. This is not a comprehensive list of all possible injuries.

UPPER EXTREMITY

Shoulder

The wide range of motion afforded by the shoulder predisposes it to instability and injury. Approximately 15% of all athletic injuries seen in the ED involve the shoulder. Shoulder dislocations account for more than half of all dislocations seen in the ED. The nature of the immature skeletal system in pediatric patients reduces the incidence of shoulder dislocations. Their joint capsule and ligaments are significantly stronger than their growth plates. Therefore children tend to have fractures of the growth plate rather than the dislocations or sprains that adult patients develop.

- *FRACTURES*

    o **Clavicular fractures** are the most common fractures of childhood. There are three characteristic clavicle fractures: fracture of the middle third, the most common; fracture of the lateral third; and the fracture of the medial third clavicle, the least common. Indirect trauma to the lateral shoulder can result in fracture at the middle third. Direct trauma to the top of the shoulder can cause fracture of the lateral third clavicle. The medial third may fracture when there is direct trauma to the anterior chest. The patient complains of pain at the fracture site and presents with the injured extremity held close to the body. Often, the shoulder will be slumped downward, inward, and forward. Complications include pneumothorax and injury to the subclavian arteries and veins and the brachial plexus, a group of nerves that supply the upper extremity.

    o **Scapular fractures** are uncommon, usually found in young men who have had high-speed auto accidents, falls, or crushing injuries. There are often other significant injuries present, and scapular injuries are therefore often missed. Patients with scapular fractures present with their arm held to the body. There is pain associated with any movement of the shoulder. Complications include hemothorax, pneumothorax, pulmonary contusion, and injury to the axillary arteries and veins and the brachial plexus.

o **Proximal humerus fractures** occur mainly in elderly patients with osteoporosis, usually resulting from a fall on an outstretched hand. The younger patient with this mechanism of injury is more likely to develop a dislocation. Often there can be a fracture-dislocation. Proximal humerus fractures also occur when there is either direct trauma to the lateral arm or an axial load transmitted through the elbow. Patients present with the arm held close to the body. Complications include axillary artery and brachial plexus injury.

- *DISLOCATIONS*

  o **Acromioclavicular joint (AC) dislocations,** or shoulder separations, are commonly caused by direct trauma to the point of the shoulder with the arm adducted. A fall on an outstretched hand may also produce this injury. Patients present with a spectrum of symptoms ranging from mild tenderness with minimal swelling over the joint to severe pain, obvious deformity, and the need to hold their injured limb close to the body with the shoulder hanging downward. Common complications are associated fractures of the clavicle or coracoid process.

  o **Glenohumeral joint dislocations** are the most common major joint dislocations. More than 95% of all shoulder dislocations are anterior dislocations. Posterior dislocations account for approximately 4% of dislocations, and inferior and superior dislocations are rare. The typical patient with an anterior dislocation is either a young man between 20 and 30 years of age or an older woman between 60 and 80 years of age. Glenohumeral joint dislocations result from either direct or indirect trauma. In the older patient the dislocation usually follows a fall on an outstretched hand, whereas in the younger patient it results from a combination of abduction, extension, and external rotation occurring during athletic activity. The patient presents with severe pain and the arm slightly abducted and externally rotated. The shoulder appears squared off, with a fullness in the anterior aspect. Common complications include injury to the axillary artery and nerve, radial nerve, or brachial plexus.

Humerous and Elbow

Injuries near the elbow run the risk of significant complications and disability. Injuries to the median nerve, ulnar nerve, radial nerve, and brachial artery may occur.

- **FRACTURES**

  o **Midshaft humerus fractures** usually result from direct trauma to the arm but may also occur as a result of a fall on an outstretched hand. This fracture is usually obvious owing to swelling and the patient's inability to use the arm. The most common complication is injury to the radial nerve. Vascular injury may also occur.

  o **Distal humerus fractures** may be supracondylar, proximal to the epicondyles, or involving the epicondyles. Supracondylar fractures usually result from a fall on an outstretched hand. The typical patient is younger than 20 years old. In young people the ligamentous structures are stronger than the bone; therefore a fracture results. The adult patient, whose bones are stronger, suffers a dislocation. The brachial artery and the median, ulnar, and radial nerves are often injured by the distal bone fragment.

  o **Elbow fractures** are actually fractures of the bones that make up the elbow joint: fractures of the distal humerus, including condylar fractures and fractures of the articular surfaces; fractures of the radial head; or fractures of the ulna's olecranon process. These injuries can result from direct trauma, a fall on an outstretched hand, or other mechanisms. Neurologic injuries of the radial, median, or ulnar nerves, as well as injury to the brachial artery, may complicate the fracture. In addition, dislocation of the elbow may be found.

- **DISLOCATIONS**

  o **Elbow dislocation** refers to the dislocation of the ulna on the humerus or the dislocation of the radius on the ulna. Associated fractures are often present because of the tremendous force required to dislocate the elbow. The most common type of elbow dislocation is a posterior dislocation resulting from a fall on an outstretched hand in an adult patient. As mentioned previously in the section on distal humerus fractures, pediatric patients usually suffer a fracture as a result of this mechanism of injury. Patients with a posterior elbow dislocation often present with the elbow flexed and a prominent olecranon. These injuries may relocate on their own. Neurovascular complications may occur.

  o **Radial head subluxation,** or "nursemaid's elbow," is a common childhood injury found most often in pediatric patients 1 to 3 years of age. This injury commonly results from a longitudinal pull on the forearm while the arm is pronated. This mechanism stretches the annular ligament, allowing the radial head to slip out of position on the humerus. The patient is reluctant to move the arm, and the arm is slightly flexed in a pronated position.

Forearm and Wrist

Injuries near the wrist lead to increased risk of injuries to the median, ulnar, and radial nerves. Eight carpal bones make up the wrist, each of which can be fractured, dislocated, or subluxed. It is often not possible to differentiate between fracture, dislocation, or subluxation without x-rays. However, it is usually possible to determine that an injury has taken place.

- *FRACTURES*

  o **Radius-ulnar fractures** usually result from direct trauma to the forearm but may also occur as a result of a fall on an outstretched hand. These fractures are often displaced because significant force is required to fracture both of these bones. Fractures of either the radius or ulna may occur alone or with dislocations at either the wrist or elbow.

  o **Colles fractures,** a fracture of the distal radius with dorsal displacement of the distal radius, is the most common wrist fracture. It occurs most frequently in adults over the age of 50 years who have fallen on an outstretched hand. The patient usually presents with the "silver-fork" deformity and pain.

- *DISLOCATIONS*

  Dislocations of the wrist, depending on the bones involved, may cause nerve impingement. These injuries may occur as a result of direct or indirect trauma.

Hand

Fractures of the bones in the hand, including fingers, are common. Complications of both fractures and dislocations can be significant because they may result in dysfunction of the hand.

Pelvis, Hip, and Femur

Pelvic fractures account for less than 5% of all fractures. These fractures and other associated injuries are a frequent cause of death in patients who have experienced trauma. The most common etiologies are secondary to motor vehicle accidents (MVAs), pedestrian accidents, or falls from heights; however, as many as one third result from minor falls among the elderly. Femur fractures also require significant force and may be associated with other injuries.

- **FRACTURES**

  o **Pelvic fractures** may be associated with hypotension owing to the significant force required to fracture the pelvis. Consideration of the patient's hemodynamic status is important. Many classification systems are used to describe these types of fractures. It is sufficient to know that there can be fractures of the individual pelvic bones, fractures that disrupt the pelvis ring (usually fractured in two places), and fractures of the weight or nonweight-bearing parts of the pelvis. Pelvic fractures may result from either direct or indirect trauma. Complications include intraabdominal, retroperitoneal, gynecologic, urologic, and neurovascular injuries.

  o **Hip fractures** are actually fractures of the proximal femur. They are characterized by shortening and external rotation of the affected limb. Certain types of hip fractures are associated with hip dislocations. Often the patient is elderly, with osteoporotic bones, and the fracture results from a minor fall. The younger patient with a fractured hip has often suffered a high-energy trauma—other associated injuries should be investigated. The femur may show evidence of significant internal hemorrhage. In addition, neurologic injury may occur.

  o **Femoral shaft fractures** are painful and accompanied by a shortened limb. Their presence may distract you from finding other significant coexisting injuries. Significant pain relief occurs when traction is applied to the fracture.

- **DISLOCATIONS**

  o **Hip dislocations** may be anterior, posterior, or central dislocations. Posterior dislocations are by far the most common, accounting for as much as 90% of all hip dislocations. In adults with normal hips, significant force is required to dislocate the hip. It most commonly occurs during an MVA, after the patient's knee strikes the dashboard, transmitting force along the femur to the hip. Hip dislocations occur with considerably less force in patients with prosthetic hips. In children a hip dislocation may occur rather than a fracture of the proximal femur. The patient with a posterior dislocation presents with a shortened, partially flexed, adducted, internally rotated leg. Neurologic injury to the sciatic nerve may occur, resulting in motor and sensory deficits in the lower leg and foot. Anterior dislocations present with abducted and externally rotated legs. Injury to the femoral vessels and nerve may accompany these injuries.

Knee and Lower Leg

Knee injuries have become more prevalent in our sports-conscious society. Most common are ligamentous or meniscal injury. The tibia is the most commonly fractured long bone.

- **FRACTURES**

  o **Patellar fractures** result from direct trauma, a fall on a flexed knee, or a forceful contraction of the quadriceps.

  o **Tibial plateau fractures** are produced by direct trauma to th e femoral knee. Although both medial and lateral plateaus may be fractured simultaneously, the lateral tibial plateau is most commonly fractured. The patient presents with a painful swollen knee and is reluctant to bend it.

  o **Tibial shaft fractures** may result from direct trauma, resulting in a fracture of the fibula as well, or from rotational or indirect forces, resulting in an isolated tibial fracture. Complications include infection (these fractures are often open), compartment syndrome (neurovascular injury caused by swelling in the compartments bounded by fascial sheets, which limits expansion of the leg with increasing edema), and injury to the peroneal nerve if the fracture is near the fibular head.

o **Isolated fibular fractures** are uncommon. Patients are often able to bear weight and walk with these isolated fractures.

- **DISLOCATIONS**

  o **Knee dislocations** are one of the few true ortho-pedic emergencies. Vascular and neurologic injury often follow. Traumatic dislocation is uncommon; however, the popliteal artery is often injured. The incidence of vascular injury is approximately 40%, with half of these patients requiring amputation. Early reduction of the dislocation is important. This injury may reduce spontaneously, but because vascular injury may have occurred, these patients should be transported to the ED.

  o **Patellar dislocations** commonly result from a twist-ing injury to the extended knee. The patella is usually dislocated laterally.

TENDON, LIGAMENT, AND MENISCAL INJURIES

- **Tears of the patellar or quadriceps tendon** may occur during strenuous contraction of the quadriceps. The injury results in the inability to actively extend the knee.

- **Injuries of the collateral and cruciate ligaments** are not uncommon. Most of these injuries are related to athletic activity. The medial collateral ligament is the most frequently injured ligament. This injury is caused by a force to the lateral aspect of the slightly flexed and internally rotated knee. The lateral collateral ligament is less frequently injured because it is often protected from a medial force by the opposite leg. The anterior cruciate ligament (ACL) may be injured from a sudden deceleration, flexion, and rotation. Injury to the posterior cruciate ligament is rare because the ligament is stronger than the ACL and the collateral ligaments. It may tear when the knee hits the dashboard in a high-speed MVA.

Cruciate injuries are often associated with an audible "pop," buckling of the knee, swelling, and pain.

- **Meniscal tears** are difficult to diagnose but are associated with a twisting motion in the flexed knee. Pain is worst during weight-bearing activities. The patient may report that the knee is locking up after the initial trauma.

Ankle and Foot

The ankle and foot bear the entire weight of the patient and are subject to significant stress. Injury results in temporary loss of function.

- *FRACTURES*

  o **Ankle fractures, or malleoli fractures,** often result from a rotational force applied to the joint while the foot is fixed in place. The most common malleolus fractured is the lateral malleolus. Significant ligamentous injury may accompany ankle fractures, leaving the joint unstable. Neruovascular compromise should be evaluated.

  o **Foot fractures** commonly result from falls and MVAs. The talus bone, responsible for support of the body and distribution of body weight, is rarely fractured. However, it has a limited blood supply and may suffer avascular necrosis if fractured or dislocated. The patient will present with pain, swelling, and deformity of the ankle. Calcaneal fractures manifest swelling and pain over both the medial and lateral aspects of the bone. A bruise may be present on the sole of the foot. Because this injury follows a fall, the paramedic must search for associated axial load injuries—fractures of the lower extremities, hip, and back.

- *DISLOCATIONS*

  o **Ankle dislocations** are usually found in combination with ankle fractures. The most common dislocation is a posterior dislocation of the talus. Ankle dislocations have significant potential for vascular compromise.

If not promptly relocated, avascular necrosis of the talus or loss of the foot may occur.

- **SPRAINS**

  o **Ankle sprains** are the most common ankle injury. Sprains of the lateral ligaments occur with the greatest frequency. The mechanism of injury is such that the ankle is internally rotated, inverted, and plantar-flexed. The medial ligaments may be sprained when the foot is everted, dorsiflexed, and externally rotated. The patient presents with pain, possibly ecchymosis, and swelling.

KEY PHYSICAL EXAMINATION FINDINGS

- *Initial assessment.*   Evaluate and treat life-threatening injuries as they are discovered.

- *Vital signs.*   Evaluate for hemodynamic instability.

- *Secondary survey.*   Perform a thorough and systematic examination once life-threatening injuries have been treated. Do not be distracted by obvious musculoskeletal injuries.

- *Lungs.*   Assess for evidence of tension pneumothorax. Evidence of blunt trauma or penetrating trauma to the shoulder, clavicle, or scapula should raise suspicion of intrathoracic injury, including pericardial tamponade, tension pneumothorax, and hemothorax.

- *Abdomen.*   Assess for evidence of penetrating and direct or indirect blunt trauma, which may indicate intraabdominal injury.

- *Pelvis and hip.*   Assess for deformity, ecchymosis, tenderness, crepitus, loss of range of motion, and soft-tissue injury.

- *Extremities.*   Assess for deformity, ecchymosis, tenderness, crepitus, loss of range of motion, length discrepancies, and soft-tissue injury. Be sure to evaluate distal neurovascular status—check distal pulses, capillary refill, and sensory and motor status.

TREATMENT PLAN

- ***Patient assessment.*** Perform an initial assessment, and institute treatment as life-threatening problems are discovered. Prompt transport to the ED is a key intervention. A rapid trauma assessment should be performed once the initial assessment and all interventions have been accomplished. Frequent reassessment of the patient with a significant mechanism of injury is necessary because of the potential for worsening of the hemodynamic status. It is often difficult for the EMS provider to differentiate between a fracture and a dislocation. Fortunately, the principles of management of these injuries are identical.

GENERAL TREATMENT GUIDELINES
PATIENT WHO IS HEMODYNAMICALLY STABLE

- **Administer O$_2$ and provide ventilatory support.**

- Management principles for treatment of suspected closed fractures and dislocations:

  o Treat all life-threatening injuries.

  o Ensure that the patient is not a "load-and-go" patient.

  o Stabilize the injury site to prevent further injury.

  o Evaluate the distal neurovascular status.

  o Controversy exists as to whether limb alignment should be sought in the field. Some experts maintain that the paramedic should "splint them where they lie" unless there is vascular compromise. In the case of vascular compromise, one attempt at limb alignment or relocation of the dislocation is recommended. Obtaining limb alignment poses the risk of causing additional soft tissue or neurovascular injury. It is often difficult, however, to adequately immobilize an angulated fracture, thereby risking further injury while transferring the patient from the accident scene to the ED. It is for this reason that some physicians recommend applying in-line traction and obtaining limb alignment.

o If relocation of a dislocated joint is attempted, consider the use of analgesia before the attempt if the patient is hemodynamically stable and alert.

o Select the appropriate immobilization device, and apply it without causing additional injury.

o Be sure to immobilize the joint proximal and distal to the injury.

o Re-evaluate the distal neurovascular status.

- **Management principles for treatment of open fractures.** Treat using the management principles previously recommended for treatment of suspected closed fractures and dislocations, except add the following steps for applying the immobilization device:

  o Irrigate the wound with sterile normal saline.

  o Apply a dry sterile dressing over the wound.

  o Apply a slight compression dressing if the wound is actively bleeding.

  o Reduce swelling by elevating the injury. Apply a cold pack to the injury to decrease pain and swelling.

- **Transport to appropriate ED.** Ensure patient comfort en route.

PATIENT WHO IS HEMODYNAMICALLY UNSTABLE

- **Administer O$_2$ and provide ventilatory support** as needed. This includes needle-chest decompression of the tension pneumothorax.

- Place patient in the **shock position** (supine with legs elevated). Use care not to aggravate other injuries.

- **Establish large-bore IV access and begin fluid resuscitation with 0.9% NaCl or lactated Ringer's solution.** If there has been inadequate response to ongoing fluid resuscitation, consider using vasopressors such as dopamine, 2 to 20 µg/kg per minute IV infusion (pediatric dosing: start at 1.0 µg/kg per minute), titrated to systolic BP greater than 90 mm Hg.

NOTE: Vasopressors are a temporary, last-ditch effort to be used only after fluid resuscitation has failed to restore stable hemodynamics. Remember, the patient is not bleeding dopamine.

- **Rapidly transport to appropriate ED.** Do not needlessly delay patient transport—expedite transport.

SECTION 1

BIBLIOGRAPHY

Buono, C. (2003). Femur fracture. In J. J. Schaider, S. R. Hayden, R. Wolfe, R. M. Barkin, & P. Rosen (Eds.), *Rosen & Barkin's 5-minute emergency medicine consult* (2nd ed., pp. 406–407). Philadelphia: Lippincott Williams & Wilkins.

Buono, C. (2003). Hip injury. In J. J. Schaider, S. R. Hayden, R. Wolfe, R. M. Barkin, & P. Rosen (Eds.), *Rosen & Barkin's 5-minute emergency medicine consult* (2nd ed., pp. 526–527). Philadelphia: Lippincott Williams & Wilkins.

Cardall, T. Y. (2003). Ankle sprain. In J. J. Schaider, S. R. Hayden, R. Wolfe, R. M. Barkin, & P. Rosen (Eds.), *Rosen & Barkin's 5-minute emergency medicine consult* (2nd ed., pp. 74–75). Philadelphia: Lippincott Williams & Wilkins.

Kennedy, A. & W. A. Carter (2003). Acromioclavicular joint injury. In J. J. Schaider, S. R. Hayden, R. Wolfe, R. M. Barkin, & P. Rosen (Eds.), *Rosen & Barkin's 5-minute emergency medicine consult* (2nd ed., pp. 28–29). Philadelphia: Lippincott Williams & Wilkins.

Manko, F. (2003). Clavicle fracture. In J. J. Schaider, S. R. Hayden, R. Wolfe, R. M. Barkin, & P. Rosen (Eds.), *Rosen*

& *Barkin's 5-minute emergency medicine consult* (2nd ed., pp. 238–239). Philadelphia: Lippincott Williams & Wilkins.

Milne, L. & A. Barkin (2003). Fractures, pediatric. In J. J. Schaider, S. R. Hayden, R. Wolfe, R. M. Barkin, & P. Rosen (Eds.), *Rosen & Barkin's 5-minute emergency medicine consult* (2nd ed., pp. 434–435). Philadelphia: Lippincott Williams & Wilkins.

Mohler, C. R. (2003). Fracture, open. In J. J. Schaider, S. R. Hayden, R. Wolfe, R. M. Barkin, & P. Rosen (Eds.), *Rosen & Barkin's 5-minute emergency medicine consult* (2nd ed., pp. 432–433). Philadelphia: Lippincott Williams & Wilkins.

Simon, R. & S. Koenigsknecht (2000). *Emergency orthopedics* (4th ed.). New York: McGraw-Hill.

Sloane, C. (2003). Elbow injuries. In J. J. Schaider, S. R. Hayden, R. Wolfe, R. M. Barkin, & P. Rosen (Eds.), *Rosen & Barkin's 5-minute emergency medicine consult* (2nd ed., pp. 356–357). Philadelphia: Lippincott Williams & Wilkins.

NOTES

CHAPTER 30

NAUSEA AND VOMITING

Jonathan S. Rubens, M.D., FACEP

PRESENTATION

Many EMS patients have nausea and vomiting as part of their symptom complex. These uncomfortable symptoms do not usually have serious sequelae, although dehydration and electrolyte abnormalities are possible. The causes of nausea and vomiting are many and come from diverse systems in the body. The history and physical examination should suggest the etiology.

IMMEDIATE CONCERNS

❶ What is the status of the patient's airway? Many patients experience nausea and vomiting. They may be at increased risk of aspiration.

❶ What is the patient's hemodynamic status? Look for and treat if there is evidence of poor perfusion.

IMPORTANT HISTORY

❷ How much has the patient vomited? Dehydration and electrolyte abnormalities are more likely with increased vomiting.

❷ Has there been any hematemesis? Patients may suffer from blood loss in addition to the loss of digestive fluids. Ask specifically about coffee-ground emesis because patients may not be aware that this indicates blood.

❷ Is there evidence of a possible bowel obstruction? Bowel obstructions do not allow gastric contents to move forward. Patients typically report abdominal pain, inability to pass gas, increasing abdominal distension, and vomiting. Often there is a history of prior abdominal surgeries or an abdominal hernia.

❓ **What is the age of the patient?** Infants and toddlers are at greater risk of dehydration with a vomiting illness. In addition, the potential causes are different for pediatric and adult patients.

❓ **Is the patient pregnant?** If the patient is of childbearing age and has a uterus and at least one ovary, pregnancy is possible. A missed or delayed menstrual period indicates a possible pregnancy. If the patient has a positive pregnancy test, find out the due date. Symptoms of an early pregnancy include amenorrhea (absent periods), breast tenderness or tingling, nausea and vomiting, and urinary frequency.

❓ **Are there any CNS symptoms?** Strokes, intracranial bleeds, head injuries, and CNS tumors can be associated with nausea and vomiting.

❓ **Are there symptoms of an acute coronary syndrome?** Inferior wall MIs often are associated with prominent GI symptoms, including nausea and vomiting. Consider obtaining a 12-lead ECG on all patients at risk of, or with a history of coronary artery disease.

❓ **Is the patient having abdominal pain?** The presence of abdominal pain and its characteristics may suggest an etiology. See chapters 1 and 2.

❓ **Does the patient have any significant past medical history?** The past medical history (PMH) may suggest an etiology or possible complications that may be caused by the vomiting.

❓ **Are there any new medications?** Nausea and vomiting are common side effects of many medications, particularly narcotic analgesics.

❓ **Are there other systemic symptoms?** Pain, fever, and neurologic symptoms such as headache, stiff neck, blurred or double vision, vertigo, and isolated weakness should be considered. Look for any history of urinary symptoms or amenorrhea or missed periods.

DIFFERENTIAL DIAGNOSIS

A list of the causes of nausea and vomiting would be exhaustive. Rather, the following major system causes should be considered for each patient:

- ***ACUTE MYOCARDIAL INFARCTION.*** Acute myocardial infarction, particularly inferior wall MIs, are sometimes associated with nausea and vomiting (see chapter 11).

- ***PERICARDITIS.*** Pericarditis may elicit these symptoms owing to diaphragmatic irritation. Patients may also have chest pain and a pericardial friction rub on auscultation.

- ***CENTRAL NERVOUS SYSTEM DISORDERS.*** All of the following can cause nausea and vomiting and are discussed in chapter 19: migraine, CVA, tumors, and hypertensive emergencies.

- ***INNER EAR DISTURBANCES.*** Vertigo and labyrinthine disorders are disturbances of sensorium involving the inner ear and positional senses. These patients often remain free of nausea and vomiting as long as they remain immobile, but with the onset of dizziness caused by any motion, they will experience these symptoms. Look for associated hearing loss and headache and focal weakness on examination as clues.

- ***ENDOCRINE.*** The CNS effects caused by the hormonal changes of early (usually first trimester) pregnancy commonly result in severe morning nausea and vomiting.

- ***DIABETES MELLITUS.*** Diabetes mellitus (DM) and its complications are frequently associated with nausea and vomiting. Elevations of blood glucose, including diabetic ketoacidosis, can result in these symptoms. Moreover, low blood glucose levels can cause nausea, diaphoresis, and syncope. Complications of this disease, including esophageal dysfunction, gastroparesis, and postural hypotension, are all known causes of nausea and vomiting. A history of DM, polyuria, polydypsia, weakness, and weight loss should be elicited. Likewise, the physical examination may reveal dehydration, the acetone breath smell associated with ketosis, or an abnormally high blood glucose level.

- **VASCULAR.** Impaired blood flow to a portion of the GI tract can cause ischemia, leading to nausea and vomiting. GI bleeding is likely as well. Black stools, bright red blood from the rectum, or hematemesis may occur. Consider the possibility of ischemia when the patient has a history of atrial fibrillation or vascular disease.

- **INFECTIOUS.** Amongst the most common causes of nausea and vomiting are viral and bacterial infections of the GI tract. These can include gastroenteritis, small intestine and colon infections, and abscesses.

- **MECHANICAL.** Nausea and vomiting may be caused by obstruction. Foreign bodies, hernias, tumors, adhesions, and strictures may be the cause.

- **PEDIATRIC DISORDERS.** Gastroesophageal reflux in infants can sometimes be mistaken for vomiting. Reflux and vomit can be differentiated by quantifying how much an infant was fed and how much was vomited. Reflux commonly occurs after each feeding and is sometimes improved with putting the child in a more erect position after feeding. Similarly, milk or food allergies can cause postprandial vomiting. Again, this is usually associated with feeding and with certain foodstuffs in particular. Obtaining a feeding history will help diagnose this type of vomiting.

Other less common causes of vomiting in children include malrotation, infections (e.g., meningitis and sepsis), and intussusception (i.e., telescoping of the intestine within itself). With intussusception, the child generally has periods of severe distress, with an intermittently tender and crampy abdomen. These episodes can last from several minutes to hours, with intervening periods during which the child appears to be in no distress at all and looks well. The passage of a "currant-jelly" or clotlike stool can also help in the diagnosis.

- **EATING DISORDERS.** Anorexia nervosa and bulimia are eating disorders caused by a disordered self-image and associated with fasting (anorexia), bingeing (bulimia), and self-induced vomiting to avoid weight gain.

- **PSYCHOLOGICAL DISORDERS.** Neurosis and irritable bowel syndrome are two psychogenic disorders that result in abnormal stimulation of the autonomic nervous system and can produce nausea and vomiting. Emotional upset, stress, and anxiety are usually precipitating factors.

- **PNEUMONIA.** Pulmonary patients with pneumonia caused by irritation of the diaphragm and pleural effusions may complain of nausea and vomiting. Look for a history of respiratory distress, tachypnea, cough with sputum production, and fever as clues. Adventitial sounds (e.g., rhonchi, rales, wheezes) may be heard on auscultation of the chest.

- **DRUGS.** Many classes of drugs, in particular nonsteroidal antiinflammatory drugs (NSAIDs), erythromycin, aspirin, and codeine, as well as chemotherapeutic agents, can cause nausea and vomiting as a result of direct irritation of the gastric lining. Likewise, many other substances (including food and bacterial toxins and pesticides) are known to have these effects on the GI system. Searching for a history of ingestion or exposure to these substances is the best way to identify these causes.

- **GASTROINTESTINAL.** See chapters 1 and 2 for a discussion of GI etiologies.

KEY PHYSICAL EXAMINATION FINDINGS

- ✅ **Initial assessment.**   Look for alterations in hemodynamic stability.

- ✅ *Vital signs.*   Although most patients have a normal or slightly elevated heart rate, some may be bradycardic as a result of vagal stimulation. Many patients with an inferior wall MI are also bradycardic. Careful monitoring of the blood pressure is needed. Patients with ruptured abdominal aortic aneurysms may be hypertensive initially and hypotensive later.

- ✅ *HEENT.*   Assess for dehydration.

- ✅ *Lungs.*   Listen to lung sounds for signs of pneumonia.

- ✅ *Abdomen.*   Look for evidence of prior surgeries, hernias, and distension. Assess for Cullen's and Turner's signs. Palpate for tenderness and masses. Percussion may help differentiate ascites from distension with air. Be alert for signs of peritonitis.

- ✅ *Extremities.*   Check for perfusion and equal pulses.

- ✅ *Skin.*   Assess for poor skin turgor.

ELECTROCARDIOGRAM

Evaluate for signs of cardiac ischemia or injury.

BLOOD GLUCOSE DETERMINATION

Assess for hypoglycemia in infants and toddlers as well as in patients with diabetes. Hyperglycemia may be found in patients with diabetic ketoacidosis or hyperosmolar hyperglycemic syndrome.

TREATMENT PLAN

GENERAL TREATMENT GUIDELINES

- *Patient assessment.* Perform a rapid and systematic initial assessment, and institute treatment as life-threatening problems are discovered. Prompt transport to the appropriate ED is a key intervention.

- **Administer O$_2$ and provide ventilatory support** as needed.

- Place the patient in a position of comfort.

- **Monitor the ECG if ischemia is suspected.**

- **Establish large-bore IV** access

- Consider the following interventions:

  o **Administer 0.9% NaCl or lactated Ringer's fluid resuscitation** if the patient presents with dehydration or shock.

  o **Treat for acute coronary syndrome if present.** See chapter 11.

  o **Administer promethazine (Phenergan) 12.5 to 25 mg IV or IM** (pediatric dose: Age > 2 years: 0.25 to 1 mg/kg IM or slow IV. Maximum dose 25 mg)

  o **Administer prochlorperazine (Compazine) 5 to 10 mg IV, IM** (pediatric dose: 0.1 mg/kg IV, IM, max 5 mg)

  o **Administer metoclopramide (Reglan) 5 to 10 mg IV, IM**

- Frequently reassess the patient's hemodynamic status.

- Frequently reassess the abdomen.

- **Transport to the appropriate ED.** Ensure patient comfort en route.

BIBLIOGRAPHY

Greenberg, M. (2003). Vomiting, adult. In J. J. Schaider, S. R. Hayden, R. Wolfe, R. M. Barkin, & P. Rosen (Eds.), *Rosen & Barkin's 5-minute emergency medicine consult* (2nd ed., pp. 1216–1217). Philadelphia: Lippincott Williams & Wilkins.

Hostetler, M. A. Vomiting, pediatric. (2003). In J. J. Schaider, S. R. Hayden, R. Wolfe, R. M. Barkin, & P. Rosen (Eds.), *Rosen & Barkin's 5-minute emergency medicine consult* (2nd ed., pp. 1218–1219). Philadelphia: Lippincott Williams & Wilkins.

Stevens, M. W. & F. W. Henretig (2000). Vomiting. In G. R. Fleisher & S. Ludwig (Eds.), *Textbook of pediatric emergency medicine* (4th ed., pp. 625–633). Philadelphia: Lippincott Williams & Wilkins.

NOTES

_____

_____

_____

_____

_____

_____

_____

_____

_____

_____

_____

_____

_____

_____

_____

CHAPTER 31

NEAR DROWNING

Gregg Margolis, M.S., NREMT-P

PRESENTATION

Drowning and near drowning can occur in any body of water. Swimming pools are the most common site of drowning. Lakes, ponds, and bathtubs are also common sites for aquatic emergencies. When responding to a near-drowning emergency, the prehospital care provider will generally find the patient with one of three presentations: without vital signs, unconscious with vital signs, or conscious. This progression generally reflects the degree of hypoxemia secondary to submersion.

IMMEDIATE CONCERNS

❗ **Is the patient in the water?** If so, an immediate plan for the safe rescue of the patient is the first concern.

❗ **Is the patient conscious?** If the patient is unconscious, immediate resuscitation and aggressive patient management, including intubation, ventilation, and oxygenation, is needed.

IMPORTANT HISTORY

❓ **Has there been any trauma involved?** If there is any possibility that the patient may have struck his or her head on the way into the water (on a diving board, etc), on the bottom, or on anything floating in the water, cervical spine precautions must be taken immediately. Any patient found unconscious in the water should be assumed to have a cervical injury until proven otherwise.

❓ **Is the patient in immediate danger?** Any patient still in the water is in immediate danger. If the patient is submerged, the patient must be recovered immediately. If the patient is found struggling on the surface, the patient is a danger to the rescuer and should be handled only by individuals trained in water rescue or lifeguarding.

❓ **Was there a loss of consciousness?** Unconsciousness is a significant finding in any near-drowning emergency. Some patients regain consciousness relatively quickly once their airway is opened and they are ventilated. Obviously, the prognosis worsens the longer the patient is unconscious.

❓ **What are the characteristics of the water?** Survival from submersion incidents is improved in clean, fresh water. Many patients, especially the young, have survived prolonged submersion in cold water. Resuscitation should be initiated in any patient who has been rescued within 60 minutes in water with a temperature below 70° F.

DIFFERENTIAL DIAGNOSIS

The assessment of the near-drowning patient is usually straightforward. Be alert for the following:

- ***TRAUMATIC INJURIES.*** Many drownings occur as divers strike the bottom of a pool or a diving board. Injuries are much more common in shallow water. You should assume that any patient found unconscious in the water has a cervical spine injury until proven otherwise.

- ***PREEXISTING MEDICAL EMERGENCY.*** Be aware that there may be a possibility of a preexisting medical problem.

- ***SCUBA DIVING INJURY.*** Consider the possibility of pulmonary barotrauma, decompression sickness, or both, in anyone who has taken a breath of pressurized gas under water.

KEY PHYSICAL EXAMINATION FINDINGS

✅ ***Mental status.*** Establish baseline level of consciousness as soon as possible.

- ☑ **Airway.** Check for airway obstruction from vomitus and fluid in the airway.

- ☑ **Breathing.** Assess the rate and work of breathing. Be sure to assess lung sounds.

- ☑ **Circulation.** Note any circulatory compromise, which is generally secondary to a respiratory insult.

- ☑ **Trauma.** Observe for signs of head injury, which indicates the need for cervical spine immobilization.

TREATMENT PLAN

- **Remove the patient from the water.** The priority in the management of the near-drowning patient is the safe removal of the individual from immediate danger. The patient has usually already been rescued by lifeguards, family, or bystanders. If the patient is still in the water, he or she should be removed as quickly as possible by trained rescuers. Be sure to consider the possibility of cervical spine trauma in any unconscious patient.

- **Secure an airway.** The swallowing of large amounts of water into the stomach makes regurgitation and aspiration a major concern in the management of near-drowning patients. If the patient is not conscious, the protection of the airway by an endotracheal tube is critical.

- **Ventilate and oxygenate the patient.** The primary insult in drowning is profound hypoxemia. As a result, hyperoxygenation with 100% oxygen is an essential component of management.

- **Provide cardiovascular support.** If the patient is pulseless, provide immediate cardiopulmonary resuscitation. Remember that the circulatory insult is secondary to hypoxemia. Provide aggressive resuscitation aimed at reversing hypoxia and respiratory acidosis.

- **Prevent heat loss.** Obviously, drowning patients are going to be wet. Water conducts heat from the body many times faster than air. As a result, you must make every attempt to keep the patient normothermic, even in warm environments. Removal of wet clothes and covering the victim with a thermal blanket should suffice in most cases. In cases of hypothermic near drowning, prevent further heat loss, but do not spend an inordinate amount of time concerning yourself with rewarming.

- Establish intravenous access with normal saline.

- Monitor electrocardiogram and treat dysrhythmias.

- **Bronchodilation.**   As a result of the bronchial irritation, many near-drowning patients suffer from considerable bronchoconstriction. Inhaled beta-2 agonists, such as aerosolized albuterol (0.5 ml in 3 ml saline), are the best short-term therapy for this situation. Remember that these agents can be nebulized directly into an endotracheal tube in the intubated patient.

BIBLIOGRAPHY

Bledsoe, B. E., R. S. Porter, & R. A. Cherry (2001). *Paramedic care: Principles and practice. Vol. 3: Medical emergencies.* Upper Saddle River, New Jersey: Prentice-Hall.

Bove, A. A. & J. A. Davis (1990). *Diving medicine* (2nd ed.). New York: W. B. Saunders.

Newman, A. B. (2001). Submersion incidents. In P. S. Auerbach (Ed.), *Wilderness medicine: Management of wilderness and environmental emergencies* (pp. 1340–1365). St. Louis, MO: Mosby.

Knopp, R. K. (1992). Near-drowning. In P. Rosen et al. (Eds.), *Emergency medicine: Concepts and clinical practice* (3rd ed.). St. Louis, MO: Mosby Year Book.

CHAPTER 32

OBSTETRIC EMERGENCIES

Thomas J. Rahilly, Ph.D.
Owen T. Traynor, M.D.

PRESENTATION

The vast majority of human births are not emergencies. The term *emergency childbirth* has been used by prehospital EMS systems to describe a labor and delivery attended to by EMTs in the field. Emergency childbirth is more accurately defined as an obstetric emergency with complications that compromise the health of the mother or infant. This chapter focuses on these situations only.

IMMEDIATE CONCERNS

❶ **Is the patient pregnant?** Obviously, no obstetric emergency is possible if the patient is not pregnant. If the patient is of childbearing age and has a uterus and at least one ovary, pregnancy is possible. A missed or delayed menstrual period indicates a possible pregnancy. If the patient has a positive pregnancy test, find out the due date. Symptoms of an early pregnancy include amenorrhea (absent periods), breast tenderness or tingling, nausea and vomiting, and frequent urination.

❶ **What is the patient's hemodynamic status?** If the patient is hemodynamically unstable, immediate resuscitation is warranted, including immediate transport, oxygen administration, large-bore IV access, and fluid resuscitation.

❶ **Is the patient in labor?** Labor is one of the most common reasons for a pregnant patient to call EMS. Find out the patient's reproductive history, including information regarding prior pregnancies and labor. Patients who have a history of short labor are likely to have progress quickly. Be prepared for a delivery.

IMPORTANT HISTORY

❷ **Is the patient reporting vaginal bleeding?** Vaginal bleeding is a common reason for a call for EMS. Some causes of vaginal bleeding, such as a ruptured ectopic pregnancy, abruptio placentae, and placenta previa, can be life-threatening. Although the amount of bleeding does not help with the diagnosis, it bears upon the hemodynamic stability of the patient. The passage of tissue may indicate a miscarriage.

❷ **Is the patient having abdominal or pelvic pain?** Pain may indicate ectopic pregnancy, miscarriage, or labor. There are nonpathologic gynecologic causes of pain, too. In addition, pregnant women suffer the same abdominal diseases as nonpregnant patients, such as appendicitis, cholecystitis, and gastritis. Consider pregnancy-related and nonpregnancy-related illnesses.

❷ **How far along is the pregnancy?** Different problems occur as the pregnancy develops. Ectopic pregnancies are found during the first trimester. Miscarriages are first or second trimester problems. Placenta previa and abruptio placentae occur during the second and third trimesters.

❷ **Has the patient had a pelvic ultrasound?** The ultrasound may provide information about the possibility of multiple births, fetal demise, threatened abortion, and placenta previa.

DIFFERENTIAL DIAGNOSIS

The differential diagnosis will be classified according to the trimester of occurrence.

FIRST TRIMESTER

- ***HYPEREMESIS GRAVIDARUM.*** Hyperemesis gravidarum is characterized by persistent nausea and vomiting that leads to dehydration, weight loss, or failure to gain weight as expected during the first trimester. It is usually at its worst during weeks 8 to 12 and resolves by week 20. Abdominal pain is not common. Consider other diagnoses when abdominal pain is present.

- **ECTOPIC PREGNANCY.** Ectopic pregnancies are pregnancies that develop outside of the uterus. Most of these pregnancies (approximately 95%) occur in the fallopian tubes. The peak time of diagnosis is between 6 and 9 weeks of gestation. The presentation can be one of profound shock if the tube ruptures. Many presentations are subtle, however. Patients report abdominal pain 95% of the time. The pain is usually poorly localized and on one side only. It can be dull and aching or sharp when it ruptures. The abdominal exam can be unremarkable if the tube has not yet ruptured. Often the ectopic pregnancy can masquerade as acute appendicitis, ruptured ovarian cyst, miscarriage, or pelvic inflammatory disease (PID). The risk factors for development of an ectopic pregnancy include a prior ectopic pregnancy, a history of PID, use of an intrauterine device (IUD), use of infertility drugs, and prior gynecologic surgery. In the past, ectopic pregnancies were all treated surgically. However, some can be treated medically using methotrexate.

- **SPONTANEOUS ABORTION.** Spontaneous abortion is commonly called a miscarriage. It can be classified as follows:

  o **Threatened abortion.** The patient has not passed the products of conception (POC). Common symptoms include vaginal bleeding, spotting, brownish vaginal discharge, and crampy suprapubic pain. The diagnosis will be made in the emergency department (ED) after evaluation, which includes a pelvic examination and possibly a pelvic ultrasound. Half of these patients will go on to have a normal pregnancy.

  o **Complete abortion.** In this case the POC have been passed. Patients commonly report significant suprapubic cramping and vaginal bleeding. Often the symptoms ease after the POC have been passed.

o **Incomplete abortion.** The patient has not expelled the entire POC and complains of moderate to severe suprapubic crampy pain and vaginal bleeding. A pelvic exam and pelvic ultrasound in the ED will help differentiate this from a complete abortion.

o **Inevitable abortion.** This occurs when the pregnancy cannot be salvaged but the POC have not yet been passed. An ED evaluation is necessary to make this diagnosis.

o **Missed abortion.** The missed abortion occurs when the fetus has died but without the passage of the POC. The patient usually reports dark vaginal bleeding. A pelvic exam and pelvic ultrasound in the ED will help make this diagnosis.

o **Septic abortion.** These patients report abdominal pain, fever, and vaginal discharge or bleeding. Their abdominal exam may reveal evidence of peritonitis.

• *MOLAR PREGNANCY.* Molar pregnancy is a pregnancy in which there is faulty fertilization, resulting in an abnormal mass of tissue. No fetus develops. In rare cases it may progress to an invasive disease, extending though the lining of the uterus into the muscular uterine wall, or to a tumor, known as a choriocarcinoma. It is difficult to distinguish clinically from an early pregnancy. Vaginal bleeding is often the reason for evaluation. Another common presentation is severe and prolonged hyperemesis gravidarum or early preeclampsia (less than 24 weeks). The uterus is usually much larger than expected, and no fetal heart tones can be detected. A pelvic ultrasound will confirm the diagnosis.

• *VAGINAL LESIONS.* Polyps and areas of inflammation may cause mild bleeding. These will be discovered during a pelvic examination in the ED. No prehospital treatment is needed.

SECOND/THIRD TRIMESTER

- ***PREECLAMPSIA AND ECLAMPSIA.*** Preeclampsia and eclampsia are classified as hypertensive disorders of pregnancy. Preeclampsia is a complication of pregnancy occurring after week 20. It consists of hypertension, edema, and protein in the urine. If seizures occur, the diagnosis becomes eclampsia. Almost 15% of the cases can occur postpartum. About 10% of patients with severe eclampsia develop HELLP syndrome (**H**emolysis, **E**levated **L**iver function tests, and **L**ow **P**latelets). One in 3 HELLP patients will develop disseminated intravascular coagulation (DIC), a life-threatening disorder characterized by systemic blood clotting followed by severe, uncontrollable bleeding. Hypertension during pregnancy is defined as 140/90 or an increase of 30/15 from baseline. Common complaints include headache and swelling of the hands, face, and legs. Patients may also present with an altered mental status and seizures. Poor urine output, right upper quadrant pain and tenderness, and visual disturbances may be seen in severe preeclampsia. Treatment is recommended when the blood pressure is equal to or greater than 160/100. Magnesium sulfate is the drug of choice for seizure prophylaxis and for severe preeclampsia and eclampsia. Diazepam (Valium) may be used when magnesium fails to control the seizures.

- ***ABRUPTIO PLACENTAE.*** Abruptio placentae is the separation of the placenta from the uterine wall. It may occur spontaneously or after trauma. It typically occurs after the twentieth week of pregnancy. Patients report vaginal bleeding, uterine cramps, and abdominal pain. Hypotension may occur secondary to blood loss. The patient may develop DIC. Abruptio placentae accounts for 15% of fetal deaths and 5% of maternal deaths. It causes approximately 30% of all vaginal bleeding in the last half of pregnancies.

- **PLACENTA PREVIA.** Placenta previa is a common cause (approximately 20% of antepartum bleeding) of bleeding in the second half of pregnancy. Placenta previa is defined as the implantation of the placenta over the cervical os (opening). It may be discovered early in pregnancy on ultrasound. Frequently, the placenta migrates from the cervical os. The placenta may cover all or part of the os. Patients frequently complain of painless vaginal bleeding. One in 5 patients has uterine cramping. In severe cases, hypotension may occur.

- **PRETERM LABOR.** Preterm labor, which occurs in up to 10% of all pregnancies, is defined as labor of significant intensity and duration to cause changes in the cervix before 37 weeks of gestation. Approximately one third of preterm labor is caused by uterine, cervical, or urinary tract infections. Treatment includes magnesium sulfate or beta agonists such as terbutaline.

LABOR COMPLICATIONS

- **ABNORMAL PRESENTATIONS.** The vertex, or head-first presentation, is the most common presentation. Breech and transverse are the most common abnormal presentations.

  - **Breech presentation.** Breech presentation requires a complicated delivery, with the buttocks or a foot as the presenting part. It is most common in preterm deliveries and decreases with gestational age. Frank breech, with the hips flexed and the knees extended is the most common breech presentation (50% to 70%). A footling, or incomplete breech, is the second most common (10% to 30%), with a foot as the presenting part. A complete breech, with both the hips and knees flexed, occurs in 5% to 10% of all breech presentations. These deliveries are best accomplished in the hospital; however, the paramedic must be prepared for a field delivery. It is possible for the baby's head to become trapped in the incompletely dilated cervix. The paramedic may be required to place a hand into the vagina to provide an airway for the baby.

o **Transverse presentation.** In a transverse presentation, the arm is the presenting part. The fetus lies transverse in the uterus. Prehospital delivery is not possible.

- **PROLAPSED CORD.** The umbilical cord can be the presenting part if it is prolapsed. This presentation is dangerous because the baby has not yet been delivered and receives its oxygenation via the cord. Prolapsed cord is more common with breech presentations, multiple gestations, prematurity, and low birth weight. The EMS treatment is to exert manual pressure through the vagina on the presenting part to decompress the cord. This procedure should be continued until a cesarean delivery can be performed.

- **UTERINE RUPTURE.** Uterine rupture is an uncommon emergency that occurs with abdominal trauma or labor. The patient reports severe abdominal pain and vaginal bleeding. Shock may occur. Treatment for shock is recommended. Risk factors include prior uterine surgeries and a history of prolonged or obstructed labor.

POSTPARTUM EMERGENCIES

- **POSTPARTUM HEMORRHAGE.** Postpartum hemorrhage (PPH) is the most common cause of maternal death. PPH is defined as loss of more than 500 ml of blood following a vaginal delivery or more than 1000 ml following a cesarean delivery. The most common cause of PPH is uterine atony, or failure of the uterus to contract adequately following delivery. Retained placenta, uterine trauma during delivery, and abnormal blood clotting are other causes. PPH may occur immediately, within the first 24 hours, or later. Prehospital management includes IV fluid resuscitation and treatment for uterine atony if present. Palpate the uterus through the abdominal wall and begin massage. If the uterus fails to contract, start oxytocin (10 to 40 units in 1 L normal saline) titrate to effect.

- **UTERINE INVERSION.**   In rare cases, the uterus may turn inside-out following the delivery. It can be caused by pulling on the umbilical cord or by trying to express the placenta from the uterus. Blood vessels that supply the uterus may be torn. Life-threatening bleeding and shock may occur. Attend first to treatment for shock. Attempt to replace the uterus by pushing the fundus of the uterus into the vagina. If the attempt fails, cover the uterus with moist dressings and transport.

KEY PHYSICAL EXAMINATION FINDINGS

Provide the woman with privacy, to the extent possible.

- ✓ *Initial assessment.* Look for signs of shock or hypertension.

- ✓ *Vital signs.* Monitor vital signs, particularly blood pressure and pulse rate. Pregnancy usually results in mild hypotension during the third trimester. A 30-mm increase in the mother's known systolic pressure should be considered suspect. A pregnant woman has an increased heart rate and may have a resting pulse rate of 100 bpm in her third trimester.

- ✓ *Skin.* Inspect for cyanosis, which indicates poor perfusion.

- ✓ *HEENT.* Observe for the presence of jugular venous distension (JVD) in the pregnant patient, which may indicate that patient is hypertensive.

- ✓ *Lungs.* Assess for evidence of pulmonary edema, a sign of preeclampsia.

⊘ **Abdomen.**   Assess for tenderness or contractions.

⊘ **Mental status.**   An altered mental status is a sensitive indicator of inadequate cerebral perfusion and fetal perfusion. Altered mental status may be found in preeclampsia and eclampsia.

⊘ **Neurologic examination.**   Note abnormal neurologic findings and the hyperreflexia of preeclampsia and eclampsia.

⊘ **Vaginal examination.**   Examine the vaginal opening for bleeding, presenting parts, or, in the case of abortion, fetal tissue.

⊘ **Extremities.**   Check the extremities for signs of edema. Although most women (about 75%) experience some edema during pregnancy, excessive or a notable increase in edema may indicate preeclampsia.

⊘ **Skin.**   The presence of easy bruising or peteclia and purpura may indicate HEILP syndrome or DIC.

ELECTROCARDIOGRAM

The woman should receive cardiac monitoring when serious signs or symptoms are present.

TREATMENT PLAN

HYPOTENSIVE PATIENT

- **Treat for shock** (see chapter 38), and follow the following guidelines for specific obstetric problems.

- **Monitor the fetal heart rate.** A fetal heart rate of less than 120 bpm indicates fetal distress. Expeditious transport to the ED is indicated, with support to the mother.

PREECLAMPSIA AND ECLAMPSIA

- **Administer O$_2$ and provide ventilatory support** as needed.

- Place the patient in the **left lateral recumbent position.**

- **Monitor the electrocardiogram, O$_2$ saturation, and fetal heart rate,** if available.

- **Establish IV** access.

- Consider the following interventions:

  o **Hydralazine, 5 mg IV** over 3 minutes. Repeat 5 mg IV every 5 minutes until diastolic blood pressure is between 90 to 100 mm Hg. Maximum total dose is 20 mg.

  o **Labetolol, 10 mg IV** over 2 minutes. May be repeated every 10 minutes at 10 to 80 mg. The maximum total dose is 300 mg.

  o **Magnesium sulfate, 2 to 4 g IV** over 5 to 10 minutes if a seizure occurs. May also be given for seizure prophylaxis. After the loading dose, run as an infusion at 2 g/hour. Magnesium causes CNS depression. Watch for decreased respiratory rate and decreased deep tendon reflexes. If CNS depression occurs or there are additional seizures or evidence of fetal distress, contact medical command for guidance. The magnesium may need to be discontinued.

- **Transport to the appropriate ED.** Ensure patient comfort en route.

SPECIFIC OBSTETRIC TREATMENT

Antepartum

- ***Hyperemesis gravidarum.*** Intravenous fluid hydration with 0.9% NaCl.

- ***Ectopic pregnancy.*** Transport expeditiously to ED.

- ***Abortion.*** Gently remove any protruding tissues. Transport to ED.

- ***Third-trimester bleeding.*** Regardless of the cause, place these patients in the left lateral recumbent position and transport to ED. Provide IV fluid resuscitation if needed.

- ***Eclampsia and preeclampsia.*** Place the patient in a left lateral recumbent position to relieve pressure on the vena cava. Anticipate seizures; medication orders may include diazepam (Valium), 5 to 10 mg slow IV, or magnesium sulfate 10%, 2 to 4 g slow IV.

Active Labor

- ***Breech presentation.*** If the delivery of the baby has begun, allow the buttocks and trunk to deliver spontaneously. While supporting the baby's body, lower the body slightly so that the remainder of the delivery is assisted by a majority of the baby's own weight. When the head is almost completely delivered (hairline is visible), gently raise the baby upward, and the head should deliver.

NOTE: If the head does not deliver within 3 minutes, place a gloved hand in the vaginal opening (palm toward the baby's face), and with your fingers, form a V on either side of the baby's nose. Exert gentle pressure against the vaginal wall to provide an oxygen supply.

- ***Leg presentation.*** This presentation is not deliverable in the field. Transport rapidly to ED.

- ***Transverse (arm) presentation.*** This presentation is not deliverable in the field. Transport expeditiously to ED.

- ***Prolapsed cord.*** A prolapsed cord is an absolute emergency. Relieve the pressure of the baby's head from the umbilical cord as you transport the mother and undelivered baby to the ED. Elevate the supine mother's hips to the extent possible. With two fingers of a gloved hand, gently push the baby back up the vagina without pushing the cord with it. Cover the vaginal opening with a sterile drape, maintain gentle upward pressure, and transport.

SECTION 1

- **Uterine rupture.** Treat for shock and expedite transport to the appropriate ED.

- **Uterine inversion.** Treat with IV fluids, and make one attempt to replace the uterus by pushing the fundus into the vagina. Expedite transport expeditiously to the appropriate ED.

Postpartum

- **Postpartum hemorrhage.** Gently massage the uterine fundus, and place the baby at the mother's breast to help control postpartum bleeding after delivery. Administer oxytocin (Pitocin), 10 to 40 units in 1 normal saline, titrated to effect.

NOTE: Make certain that all fetuses have been delivered before you even consider oxytocin.

BIBLIOGRAPHY

Della-Giustina, D. (2003). Hyperemesis gravidarum. In J. J. Schaider, S. R. Hayden, R. Wolfe, R. M. Barkin, & P. Rosen (Eds.), *Rosen & Barkin's 5-minute emergency medicine consult* (2nd ed., pp. 550–551). Philadelphia: Lippincott Williams & Wilkins.

Sapiro, E. M. (2003). Preeclampsia/eclampsia. In J. J. Schaider, S. R. Hayden, R. Wolfe, R. M. Barkin, & P. Rosen (Eds.), *Rosen & Barkin's 5-minute emergency medicine consult* (2nd ed., pp. 892–893). Philadelphia: Lippincott Williams & Wilkins.

Walker, J. (2003). Labor. In J. J. Schaider, S. R. Hayden, R. Wolfe, R. M. Barkin, & P. Rosen (Eds.), *Rosen & Barkin's 5-minute emergency medicine consult* (2nd ed., pp. 626–627). Philadelphia: Lippincott Williams & Wilki.

Zigman, A. J. (2003). Abortion, spontaneous. In J. J. Schaider, S. R. Hayden, R. Wolfe, R. M. Barkin, & P. Rosen (Eds.), *Rosen & Barkin's 5-minute emergency medicine consult* (2nd ed., pp. 14–16). Philadelphia: Lippincott Williams & Wilkins.

CHAPTER 33

OBSTRUCTED AIRWAY

Mike Yee, B.S., EMT-P

PRESENTATION

Airway obstruction is one of the most readily treatable yet immediately life-threatening emergencies faced by pre-hospital providers. Patients may present with any degree of obstruction, from simple hoarseness cleared with a cough to complete obstruction requiring a surgical airway, such as cricothyrotomy. Significant airway obstruction can occur at any time. Early recognition and treatment is essential to successful outcome. It is therefore important to distinguish this problem from more serious conditions that cause sudden respiratory failure but are treated differently.

IMMEDIATE CONCERNS

- ❗ **What is the status of the patient's airway?** The assessment must be more sophisticated than merely noting whether the airway is open, it must consider whether the airway will remain open and whether aspiration is a danger. Airways that are endangered must be secured and protected. Positioning of the airway, suctioning, and the use of oropharyngeal or nasopharyngeal airways, as well as endotracheal intubation, should be accomplished early.

- ❗ **Is the airway obstructed?** If the patient is not ventilating or cannot be mechanically ventilated, then airway obstruction is present. The mechanism causing the obstruction must be promptly discovered. Sudden onset of obstruction is likely to be caused by a foreign body. However, anaphylaxis may occur suddenly as well. A history of fever, chills, or sore throat may point to an infectious etiology; croup and epiglottitis must be considered. The cause is usually readily apparent. If a foreign body obstruction is responsible, BLS airway obstruction techniques should be employed. If an anatomic obstruction—perhaps caused by angioneurotic edema, infection in the upper airway, or obstruction by a mass or expanding hematoma—is present, the BLS airway obstruction techniques will not be helpful. When it is not possible to know the mechanism of the obstruction, employing the BLS airway obstruction techniques is recommended; foreign body obstruction is more common and is likely to be relieved by these techniques.

● **Is the airway obstruction complete or partial?** Complete obstructions and partial obstructions with poor air exchange are best managed as discussed previously. Partial obstructions with good air exchange are best managed by having the patient continue to cough forcefully and expel the foreign body. Patients with good air exchange must be monitored; the potential for worsening is great.

IMPORTANT HISTORY

❷ **Does the patient have a history that suggests a decreased ability to protect the airway?** Patients who have a depressed mental status are often at increased risk of aspiration. The use of alcohol and other central nervous system depressants also increases the risk of foreign body obstruction.

❷ **Does the patient have a history of oral or throat cancer?** Airway obstruction may result from a tumor obstructing the airway, bleeding, or swelling.

❷ **Is there a history of sore throat or fever?** The presence of sore throat should alert you to the possibility of croup or epiglottitis, particularly in children.

DIFFERENTIAL DIAGNOSIS

The differential diagnoses presented here are causes of obstruction of the upper airway and therefore do not include lower respiratory causes of respiratory distress, such as pneumothorax, hemothorax, pneumonia, and so forth.

- **FOREIGN BODY OBSTRUCTION.** Approximately 3,000 deaths occur each year in the United States by choking. Most of these deaths are in children younger than 4 years of age. In adults the history of a foreign body aspiration is usually readily available from the patient or from bystanders. With children, you should consider the possibility of foreign body aspiration in any patient who presents with ongoing respiratory distress or resolved respiratory distress. The child may have a history of a sudden onset of respiratory distress with choking and cough, followed by an absence of symptoms and then by delayed stridor or wheezing. This cycle occurs when the foreign body is not cleared from the airway but passes distally into the smaller airways. In children a foreign body may also lodge in the esophagus, causing stridor.

- **CROUP.** Croup is usually a relatively benign viral illness occurring in patients 6 months to 3 years of age. The patient usually presents after several days of an upper respiratory infection with a barking cough, stridor, and dyspnea. The patient often improves with humidified or nebulized oxygen. (See chapter 13.)

- **EPIGLOTTITIS.** In children, epiglottitis is a life-threatening emergency. The typical patient is between 2 and 7 years of age and presents with several hours of worsening sore throat, high temperature, drooling, and stridor. The patient is often sitting quietly, with the neck slightly extended and chin forward. No attempt should be made to examine the airway: Laryngospasm and complete obstruction may occur. Should a complete obstruction occur, the patient with epiglottitis is usually able to be ventilated with a bag-valve-mask device. Epiglottitis may occur in teenagers and adults, with the development of the disease occurring over a period of days. These patients are less likely to develop complete obstruction acutely. (See chapter 13.)

- **ANGIONEUROTIC EDEMA.** Angioneurotic edema is characterized by a sudden onset of edema due to an allergic reaction in the upper airway, which may involve the uvula, tongue, palate, epiglottis, or larynx. It most commonly occurs in patients who have a history of allergies. It should be treated in a fashion similar to anaphylaxis.

- **TRAUMATIC OBSTRUCTION.** Traumatic obstruction may occur after direct trauma to the neck or throat. A direct injury to the larynx may cause paralysis of the vocal cords, leading to obstruction.

- **CHEMICAL OR THERMAL INJURY.** Chemical or thermal injury to the airway may cause obstruction secondary to the soft-tissue injury and swelling.

- **ABSCESSES.** Abscesses located in the upper airway, such as retropharyngeal and peritonsillar abscesses, may cause obstruction secondary to swelling and mass effect. The history is usually one of prior infection, either upper respiratory infection or tonsillitis, and possibly fever, drooling, and trismus (a painful spasm of the muscles of mastication or chewing).

- **TUMORS AND CYSTS.** Tumors and cysts of the upper airway may manifest as airway obstruction. Although these are generally chronic and slow growing, they may manifest as an acute obstruction.

KEY PHYSICAL EXAMINATION FINDINGS

- ✅ **Initial assessment.** Be alert for upper airway compromise; stridor or hoarseness may be present. Respirations may be ineffective. Look for the universal choking sign. Assess the patient's ability to cough or speak.

- ✅ **Vital signs.** Assess for the presence of tachycardia and tachypnea.

- ✅ **Skin.** Inspect for generalized erythema (redness), pruritus (itching), urticaria (hives), and angioedema (swelling of the hands, face, neck, and upper airway). Flushing, cyanosis, chills, and diaphoresis may occur.

⊘ **HEENT.** Note the presence of drooling, trismus (inability to open mouth as a result of spasm), stridor, or angioneurotic edema. Do not attempt to examine the airway of pediatric patients suspected of having epiglottitis.

⊘ **Neck.** Examine the neck for enlarged lymph nodes or masses or any evidence of trauma.

⊘ **Lungs.** Check breath sounds for signs of broncoconstriction—wheezing and prolonged expiratory phase. A foreign body that has moved into the smaller airways may result in localized wheezing rather than the diffuse wheezing found in asthma or anaphylaxis. Look for retractions and use of respiratory accessory muscles.

⊘ **Mental status.** Check for impaired mentation and altered consciousness, which may indicate significant respiratory compromise and the need for immediate respiratory support.

TREATMENT PLAN

The goals of the treatment plan are to relieve the obstruction, if possible, and to improve the oxygenation of the patient. Frequent reassessment of the patient with an airway obstruction is necessary because of the potential for worsening of the respiratory status. Be prepared—potential for respiratory arrest and cardiac arrest exists.

GENERAL TREATMENT GUIDELINES

- **Administer O_2 and provide ventilatory support** as needed. This includes relieving upper airway obstructions, suctioning, or endotracheal intubation if indicated. Protect cervical spine as necessary.

- If BLS treatments are not effective, transport expeditiously to the ED.

Foreign Body Obstruction

- Follow AHA guidelines for relieving foreign body obstructions. BLS techniques will likely be effective.

- If BLS techniques are ineffective, perform direct laryngoscopy, and if a foreign body is visualized, use the Magill forceps to remove the object.

- If a foreign body is not visualized or cannot be removed from the airway, attempt endotracheal intubation and ventilation.

- If ventilation is not possible after endotracheal (ET) intubation, consider expeditious transport and transtracheal jet insufflation, cricothyrotomy, or advancing the ET tube to push the obstruction into the right mainstem bronchus. Withdraw the tube to a point above the carina, thus allowing both lungs to be ventilated.

Epiglottitis: Pediatric Patients

- **Do not do anything that may precipitate complete obstruction.** Do not examine the airway or draw blood. Transport the child in a comfortable position, with the parent present.

- **Provide supplemental O$_2$** and use blowby O$_2$ rather than a mask to provide less noxious stimuli.

- **Transport expeditiously to the appropriate ED.** Do not needlessly delay patient transport. Ensure patient comfort en route.

- **If air exchange is inadequate, ventilate the patient.** Do not attempt endotracheal intubation unless mechanical ventilation is impossible. A surgical airway may be required if ET intubation is impossible—consider needle cricothyrotomy. (See chapter 13.)

Epiglottitis: Adult Patients

- **Provide supplemental O$_2$.**

- **Transport expeditiously to the appropriate ED.** Do not needlessly delay patient transport. Ensure patient comfort en route.

- **If air exchange is inadequate, ventilate the patient.** Attempt endotracheal intubation if indicated. A surgical airway may be required if endotracheal intubation is impossible—consider needle cricothyrotomy.

Croup

- Provide supplemental humidified oxygen.

- Transport in a comfortable position.

- If patient is in distress, **administer 3 ml of nebulized 0.9% NaCl**—this is often treatment enough and prevents rebound after racemic epinephrine.

- Consider **nebulized racemic epinephrine, 0.25 to 0.5 ml in 2.5 ml of 0.9% NaCl.** Dose may be repeated every 20 to 30 minutes.

- **If air exchange is inadequate, ventilate the patient.** Do not attempt endotracheal intubation unless mechanical ventilation is impossible. A surgical airway may be required if endotracheal intubation is impossible—consider needle cricothyrotomy. (See chapter 13.)

SECTION 1

BIBLIOGRAPHY

Aufderheide, T. P., Stapleton, E. R., Hazinski, M. F., et al. (2002). *The ABCs: Techniques of adult CPR, heartsaver AED for the lay rescuer and first responder.* Dallas, TX: American Heart Association.

Bledsoe, B. E., R. S. Porter, R. A. Cherry (2000). *Paramedic care: Practice and principles* (vol. 1, pp. 576–577). Saddle Run, N.J.: Brady.

CHAPTER 34

OVERDOSES AND POISONINGS

Daniel E. Brooks, M.D.

PRESENTATION

With over 2.3 million reported human exposures to drugs and chemicals last year, poisonings are both common and diverse. Poisoned patients present in many ways, depending on the substance or substances and the time since exposure or ingestion. Patients may be asymptomatic and cooperative, agitated, comatose, or in cardiovascular shock. Furthermore, the patient's condition can deteriorate rapidly.

IMMEDIATE CONCERNS

❶ **Is the scene safe?** Always consider that the scene may hold an exposure risk for you, EMS personnel, or other people. Carbon monoxide can pose a risk to anyone exposed to it for long enough. Other industrial toxins, such as arsine gas, can lead to immediate collapse. Always consider scene safety for yourself and other persons who may subsequent enter the area and contact other agencies, police, and fire departments.

❶ **Is the patient stable?** Rapidly determine the level of consciousness and initial vital signs. Primary objectives include ensuring a stable airway, assisting with oxygenation or ventilation as needed, and establishing IV access.

IMPORTANT HISTORY

❷ **Identifying the toxin.** Rapidly identifying the exact drug(s) or toxin(s) to which the patient was exposed can improve survival. Prehospital personnel may be able to determine the toxin with just a quick evaluation of the scene. Look for prescription and over-the-counter pill containers, industrial products, or illicit drug paraphernalia. Interview available friends and family about recent events, drug use, and any other medical or psychiatric history. These facts can help determine the events surrounding the poisoning and expedite optimal management.

❷ **Was anything else ingested?** Try to identify other potential medications or toxins that the patient may have ingested or been otherwise exposed to. Often, several medications are involved but only one empty pill bottle is found. Concomitant alcohol or drug abuse can alter the patient's signs and symptoms.

DIFFERENTIAL DIAGNOSIS

The differential diagnosis of the poisoned patient is extensive. An awareness of several toxicologic syndromes, or toxidromes, is helpful. A quick but thorough history of recent events and accurate physical examination may aid in diagnosis. Overall, it is most important to consider that a poisoning may be responsible for a patient's condition. This is particularly important when the available facts (e.g., empty pill containers, intoxication, pin-point pupils) do not support the initial complaint or patient history.

IMPORTANT TOXIDROMES

- **SYMPATHOMIMETIC SYNDROME.** Sympathetic agents, such as cocaine, amphetamines, and caffeine, can lead to overactivation of the central nervous system (CNS), cardiovascular system, and respiratory system. Signs and symptoms include tachycardia, hypertension, agitation, hyperthermia, tremor, and seizures.

- **ANTICHOLINERGIC SYNDROME.** Medications and chemicals that inhibit acetylcholine can lead to an anticholinergic syndrome following toxic exposures.

Signs and symptoms include tachycardia, flushed skin, mumbling speech, visual hallucinations, and mydriasis (dilated pupils).

- **CHOLINERGIC SYNDROME.** Drugs and toxins that inactivate acetylcholinesterase, the enzyme that breaks down acetylcholine in the nervous system, can lead to a cholinergic crisis. Organophosphate insecticides and nerve agents such as sarin are two examples of cholinesterase inhibitors. Signs and symptoms of a cholinergic crisis or syndrome include copious airway secretions, salivation, defecation, emesis, and miosis (constricted pupils). Rapid control of airway secretions with the aggressive use of atropine (an anticholinergic medication) can prevent death from secretions and airway compromise.

- **ALCOHOL WITHDRAWAL SYNDROME.** Ethanol (alcohol) is a CNS depressant through its agonist effects on GABA (gamma aminobutyric acid), the main inhibitory neurotransmitter in the CNS. Withdrawal from ethanol and other GABA agonists, such as benzodiazepines and barbiturates, has life-threatening consequences. Patients may present with signs and symptoms that mimic other toxic syndromes. Signs and symptoms include tachycardia, hypertension, fever, agitation, delirium, tremor, and seizures.

- **OPIOID SYNDROME.** Drugs such as morphine, heroin, meperidine (Demerol), and oxycodone (Oxycontin) lead to the classic signs of opioid toxicity: CNS depression, respiratory depression, and miosis. The adulteration of illicit opioids with other drugs may lead to a mixed picture, with only some signs or symptoms of opioid toxicity. The administration of naloxone to nonintubated patients can help determine whether a patient is suffering from opioid toxicity.

- **SEDATIVE-HYPNOTIC SYNDROME.** Sedative-hypnotics, such as ethanol, result in CNS depression by activating GABA within the CNS. Some of these medications include benzodiazepines, barbiturates, ethanol, zolpidem, and baclofen. Signs and symptoms include CNS and respiratory depression, ataxia, slurred speech, and hypotension.

COMMON INGESTIONS

- **ACETAMINOPHEN (TYLENOL).** Acetaminophen toxicity initially causes nausea, vomiting, and liver dysfunction. Determining the time and amount of ingestion is very important. Prehospital care should include fluid resuscitation and gathering information about the ingestion (e.g., substance(s), amount, and timing).

- **SALICYLATE (ASPIRIN).** Salicylate toxicity can rapidly progress to seizures and death. Fluid resuscitation should be initiated if the patient has any evidence of dehydration (e.g., vomiting, tachycardia, dry mucous membranes). Patients with significant CNS depression or inadequate ventilation should be intubated and hyperventilated during transportation to the nearest emergency department (ED).

- **BETA BLOCKERS.** Patients who intentionally ingest beta blockers are at risk for severe bradycardia and hypotension. Other antihypertensives medications, such as calcium channel antagonists, can lead to hypotension with a normal or fast heart rate. Close attention should be paid to vital signs and mental status.

- **TRICYCLIC ANTIDEPRESSANTS.** Tricyclic antidepressants (TCAs), such as amitriptyline and other antidepressant and antipsychotic medications, are associated with CNS depression, hypotension, and cardiac dysfunction. TCA toxicity can lead to seizures and wide complex tachydysrhythmia, both of which are controlled with IV boluses of sodium bicarbonate.

- **ORAL HYPOGLYCEMICS.** Oral hypoglycemic agents (e.g., glyburide) can lead to profound hypoglycemia, even after an accidental ingestion of several tablets. The onset of action can be delayed for several hours so **all** patients should be transferred to an ED for evaluation and monitoring. Patients should have an IV established and a blood glucose level determined. Closely monitor for signs and symptoms of hypoglycemia (e.g., tachycardia, diaphoresis, altered sensorium).

SPECIAL PATIENT POPULATIONS

Patients with significant comorbidities, such as congestive heart failure or renal failure, as well as elderly and pediatric patients, are all at increased risk for toxic effects from poisonings. Also, poisoned patients may have an underlying psychiatric disorder that interferes with obtaining an accurate history, performing a physical examination, or determining harmful intent. A low threshold to transport for ED evaluation should be used when evaluating any patient that falls into one of these at-risk populations.

KEY PHYSICAL EXAMINATION FINDINGS

✓ *Initial assessment.* Look for alterations in mental status, respiratory compromise, and hemodynamic instability. Note abnormal odors on body or clothing.

✓ *Vital signs.* An accurate record of several vital sign measurements helps develop a timeline that may assist with subsequent ED management.

✓ *HEENT.* Examine pupils for responsiveness and equality. Note if there are excess secretions or if the mucous membranes are dry. Assess for odors on breath.

✓ *Lungs.* Listen to lung sounds for signs of pulmonary edema.

✓ *Extremities.* Assess for track marks and cyanosis.

ELECTROCARDIOGRAM

Evaluate for arrhythmias, increased QT intervals, and ischemia.

DIAGNOSTIC TESTS

Evaluate oxygen saturation and serum glucose.

TREATMENT

- ***Patient assessment.*** The identification and correction of abnormal vitals signs is the priority of prehospital personnel dealing with the poisoned patient. Other important issues include determining and correcting hypoglycemia, sedating the agitated patient, administering naloxone to the nonintubated patient with CNS and respiratory depression, applying noninvasive cooling measures (e.g., removal of outer garments, application of ice packs, use of air-conditioning during transport) for the hyperthermic patient, and rewarming a hypothermic patient. Poisoned patients may experience a rapid and dramatic change in their condition caused by the clinical onset of the drug effects. These effects may be delayed for several hours after the ingestion of sustained-release medications. Further treatment options and the use of chemical restraint (benzodiazepines) may be explored by consulting the physician at your base command or a regional poison control center (800-222-1222).

- **Administer O$_2$ and provide ventilatory support** as needed.

- Place the patient in a **head-elevated position,** unless spinal immobilization is needed.

- **Monitor the electrocardiogram and O$_2$ saturation.**

- **Establish large-bore IV** access.

- Consider the following interventions:

    o If an opiate overdose is suspected: naloxone (Narcan) 0.2 to 2 mg IV/IM/IN. Titrate to respiratory rate. May be repeated as needed.

    o If hypoglycemia is suspected, D50, 25 g IV.

o If hemodynamically unstable, normal saline or lactated Ringer's IV fluid resuscitation.

- Frequently reassess the patient's hemodynamic and neurologic status.

- **Transport to the appropriate ED.** Ensure patient comfort en route.

BIBLIOGRAPHY

Watson, W. A., T. L. Litovitz, G. C. Rodgers, et al. (2003). 2002 annual report of the American Association of Poison Control Centers toxic exposure surveillance system. *American Journal of Emergency Medicine, 21,* 353–421.

Ford, M. D. & K. A. Delaney. (2001). Initial approach to the poisoned patient. In M. D. Ford, K. A. Delaney, L. J. Ling, & T. Erickson (Eds.), *Clinical toxicology* (pp. 1–5). New York: W. B. Saunders, 2001.

O'Neil Davis, D. & P. M. Wax. (2001). Focused physical examination/toxidromes. In M. D. Ford, K. A. Delaney, L. J. Ling, & T. Erickson (Eds.), *Clinical toxicology* (pp. 21–33). New York: W. B. Saunders, 2001.

Goldfrank, L. R., N. W. Flomenbaum, N. A. Lewin, et al. (1998). Principles of managing the poisoned or overdose patient: An overview. In L. R. Goldfrank, N. E. Flomenbaum, N. A. Lewin, et al. (Eds.), *Goldfrank's toxicological emergencies* (6th ed., pp. 31–35). New York: Appleton & Lange.

NOTES

_____

_____

_____

_____

CHAPTER 35

PALPITATIONS

Francis X. Guyette, M.D.

PRESENTATION

Patients with palpitations complain of a forceful or irregular heartbeat. It is usually caused by a change in rate, rhythm, or forcefulness of contraction. This sensation may be associated with anxiety, shock, syncope, chest pain, shortness of breath, nausea, diaphoresis, or lightheadedness.

IMMEDIATE CONCERNS

❶ Is the patient stable? Patients who are unstable require immediate intervention. As always, resuscitation requires ABCs but in this case, "D" (for defibrillation) may be equally important. The patient should be placed on the monitor immediately because treatment with electricity may be necessary. The patient may also require treatments such as oxygen, fluids, vagal maneuvers, and adenosine.

IMPORTANT HISTORY

❷ Has this ever happened before? Patients will often be able to say whether they have a history of palpitations as a result of arrhythmias, such as atrial fibrillation or flutter. Patients may also have information regarding medical conditions that predispose them to abnormal heart rhythms, such as coronary artery disease, congestive heart failure (CHF), or Wolff-Parkinson-White syndrome. The patient can also provide information regarding the frequency and duration of the palpitations.

❓ **What were the circumstances of the event?** Episodes that occur independent of activity or excitement may be found in atrial fibrillation or flutter, fever, hypoglycemia, anemia, hyperthyroidism, and anxiety states. Episodes that occur when the patient stands may be associated with orthostatic hypotension. Perimenopausal woman may feel palpitations accompanied by flushing and sweating.

❓ **What were the associated symptoms?** Syncope and lightheadedness are particularly worrisome because they may indicate shock and instability. Palpitations in the presence of chest pain, dyspnea, or nausea could be the result of angina or CHF. Patients with wheezing or cough may have palpitations associated with chronic lung disease.

❓ **What medications is the patient taking?** Medications to treat abnormal heart rhythms and cardiac disease are important (Digoxin, antiarrhythmics, and hypertension medications). Anticoagulants (Coumadin) are commonly prescribed to patients with atrial fibrillation. Pulmonary medications such as albuterol and theophylline may cause palpitations. Cold remedies and diet pills that contain pseudoephedrine or dextromethorphan can also cause palpitations. Other stimulants that can cause palpitations include caffeine, cocaine, amphetamines, and herbal medications such as ginko biloba and ephedra.

❓ **Does the patient have risk factors for cardiac disease?** A history of cardiac disease, age over 40, hypertension, diabetes, high cholesterol, smoking, male sex, and a family history of cardiac disease are the classic risk factors.

DIFFERENTIAL DIAGNOSIS

The following causes of palpitations are more likely to result in hemodynamic instability and require prehospital therapy. ,

- **Atrial fibrillation.** In atrial fibrillation (AF), an irregularly irregular rhythm occurs in which the P wave is randomly conducted into a narrow QRS complex.

- **Bradycardias.** It is unusual for slow heart rhythms to be perceived as palpitations. These rhythms may require atropine or pacing.

- **Multifocal premature ventricular complexes.** Multifocal premature ventricular complexes (PVCs) feature three or more ventricular beats with different morphologies (shapes). Although this rhythm is usually stable, it has the potential to degrade into ventricular fibrillation or ventricular tachycardia.

- **Supraventricular tachycardia.** Supraventricular tachycardia **(SVT)** features a regular narrow complex rhythm usually between 100 and 180 beats per minute. Although it can usually be treated with vagal maneuvers and adenosine it to may require electricity if the patient decompensates.

- **Ventricular fibrillation.** Ventricular fibrillation (VF) features an irregular wide complex rhythm that produces no cardiac output. This rhythm must be defibrillated immediately.

- **Ventricular tachycardia.** Ventricular tachycardia (VT) usually entails a regular wide complex rhythm that may be stable at first and then quickly degrade. This rhythm is also treated with electricity.

Stable causes of palpitations. Although any abnormal rhythm may result in an unstable patient, the following rhythms tend to remain stable and allow for more conservative treatment.

- **Atrial flutter.** Atrial flutter (Af) features a narrow complex rhythm wherein only a fraction of the P waves are conducted, resulting in a sawtooth pattern.

- **Extrasystoles.** Extrasystoles are extra, often premature complexes, such as premature atrial contractions (PACs), premature junctional contractions (PJCs), and premature ventricular contractions (PVCs). These pose little danger and generally require no prehospital therapy.

- **Multifocal atrial tachycardia.** Multifocal atrial tachycardia (MAT) features a regular rhythm with a rate greater than 100 and P waves of at least three different morphologies. This rhythm is often caused by pulmonary disease.

- **Sinus tachycardia.** Sinus tachycardia is a common, narrow complex, regular rhythm with a rate greater than 100. It is often caused by dehydration, hypoxia, infection, blood loss, stress, or pain.

KEY PHYSICAL EXAM FINDINGS

✅ *Initial assessment.* Look for alterations in mental status, respiratory compromise, and hemodynamic instability.

✅ *Vital signs.* Careful monitoring of the heart rate and BP is needed.

✅ *Lungs.* Listen to lung sounds for signs of pulmonary edema.

✅ *Heart.* Assess heart sounds for rhythm and murmurs.

✅ *Extremities.* Assess for edema and capillary refill in the extremities.

ELECTROCARDIOGRAM

Continuous electrocardiogram (ECG) monitoring may reveal the source of the palpitation. A 12-lead ECG may reveal evidence of ischemia.

TREATMENT PLAN

- **Rapidly assess for hemodynamic instability.** Frequent reevaluation and continuous ECG monitoring may be needed. Hemodynamically unstable patients who do not have a significant arrhythmia may be treated following the guidelines in chapter 38.

- **Administer O₂ and provide ventilatory support** as needed. Protect cervical spine as indicated.

- **Establish IV access** if needed.

- Treat arrhythmias according to ACLS guidelines. See chapter 6, chapter 44, or chapter 8.

- **Transport to the appropriate emergency department.** Expedite the transport of unstable patients.

SECTION 1

BIBLIOGRAPHY

(2000). Arrhythmias. In R. O. Cummins (Ed.). *Advanced cardiac life support* (pp. 3.3–3.20). Dallas, TX: American Heart Association.

Sanders, M. J. Cardiology. (2001). In M. J. Saunders & K. McKenna *Mosby's paramedic textbook* (2nd ed., pp. 768–770). St. Louis, MO: Mosby.

Votey, S. R., M. Herbert, & J. R. Hoffman (2001). Tachyarrhythmias. In A. Harwood-Nuss, A. B. Wolfson, C. H. Linden, S. Moore, & R. H. Stenklyft (Eds.), *The clinical practice of emergency medicine* (3rd ed., pp. 685–694). Philadelphia: Lippincott Williams & Wilkins.

NOTES

_____

_____

_____

_____

_____

_____

CHAPTER 36

RAPE AND SEXUAL ASSAULT

Sally Kuzniewski, R.N., SPNE

PRESENTATION

Patients who have experienced the trauma of rape or sexual assault may present in a variety of ways. Physical trauma may be evident, along with emotional trauma, which is common in these situations. In some cases, emotional trauma may be the only presenting problem. Prehospital EMS providers may be thrust into the role of mediator, buffer, or confidant. They may even be subject to violent aggression on the part of the victims or their families.

IMMEDIATE CONCERNS

As always, the safety and well-being of the EMS team should remain paramount. Even though a patient may be visible and in need of immediate care, rescuers must ensure that they do not inadvertently become victims in a hostile or violent situation.

❶ When dealing with the concerns of the victim, confidentiality and modesty should always be considered. The care of the patient always takes precedence and should never be compromised to gather information on possible suspects or perpetrators. The primary investigation of the incident is the responsibility of law enforcement agencies.

❶ Injuries associated with sexual assault vary widely. They can be as subtle as slight pain or discomfort or as grossly evident as either debilitating or disfiguring trauma. The victim's injuries may not be obvious or visible on first inspection. Some victims may deny the injuries and relate untruthful information regarding the occurrence.

You must develop and foster rapport with the victim to gain the victim's confidence so that accurate information can be obtained.

❶ The process of helping this patient progress from being a victim to becoming a survivor begins in the field by the first responders.

IMPORTANT HISTORY

Unfortunately, rape and sexual abuse are not confined only to the adult population. Rape and sexual abuse can occur in infants, children, adolescents, and the elderly. Rape and sexual abuse are not the province of any one sex or race. The history offers the best indication that rape or sexual abuse has occurred. The prehospital provider may be in the best position to observe the patient at the scene of the rape or abuse.

EMS personnel can use their training to identify the abused patient if they take the time to observe all of the elements of a possible rape or sexual abuse case. Take care to record any information about the incident that may assist the victim and law enforcement officials at a later time. Begin the "chain of evidence" by preserving any and all evidence. Keep in mind that if the incident results in an arrest and subsequent trial, you may be called to provide testimony. Remember, never jump to conclusions, either "pro" or "con." Be supportive, but remain neutral and concentrate primarily on the physical and emotional care of the patient. Pay particular attention to these five areas:

1. ***Recurring injuries.*** "Hospital shopping" (i.e., when patients do not frequent the same hospital or medical facility for fear of detection of possible abuses) usually becomes obvious. An astute EMS provider will recognize this type of activity. Naturally, the fearful victim should be carefully evaluated, whether it is the parent of an infant, a juvenile, an adult, or an elderly person who cannot explain the injuries, especially if the injuries are not consistent with the scenario

as it is reported. Without being accusatory, follow local protocols and statutes for reporting these incidents. Avoid confrontation with either the patient or bystanders.

2. ***Abuses committed by an "unknown" person.*** Too often, abuse is ongoing and committed by a family member or someone close to the victim. It goes without saying that neighbors, friends, relatives, immediate family, or even parents can perpetrate rape or sexual abuses. Therefore always maintain an open mind. The investigation of any crime is not the responsibility of the EMS system. Assisting the investigators, however, is both a moral requirement and, in many states, a legal one.

3. ***Withdrawal or hostility.*** A person who has been subjected to these types of assaults may be hostile to your inquisition. A child may completely regress and may not be able to relate the facts of the incident. Keep in mind that your actions and words play a great part in whether you can successfully initiate a dialogue with the patient. Be firm, professional, and caring. Maintain an acute awareness of your attitude and demeanor, as well as that of the entire EMS team. Using a nonjudgmental, supportive approach will facilitate your interaction with the patient. Provide a secure environment for the patient, removing the patient from public view. Avoiding further exposure will prevent more embarrassment. Be sensitive and empathetic when in contact with a victim of any crime.

4. ***Confidentiality.*** When the victim begins to trust you and the other members of the EMS team, vast amounts of pertinent information may be volunteered. Your duty is to listen and reassure the victim and to provide appropriate treatment. These persons may have certain legal rights to privacy during conversations with medical providers. As with any patient contact, never discount voluntary information. Often, the victim in these cases will seek the assistance of a professional group or person; you may be that person, so be fair, honest, and concerned. This is considered an "immediate outcry," which is often therapeutic in nature.

5. ***Need for emotional support.***   In the case of a violent confrontation, some victims may seek out a mentor, someone to whom that victim can relate. Do not consider the victim's requests to seek an "equal" (i.e., someone of the same sex or gender) as a personal insult. What the victim may need most at this point is a confidant, not a medical provider. This preference is common and in some cases can be a great asset to the well-being of the patient. Allow the process of regaining control to start in the field. Let the patient decide whether he or she would like to sit or lie on a stretcher. Let the patient decide whether he or she wants someone to be contacted.

INJURIES

Injuries resulting from rape and sexual abuse incidents vary on a case-by-case basis and may include any of the following:

● ***Physical trauma.***   Lacerations, punctures, avulsion, traumatic amputations, and, in some isolated cases, human or animal bite injuries may be observed. Each injury should be carefully evaluated and treated. Objects inserted into a body cavity can cause injury and may become foreign bodies in the anatomic structure.

● ***Emotional injuries.***   Emotional injuries are usually prevalent in this type of incident. As described previously, they can vary from slight to extreme in nature. Never discount the victim's emotional status.

● ***Respiratory status.***   The patient's respiratory system should never be overlooked. As always, ABCs must be assessed initially and as required thereafter for every patient.

PATIENT–EMS PROVIDER INTERACTION

Your demeanor and attitude will be tested regularly when dealing with victims of rape and sexual abuse. The following forms of sexual abuse, which apply to both male and female victims, are among the most common:

- **Rape:** unwanted sexual intercourse by another participant.

- **Sodomy:** unwanted, and often aggressive, deviant sexual activity in which the victim is forced to conduct acts of deviant sexual activity or is the recipient of such activity (e.g., the forceful insertion of the penis into the mouth of another person).

- **Sexual abuse:** the unwanted feeling, fondling, or probing of the genitalia by a second person.

Sexual abuse, however, is not limited to the genitalia. It can also encompass the other "private parts" of the victim that do not meet the definition of sodomy.

TREATMENT PLAN

Although the patient must be treated for any injury associated with rape or sexual abuse, care should be taken to preserve any evidence that will be required by law enforcement authorities. Injuries may include rectal bleeding and painful itching or swollen genitals. Sodomy victims may also have injuries to the mouth and eyes. You must ensure that you are properly protected from any sexually transmitted diseases that may be present.

- *Monitor ABCs.* Trauma to the mouth can compromise the airway. Patients in respiratory distress should receive oxygen. The emotional trauma of a sexual assault can result in cardiovascular emergencies.

- *Treat lacerations.* Apply direct pressure and sterile packing, provide intravenous cannulation, administer oxygen therapy, and transport to the appropriate ED.

- *Treat avulsions.* As lacerations, skin flaps should not be removed; if intact, apply and secure sterile dressings.

- *Manage amputations.* Follow local trauma protocol for the amputated part.

- **Treat puncture wounds.**   Follow the same procedure as for the treatment of lacerations. Evaluate the site for impaled objects; secure any objects in place without removing.

- **Provide emotional support.**   Assist the victim. Be supportive and empathetic. Continue to monitor and support the patient during transport to the medical facility.

- **Evaluate fractures at the injury site.**   Is the fracture consistent with the reported incident? Stabilize and immobilize as necessary.

SPECIAL CONSIDERATIONS

Although the primary function of an EMS provider is the protection of the victim while providing prehospital medical care, the following are a few things to remember:

- In the case of rape, have the victim refrain from showering or washing before the hospital physical examination. Because this is a natural reaction after a rape, a great deal of sensitivity is required. Valuable medical and forensic information and evidence can be destroyed if the victim is permitted to engage in any personal hygiene activities.

- Avoid rinsing mouth or brushing teeth. Discourage urination, defecation, or douching.

- It is also a good idea that the clothing worn at the time of the incident be retained and transported to the hospital with the victim in a brown paper bag; do not use plastic. This precaution will preserve evidence.

CRIMINAL REPORTING

As for all other incidents, EMS providers are required to complete pertinent forms and necessary paperwork to document the complaint of a sexual assault. In the case of rape or sexual abuse, the professional healthcare provider may be duty bound in some jurisdictions to report the incidence of sexual assault to the authorities. However, it is not usually a requirement that the EMS provider do so. Most EMS personnel, however, take the responsibility and initiative to report to local authorities what they believe to be true abuse, either formally or informally. The criminal reporting requirements vary according to state and local statutes. EMS providers must keep abreast of the laws pertaining to their EMS system.

BIBLIOGRAPHY

Bledsoe, B. E., R. S. Porter, & R. A. Cherry (Eds.) (2003). *Essentials of paramedic care* (pp. 1862–1865). Englewood Cliffs, N.J.: Prentice-Hall.

Newberry, L. (2003). Sexual assault. In L. Newberry (Ed), *Sheehy's emergency nursing: Principles and practice* (5th ed.). St. Louis, MO: Mosby.

New York State Penal Law Sections: 130.00; 130.05; 130.16; 130.25–35; 130.38–40; 130.45–70, Looseleaf Law Publications, 1993 Edition, Chapters 1–717 of the Regular Session of the State Assemply.

Patel, M. (2001). Management of sexual assault. *Emergency Medicine Clinics of North America, 19*, 817–831.

NOTES

_____

_____

_____

_____

_____

_____

_____

CHAPTER 37

SEIZURE

Micelle Haydel, M.D.

PRESENTATION

Seizures are a condition in which abnormal electrical discharges of neurons in the brain cause paroxysmal events in the rest of the body. The patient exhibits these paroxysmal events by a disturbance of movement, altered mental status, alteration in sensation, or behavior change. Complications of seizures include death from anoxia and aspiration, trauma caused by loss of consciousness, encephalopathy caused by hypoxia, acute renal failure caused by muscle breakdown (rhabdomyolysis), and respiratory arrest caused by medications.

IMMEDIATE CONCERNS

- **Does the patient have a patent airway?** When a patient's level of consciousness is decreased, the patient is not able to adequately maintain a patent airway, and a nasopharyngeal airway should be inserted. The patient may not be able to clear secretions and should be positioned on the side, with suction equipment easily accessible.

- **Is the patient ventilating adequately?** The period of apnea is usually short and resolves spontaneously; however, supplemental oxygen by nonrebreather mask or bag-valve-mask (BVM) device is necessary because ventilations during a seizure are usually ineffective and may result in hypoxia.

- **Does the patient have adequate circulation?** Seizures can be associated with circulatory collapse and, if the patient is hemodynamically unstable, intravenous access and immediate resuscitation are warranted.

❶ **Is the patient's safety maintained?**   During any phase of seizure activity, the patient is not able to provide for personal safety. Move any potentially hazardous objects away from the patient. Bite blocks may be used to prevent the patient from biting the tongue.

NOTE: A bite block should never be forcefully inserted into a seizing patient's mouth.

❶ **How long has this seizure lasted?**   If the patient is still seizing when the EMS providers arrive, it is important to find out how long the seizure has lasted and whether this is a second seizure. Status epilepticus must be suspected if the patient has had two or more seizures without regaining consciousness or if the seizure has lasted for longer than 30 minutes.

IMPORTANT HISTORY

❷ **Has the patient ever had a seizure before?**   Seizures commonly occur in a patient with a known seizure disorder who is not adequately controlled on medications. Patients with a known seizure disorder may have a medical alert tag or bracelet that may help you determine whether this seizure is different from other seizures. Remember, however, that medical alert devices are useful but not always definitive.

❷ **Is the patient taking seizure medications as prescribed?**   Commonly, seizures (including status epilepticus) occur in a patient who is noncompliant with medications or needs adjustment of medication dosage or intervals. Common seizure medications include phenytoin (Dilantin), phenobarbital (Luminal), ethosuximide (Zarontin), carbamazepine (Tegretol), valproic acid (Depakene), clonazepam (Klonopin), felbamate (Felbatol), lamatrigine (Lamictal), primidone (Mysoline), gabapentin (Neurontin), and topiramate (Topamax).

DIFFERENTIAL DIAGNOSIS

SEIZURE VERSUS SYNCOPE

Seizures and syncope are frequently difficult to differentiate, even when witnessed. Seizures typically involve tongue-biting, incontinence, and a period of postictal confusion, which is not commonly found in syncope.

SEIZURES: CLINICAL MANIFESTATIONS

* ***GENERALIZED SEIZURES*** (also known as grand mal or tonic-clonic) are characterized by a loss of consciousness, apnea, incontinence, and alternating contraction and relaxation of the extremities. Generalized seizures end with a postictal phase characterized by a period of flaccidity, followed by the level of consciousness changing from confused, and often combative, then slowly returning to normal.

* ***FOCAL SEIZURES*** (also known as petit mal or partial) are manifested as limited muscle contra ctions or sensory disturbances but do not include complete loss of consciousness.

* ***JACKSONIAN SEIZURES*** start as a focal seizure of an extremity that moves proximally and typically leads to a generalized seizure.

* ***STATUS EPILEPTICUS*** is repetitive, generalized seizure activity without full recovery of consciousness or seizure activity lasting over 30 minutes.

SEIZURE ETIOLOGIES

* ***PRIMARY SEIZURES (EPILEPSY).*** Patients with unprovoked, intermittent, recurring seizure activity have epilepsy or primary seizures. The most common cause of seizures in a patient with epilepsy is subtherapeutic medication levels.

- **SECONDARY SEIZURES (REACTIVE).**   Secondary seizures are predictable responses to toxins, or environmental or pathophysiological events and must be considered in all patients with seizures, even those with known epilepsy.

- **HYPOXIC SEIZURES.**   Seizures can be caused by inadequate airway or ventilation. As in any situation, airway, breathing, and circulation are the priority.

- **METABOLIC SEIZURES.**   Seizures can be caused by alterations in electrolytes, such as glucose, sodium, magnesium, and calcium. A low glucose count is the most common cause of metabolic seizures. Patients with diabetes may wear a medical alert tag or bracelet, but all patients with seizures should have their glucose level checked.

- **ALCOHOL OR DRUG-INDUCED SEIZURES.**   Seizures are often associated with alcohol intoxication or withdrawal. Pertinent history of alcohol or drug abuse or signs of overdose should be obtained. Common drugs causing seizures include overdose of cyclic antidepressants, cocaine, lead, strychnine, and camphor.

- **INTRACRANIAL INSULTS.**   Seizures can be caused by infections, trauma, strokes, or tumor in the central nervous system.

- **FEBRILE SEIZURES OF CHILDHOOD.**   Children who have underlying systemic infections and fevers can have febrile seizures. These are usually self-limiting, but because complications can occur, they should be treated like other seizure disorders.

- **ECLAMPSIA (TOXEMIA OF PREGNANCY).**   Pre-eclampsia (hypertension after 20 weeks' gestation, edema, and proteinuria) occurs in about 5% of pregnancies and may lead to life-threatening eclampsia, which is a seizure or coma in the preeclamptic patient. Seizures during pregnancy are life-threatening to the mother as well as to the baby, and transportation for definitive care should be expedited. Magnesium sulfate is used for treatment or prevention of seizures in the patient with severe pre-eclampsia (continuous magnesium sulfate infusions may have been instituted before interhospital transfers). Magnesium overdose causes respiratory depression and cardiac standstill, which are treated with calcium chloride.

KEY PHYSICAL EXAMINATION FINDINGS

- *Initial assessment.* Airway, breathing, and circulation are the priority in all patients, including the actively seizing patient. Life-threatening complications must not be neglected because of the distracting seizure activity.

- *Head and neck.* Cervical spine precautions should be taken if a potential injury is suspected. In addition to noting any scalp or head trauma, look for buccal or tongue lacerations.

- *Extremities.* Musculoskeletal injuries, especially shoulder dislocations, are common as a result of falls secondary to seizures.

- *Neurologic examination.* Assess level of consciousness. Serial mental status examinations are required in all patients. Look for any progressive decline in mental status and for any focal weakness.

TREATMENT PLAN

- *Patient assessment.* Perform a rapid and systematic primary survey, and institute treatment as life-threatening problems are discovered. Frequent reassessment of any patient with an altered mental status is necessary because of the potential for respiratory compromise and worsening of the neurologic status.

- Administer **O₂** and provide **ventilatory support** as needed. This may include insertion of nasopharyngeal airways and endotracheal intubation. Monitor O₂ saturation with pulse oximetry if available.

SECTION 1

- Place patient in the semirecumbent or left, lateral decubitus position to reduce the aspiration risk in patients with a compromised gag reflex or depressed consciousness.

- Establish **IV access.**

- If the patient continues to have generalized seizure activity, the prehospital drug of choice is a **benzodiazepine:** diazepam (Valium), 5 to 10 mg IV; lorazepam (Ativan), 2 mg IV; or midazolam (Versed), 1 to 2 mg IV. Dosing may be repeated every 10 to 15 minutes, but all can cause respiratory depression, hypotension, and decreased levels of consciousness. Pediatric dosing: diazepam, 0.2 to 0.5 mg/kg slow IVP; lorazepam, 0.1 mg/kg slow IVP; and midazolam, 0.05 mg/kg slow IVP. Diazepam may be administered rectally, endotracheally, or intraosseously. Midazolam may be administered intramuscularly or rectally.

- As with any patient with an altered mental status, consider the administration of the following agents:

  o **Naloxone** (Narcan), **0.4 to 2.0 mg IV bolus.** Dose may be repeated in 2 to 3 minutes.

  o **Thiamine, 50 mg IV and 50 mg IM.** Give 100 mg IM if IV cannot be established.

  o **50% dextrose, 25 g IV** if the patient is hypoglycemic or if hypoglycemia is suspected in a patient with diabetes.

- Treat symptomatic arrhythmias as indicated. (See chapters 6 and 44, for specific options.)

- If a specific etiology of the seizure is suspected (e.g., hypoglycemia, arrhythmia, hypoxia, fever), treat the underlying illness as well.

- **Treat non–life-threatening injuries** (i.e., control of bleeding and splinting of fractures).

- **Transport to appropriate emergency department.** Ensure patient comfort en route.

BIBLIOGRAPHY

Pollack, C. V. & E. S. Pollack. (2002). Seizures. In J. Marx, R. Hockberger, & R. Walls (Eds.), *Rosen's emergency medicine: Concepts and clinical practice* (5th ed., pp. 1445–1455). St. Louis, MO: Mosby.

Viola, C. C. (2000). Seizures and status epilepticus in adults. In J. E. Tintinalli, G. D. Kelen, & J. S. Stapczynski (Eds.), *Emergency medicine: A comprehensive study guide* (5th ed., pp. 1463–1470). New York: McGraw-Hill.

SECTION 1

NOTES

_____

_____

_____

_____

_____

_____

_____

_____

_____

_____

_____

_____

_____

CHAPTER
38
SHOCK

Owen T. Traynor, M.D.

PRESENTATION

Shock is often defined as a state of inadequate tissue perfusion. It may result in acidosis, derangements of cellular metabolism, potential end-organ damage, and death. Although there are many possible causes of shock, it is helpful to think of the following classes of shock:

- Hypovolemia—caused by hemorrhage, burns, or dehydration

- Distributive shock—maldistribution of blood, caused by poor vasomotor tone in neurogenic shock, sepsis, anaphylaxis, severe hypoxia, or metabolic shock

- Pump failure—caused by necrosis of the myocardial tissue or by arrhythmias

- Obstructive shock—caused by impairment of cardiac filling, found in pulmonary embolism, tension pneumothorax, or cardiac tamponade

Early in the shock process, patients are able to compensate for the decreased perfusion by increased stimulation of the sympathetic nervous system, leading to tachycardia and tachypnea. Later, compensatory mechanisms fail, causing a decreased mental status, hypotension, and death. Early cellular injury may be reversible if definitive therapy is delivered promptly. It is not always possible for the advanced EMT to provide this level of care. Therefore early transportation to the appropriate emergency department (ED) is required. Most studies that examine the outcome of patients who experience shock secondary to trauma find that the most significant predictor of outcome is the time spent on the scene. Longer on-scene time is directly related to a higher degree of mortality. Although not always considered to be so, prompt transport is a highly effective treatment modality and should remain a high priority in the patient care plan. The prehospital standard of care for the patient in shock is rapid assessment, aggressive treatment of life-threatening injury or illness, and expeditious transport to the appropriate ED.

IMMEDIATE CONCERNS

❶ **What is the patient's hemodynamic status?** If the patient is hemodynamically unstable, immediate resuscitation is warranted, including immediate transport, oxygen administration, establishment of large-bore IV access, and possibly fluid resuscitation. If the patient is in compensated shock, prompt transport, as well as the previous treatments, is necessary. Those patients in cardiogenic or arrythmogenic shock require electrocardiogram (ECG) monitoring and may require pharmacologic or electrical therapy.

❶ **What is the patient's mental status?** Anxiousness, agitation, or confusion may indicate inadequate cerebral perfusion. Continued resuscitation and prompt transport are indicated.

❶ **Does the patient have a tension pneumothorax?** Immediate needle decompression of the chest is warranted and should result in significant rapid improvement. Continued resuscitation and prompt transport are indicated.

❶ **Is there evidence of uncontrollable bleeding?** Some evidence suggests that patients with uncontrollable hemorrhage might benefit from being treated without the traditional IV fluid resuscitation. This concept is presently controversial, but its premise is that IV fluids may actually increase the rate of bleeding. Proposed mechanisms for the increased bleeding include hydraulic acceleration of bleeding caused by elevated blood pressure, dislodgment of soft clots, and dilution of clotting factors. Proponents of this theory suggest withholding preoperative IV fluids in patients with uncontrollable bleeding.

IMPORTANT HISTORY

❷ **What is the mechanism of injury?** Knowledge of the mechanism of injury allows you to look for and treat hidden injuries such as spinal injury, cardiac tamponade, tension pneumothorax, fractures, pelvic injury, and intraabdominal injuries. Be sure to consider the medical causes of shock in patients who do not present with a traumatic mechanism of injury. Examples of these causes are myocardial infarction, anaphylaxis, arrhythmias, gastrointestinal (GI) bleeding, ruptured or leaking abdominal aortic aneurysm (AAA), ectopic pregnancy in women of child-bearing age, and severe hypoxia.

❷ **Does the patient complain of any specific symptoms?** Obtaining a medical history is still important. The treatment of the patient whose chest pain is a result of a minor motor vehicle accident may be markedly different than the treatment of the patient whose chest pain is the result of trauma to the chest.

❷ **Is the patient taking any new medications?** A patient's hypotension may be a result of a new antihypertensive agent.

DIFFERENTIAL DIAGNOSIS

HYPOVOLEMIC SHOCK

• *HEMORRHAGIC SHOCK.* In the context of severe trauma, acute blood loss is usually obvious; however, patients can lose a great deal of blood into the thoracic, abdominal, and pelvic cavities. A thorough examination of the patient can be a life-saving measure in itself. GI bleeding may be less obvious if it has been gradual; ask about melena, hematemesis, and hematochezia. Consider the diagnosis of ectopic pregnancy in all women of childbearing age who complain of abdominal or pelvic pain. Patients with burns lose massive amounts of fluids and can easily be hypovolemic.

- ***OTHER FLUID LOSSES.*** Severe diarrhea, vomiting, diuresis, or some combination of these features may lead to dehydration and hypovolemia.

DISTRIBUTIVE SHOCK

Distributive shock may result from poor vascular tone or the maldistribution of blood. Specific examples of this type of shock include sepsis, anaphylaxis, severe acidosis, or central nervous system (CNS) injury in the case of spinal shock.

PUMP FAILURE

Pump failure may result from any illness or injury that causes a decrease in the heart's ability to pump, such as heart wall damage from an acute myocardial infarction (AMI) or arrhythmias. The common pathway is a drop in cardiac output that causes decreased tissue perfusion. If any arrhythmia is the cause, then treatment of the arrhythmia may result in a dramatic improvement in the patient's hemodynamic status. Cardiogenic shock is a clinical syndrome characterized by hypotension and inadequate perfusion in the setting of an injury to the heart; most often, an AMI is the underlying cause. It is generally agreed that when 40% or more of the left ventricle is infarcted, the heart has difficulty maintaining an adequate cardiac output. This condition is manifested by hypotension. The patient in cardiogenic shock has a poor prognosis, with a mortality rate greater than 80%. This poor prognosis is due, in part, to the failure of the normal compensatory mechanism, mediated by the sympathetic nervous system, to compensate for poor perfusion (tachycardia and increased peripheral vascular resistance). In addition, an increased workload on the heart and, therefore, an increase in myocardial oxygen demand exacerbate the shock syndrome. The increase in oxygen demand may increase the infarct size and further decrease myocardial function; thus the prognosis is poor.

OBSTRUCTIVE SHOCK

Obstructive shock results from impaired filling of the heart. There are three major causes:

- **TENSION PNEUMOTHORAX.** A tension pneumothorax usually results from trauma. It may, however, result from a spontaneous pneumothorax. Physical examination findings may include absent or diminished breath sounds, tracheal deviation away from the tension pneumothorax, and jugular vein distension (JVD).

- **PERICARDIAL TAMPONADE.** Pericardial tamponade may result from penetrating or blunt trauma to the chest. It may develop over a period ranging from minutes to approximately 1 week. Muffled heart tones, together with JVD and narrowed pulse pressure (known as Beck's triad), may be found in pericardial tamponade. Several atraumatic causes also exist, including pericardial effusions resulting from renal disease, acute leukemias, lymphomas, breast cancer, lung cancer, and ovarian cancer.

- **PULMONARY EMBOLISM.** Pulmonary embolism is an important cause of obstructive shock. Risk factors include a history of atrial fibrillation, obesity, pregnancy, prolonged immobilization, trauma, oral contraceptive use, surgery, and cancer. Common symptoms include chest pain in 88% of patients, dyspnea in 84% of patients, and cough in 53% of patients. Common physical findings include tachypnea (respiratory rate greater than 16 breaths per minute) in 92% of patients, tachycardia (heart rate greater than 100 bpm) in 44% of patients, and temperature of approximately 100° F in 43% of patients.

KEY PHYSICAL EXAMINATION FINDINGS

✔ **Initial assessment.** Look for signs of shock.

- ***Vital signs.*** Assess for tachycardia and tachypnea, which usually precede hypotension. Hypotension is a late sign of shock.

- ***Skin.*** Inspect for temperature, appearance, and signs of moisture or dryness. Skin is usually cool, pale, and moist in the patient who has experienced shock. However, the skin may be warm and dry in the patient with spinal or septic shock. Hives may be present in patients with anaphylaxis.

- ***Neck.*** Check for the presence of JVD. In the shock patient, JVD may indicate an obstructive shock—consider tension pneumothorax, pericardial tamponade, and massive pulmonary embolism. Assess for tracheal deviation.

- ***Lungs.*** Assess for evidence of tension pneumothorax. Evidence of blunt trauma or penetrating trauma should raise suspicion of intrathoracic injury, including pericardial tamponade, tension pneumothorax, and hemothorax.

- ***Heart.*** Assess for muffled heart tones.

- ***Abdomen.*** Assess for evidence of penetrating or blunt trauma, which may indicate intraabdominal injury. In addition, check for the pulsatile abdominal mass found in patients with an AAA.

- ***Peripheral pulses.*** Check for peripheral pulses. They may be absent as perfusion decreases. Radial pulses are usually present when the systolic BP is greater than 80 mm Hg, femoral pulses indicate a systolic BP greater than 60 mm Hg, and carotid pulses indicate a systolic BP greater than 50 mm Hg. Unequal pulses may be found in the patient with an AAA.

- ***Mental status.*** An altered mental status is a sensitive indicator of inadequate cerebral perfusion.

- ***Neurologic examination.*** Assess for head or spinal trauma.

ELECTROCARDIOGRAM

Cardiac monitoring is most helpful when treating shock caused by pump failure; however, all shock patients should be monitored.

TREATMENT PLAN

- *Patient assessment.* Perform a rapid and systematic initial assessment, and institute treatment as life-threatening problems are discovered. Prompt transport to the appropriate ED is a key intervention. A focused physical examination should be performed once the initial assessment and all initial survey interventions have been accomplished. Frequent reassessment of patients in shock is necessary because of the potential for worsening of their hemodynamic status. Be prepared—potential for cardiac arrest exists.

- *Communications.* Consult with a medical control physician for guidance and institution of appropriate orders, as well as for notification of the receiving ED. Such consultation may prove invaluable in the care of the patient in shock.

GENERAL TREATMENT GUIDELINES:
PATIENT WHO IS HEMODYNAMICALLY STABLE

- Administer **O₂** and **provide ventilatory support** as needed. This includes needle-chest decompression of the tension pneumothorax if indicated.

- Place patient in the **shock position** (supine with legs elevated). Protect the cervical spine as indicated.

- **Treat nonlife-threatening injuries** (e.g., control bleeding, splint fractures).

- Establish **large-bore IV access with 0.9% NaCl or lactated Ringer's solution.**

- **Transport to appropriate ED.** Ensure patient comfort en route.

GENERAL TREATMENT GUIDELINES:
PATIENT WHO IS HEMODYNAMICALLY UNSTABLE

- Administer **O₂** and **provide ventilatory support** as needed. This includes needle-chest decompression of the tension pneumothorax.

- Place patient in the **shock position** (supine with legs elevated).

- Establish **large-bore IV access with 0.9% NaCl or lactated Ringer's solution and begin fluid resuscitation.** Controversial therapy note: Some EMS experts recommend withholding IV fluid resuscitation in the context of penetrating trauma with uncontrollable hemorrhage unless the patient is in extremis. If transportation is delayed or the patient does not respond adequately to 2 to 3 liters of crystalloid infusion, consider infusing colloid solutions, such as plasmanate or hespan. If response to ongoing fluid resuscitation is inadequate, consider using vasopressors such as dopamine 2 to 20 μg/kg per minute IV infusion (pediatric dosing: start at 1 μg/kg per minute), titrated to systolic blood pressure greater than 90 mm Hg. Vasopressors are a temporary last-ditch effort to be used only after the patient does not respond to fluid resuscitation.

- **Expeditiously transport to appropriate ED.** Do not needlessly delay patient transport—expedite transport.

SPECIFIC TREATMENT GUIDELINES
Anaphylaxis

The patient experiencing anaphylactic shock should be treated using the previous guidelines, with the addition of the following therapeutic modalities:

SECTION 1

- **Maintain a patent airway.** A high flow of oxygen via non-rebreathing face mask is indicated. Immediate endotracheal intubation may be required but may be extremely difficult if angioedema or severe laryngospasm is present. Use caution to prevent trauma during the attempted intubation.

- Administer **epinephrine, 0.3 to 0.5 mg of a 1:1000 solution SC** (pediatric dose: 0.01 mg/kg SC, not to exceed 0.5 mg) if the patient is hemodynamically stable, or

- Administer **epinephrine, 0.3 to 0.5 mg of 1:10,000 solution IV** (pediatric dose: 0.1 mg/kg IV, not to exceed 0.5 mg) if the patient is hemodynamically unstable. Dose may be repeated every 5 minutes.

- Administer **diphenhydramine (Benadryl), 10 to 50 mg slow IV bolus or deep IM injection** (pediatric dose: 2 to 5 mg/kg IV or deep IM, usual dose is 10 to 30 mg).

- Administer **hydrocortisone, 100 to 500 mg IV or IM** (pediatric dose: 0.16 to 1.0 mg/kg IV or IM), or

- Administer **methylprednisolone (Solumedrol), 100 to 200 mg IV or IM** (not recommended for prehospital use in pediatric patients).

- Provide **aerosolized albuterol, (0.5 ml in 3 ml saline)** to manage bronchospasm.

- **Transport expeditiously to appropriate ED.** Do not needlessly delay patient transport. Ensure patient comfort en route.

Pericardial Tamponade

- Treat patients with tamponade using the previous general shock treatment guidelines. A surgical procedure, pericardiocentesis, is necessary to relieve the tamponade. Pericardiocentesis should only be performed by a physician skilled in its use. You should begin fluid resuscitation and transport to the appropriate ED.

Cardiogenic Shock

- The most effective means of managing cardiogenic shock is to prevent it by attempting to limit the infarct size in patients with AMIs. Treat tachycardias, symptomatic bradycardias, and hypertension occurring in the context of an AMI. The administration of O_2, nitrates, analgesia, beta blockers, and aspirin is instrumental. These modalities are covered in chapter 11.

- Administer **O_2** and **provide ventilatory support** as needed. Endotracheal intubation may be required.

- Establish **IV access.** Although most patients in cardiogenic shock have pulmonary edema, those who do not may benefit from small 0.9% NaCl fluid boluses.

- If a fluid challenge is not effective or not indicated, vasopressors should be given. Managing the patient's hypotension and hemodynamic status is difficult without the benefit of the Swan-Ganz catheter and arterial lines available in intensive care units. The following two modalities are commonly used:

- **Dobutamine, 2.5 to 10 µg/kg per minute IV infusion** (not recommended for prehospital use in pediatrics), titrated to systolic BP greater than 90 mm Hg.

- If the response is inadequate, add **dopamine, 2 to 20 µg/kg per minute IV infusion** (pediatric dosing: start at 1 µg/kg per minute), titrated to systolic BP greater than 90 mm Hg, or

- **Transport expeditiously to appropriate ED.** Do not needlessly delay patient transport—expedite transport. Ensure patient comfort en route.

Arrhythmogenic Pump Failure

- Treat the patient with shock secondary to a tachycardia or a bradycardia as outlined in chapters 6 and 44.

BIBLIOGRAPHY

Pepe, P., et al. (2002). Prehospital fluid resuscitation of the patient with major trauma. *Prehospital Emergency Care, 6,* 81–91.

Shapiro, N. (2003). Shock. In J. J. Schaider, S. R. Hayden, R. Wolfe, R., M. Barkin, & P. Rosen (Eds.), *Rosen & Barkin's 5-minute emergency medicine consult* (2nd ed., pp. 1016–1019). Philadelphia: Lippincott Williams & Wilkins.

NOTES

_____

_____

_____

_____

_____

_____

_____

_____

_____

_____

_____

_____

_____

_____

_____

CHAPTER 39

SICKLE CELL CRISIS

Owen T. Traynor, M.D.

PRESENTATION

Sickle cell disease, a genetic disease that produces abnormal hemoglobin, affects approximately 8% of all black persons in the United States. A single amino acid substitution in the hemoglobin molecule accounts for the change in behavior of the molecule, leading to abnormally shaped (sickle-shaped) red blood cells. The sickling occurs under conditions that cause deoxygenation of the hemoglobin. When the red blood cells become sickle-shaped, they can no longer easily pass through capillaries, causing the formation of thrombi and subsequent destruction (hemolysis) of the red blood cell. Multiple thrombi and hemolysis lead to ischemia, infarction, and anemia. Because multiple organs are typically involved, the presentation varies from completely asymptomatic to severe pain, dyspnea, blindness, poor healing, infection, and severe anemia.

IMMEDIATE CONCERNS

❶ **What is the patient's respiratory status?** Multiple thrombi in the pulmonary vasculature can cause a clinical picture consistent with pulmonary embolism. Patients with sickle cell disease also have an impaired immune system that predisposes them to pulmonary infections. Severe anemia may also lead to dyspnea. Pulse oximetry should be employed, as well as the administration of supplemental oxygen. The increase in oxygenation may help the sickled cells return to their normal shape.

❶ **What is the patient's mental and neurologic status?** Central nervous system manifestations occur primarily as a result of vascular occlusion. Severe anemia, narcotic overdose, or withdrawal also may be responsible for an altered mental state.

❷ **Are the patient's current complaints similar to a previous sickle cell crisis?** Different presenting complaints may indicate that something other than a sickle cell crisis may be responsible. Patients with sickle cell disease are at risk for most of the diseases that affect patients without sickle cell disease.

❷ **Are there any crisis precipitating factors present?** Often, these crises are preceded by infection: pneumonias, urinary tract infections, and pharyngitis. Dehydration, exposure to cold, acidosis, and trauma may also predispose toward a crisis.

This section focuses on sickle cell disease and its manifestations. Remember, however, that patients with sickle cell disease can have myocardial infarctions, appendicitis, strokes, and other serious illnesses. Consult the medical control physician to help differentiate clinical situations.

Sickle cell disease is a genetic disease of hemoglobin. Genes for hemoglobin are contributed by both parents. When both parents contribute the sickle cell gene to their offspring, sickle cell anemia is present. When a person receives only one sickle cell gene, he or she is said to carry the sickle cell trait. The final class of sickle cell variants are those patients who have one sickle cell gene and one gene for another abnormal hemoglobin.

- ***SICKLE CELL ANEMIA.*** Patients with sickle cell disease have two genes for sickle cell hemoglobin and therefore have the most severe disease of the sickle cell spectrum. During a severe crisis, more than 75% of the hemoglobin may be in the sickle state. This form of sickle cell disease is, in most cases, discovered during childhood (before the age of 15 years).

- **SICKLE CELL TRAIT.** Patients with sickle cell trait have one normal hemoglobin gene and one sickle cell gene, resulting in partial expression of the abnormal gene. Less than 50% of the circulating hemoglobin are abnormal, and therefore the amount of sickling hemoglobin is low. These patients do not have severe crises or anemia.

- **SICKLE CELL TRAIT AND ANOTHER ABNORMAL HEMOGLOBIN TRAIT.** Patients with sickle cell trait and another abnormal hemoglobin trait may be without significant crises or may have severe manifestations depending on the type of abnormal hemoglobin present. Diagnosis may be delayed until these patients are in their 20s or 30s.

Four types of crisis are found in sickle cell disease:

1. **Vasoocclusive** crises are caused by the formation of multiple thrombi within capillary beds. Vasoocclusive crises are by far the most common type of crisis. Symptoms include constant pain, weakness, and anxiety. The pain commonly occurs in bones, joints, abdomen, back, and chest. The pain may be mild or severe, lasting hours or longer. It may be alleviated through the administration of oxygen, IV fluids, and pain medicine. Narcotic analgesia is often required.

2. **Hemolytic** crises are caused by the premature destruction of red blood cells. Patients in hemolytic crises exhibit symptoms of anemia and jaundice.

3. **Aplastic** crises are characterized by inadequately low red and white blood cell counts. This inadequacy results from bone marrow suppression caused by concurrent infection or folic acid depression.

4. **Sequestration** crises result from the entrapment of blood cells within the liver and spleen. Patients in sequestration crises exhibit abdominal pain and an enlarged liver or spleen. In addition, their white and red blood cell counts

are low. Children in a sequestration crisis may even be in shock.

Complications of sickle cell disease include the following:

- Increased risk of cerebrovascular accident (CVA)

- Pulmonary embolism

- Hepatitis secondary to transfusions

- Hepatic infarction

- Chronic anemia

- Narcotic dependence

- Blindness

- Pulmonary infarcts

- Vascular occlusion

- Hematuria

- Predisposition to infection

- Priapism

- Congestive heart failure

- Pulmonary infections

- Splenic infarction

- Bone infarctions, osteomyelitis (bone infections)

- Seizures

- Mild dehydration secondary to decreased ability to concentrate urine

KEY PHYSICAL EXAMINATION FINDINGS

✅ *Initial assessment.* Be alert for respiratory compromise. Look for signs of inadequate perfusion.

- ✅ *Vital signs.* Assess for the presence of tachycardia, tachypnea, fever, and hypotension.

- ✅ *Lungs.* Assess breath sounds for pneumonia.

- ✅ *Abdomen.* Look for enlarged, tender liver or spleen.

- ✅ *Extremities.* Assess for inadequate circulation, swelling, or trauma.

- ✅ *Mental status.* Assess for altered mental status and neurologic deficits, which may indicate central nervous system (CNS) involvement, severe anemia, narcotic abuse, or withdrawal.

TREATMENT PLAN

- *Patient assessment.* Perform a rapid and systematic initial assessment, and institute treatment as life-threatening problems are discovered. Prompt transport to the appropriate emergency department (ED) is a key intervention. A secondary survey should be performed once all the primary interventions have been accomplished. When appropriate, be sure to consider alternative diagnoses, such as ischemic heart disease, CVA, and acute abdomen.

- Administer **supplemental O_2** to prevent or reduce additional sickling. Nasal cannula oxygen may be given to all patients in nonhypoxic sickle cell crisis. Give high-flow O_2 to hypoxic patients.

NOTE: Normal pulse oximetry readings may give a false indication of the patient's true O_2 level because the hemoglobin count is abnormally low.

- If the patient is hemodynamically unstable, place in the **shock position** (supine with legs elevated).

- Establish a **large-bore IV with 0.9% NaCl or lactated Ringer's solution.** Fluid resuscitation is a key component

SECTION 1

of ED treatment because many of these patients are mildly dehydrated. Fluid resuscitation, however, is often not needed in the prehospital phase.

- Analgesics will likely be used in the ED. Meperidine (Demerol) and morphine are most commonly used. Field use is uncommon, however.

- **Transport to appropriate ED.**

BIBLIOGRAPHY

Bowman, S. (2003). Sickle cell disease. In J. J. Schaider, S. R. Hayden, R. Wolfe, R., M. Barkin, & P. Rosen (Eds.), *Rosen & Barkin's 5-minute emergency medicine consult* (2nd ed., pp. 1024–1025). Philadelphia: Lippincott Williams & Wilkins.

Yale, S. H. (2000). Approach to the vaso-occlusive crisis in adults with sickle cell disease. *American Family Physician, 61,* 1349–56, 1364–4.

NOTES

_____

_____

_____

_____

_____

_____

_____

_____

_____

_____

CHAPTER 40

SMOKE INHALATION

Bernard Beckerman, M.D., FACEP

PRESENTATION

Patients suffering from smoke inhalation may present in many different ways. At one extreme are those found in cardiorespiratory arrest. At the opposite extreme are patients with mild conjunctival and upper airway irritation with no respiratory insufficiency. Members of the latter group may rapidly become asymptomatic after removal from the source of the smoke.

IMMEDIATE CONCERNS

❶ **Is the scene safe?** Safety of the rescuers is of prime importance. Extrication of the patient is best accomplished by those who are trained and equipped for fireground operations.

❶ **Is the patient's airway at risk?** The presence of severe burns to the lower face and anterior neck may cause upper airway edema. Early intubation should be considered. Patients who have been in a fire in a confined space and those with an altered mental status, singed nasal hair, hoarseness, and carbonaceous sputum may be at increased risk of upper airway edema caused by inhalation of superheated gases and should be considered for early intubation. Of course, those with obvious upper airway compromise, such as stridor, should be intubated.

❶ **What is the cardiorespiratory status of the patient?** If severe respiratory distress is a presenting symptom, then complete cardiorespiratory collapse may be imminent and immediate resuscitative efforts must be started.

● **What is the mental status of the patient?** A clear mental status examination in a patient after smoke inhalation gives you the opportunity to carefully plan for the patient's evaluation and treatment. Confusion, combativeness, and lethargy, or some combination of those features, are indications that a more severe exposure has occurred, and immediate action is necessary, particularly airway management.

IMPORTANT HISTORY

● **Is there evidence of carbon monoxide poisoning?** Carbon monoxide (CO) is a product of incomplete combustion, so many fire victims will be at risk of CO poisoning. The diagnosis will be confirmed after a blood gas has been obtained. Clinical features can be mild, such as mild headache, dyspnea on exertion, irritability, and fatigue. Higher levels can cause altered mental status, dyspnea at rest, myocardial ischemia, tachycardia, and seizures. Recall that the pulse oximeter cannot differentiate carboxyhemoglobin from oxyhemoglobin. Therefore the pulse oximeter's reading will be the sum of the carboxyhemoglobin plus the oxyhemoglobin saturation. High-flow oxygen should be applied as soon as the diagnosis is considered. Consider hyperbaric oxygen, if available, for those with an altered mental state, myocardial ischemia, loss of consciousness, or pregnancy.

● **Is the patient in a high-risk group?** Children and the elderly are at greater risk of serious injury. Those with comorbid illness, such as chronic obstructive pulmonary disease (COPD), congestive heart failure (CHF), coronary artery disease, tolerate smoke inhalation poorly.

● **Has the patient been exposed to unusual chemicals in the fire?** If the fire is in an industrial context, it may be possible to identify chemicals that cause injury to the respiratory tract and those that may cause systemic illness. Many of the chemicals found in residential fires can cause bronchospasm, laryngeal edema, and pulmonary edema. These problems may be delayed several hours. Cyanide has been found in the smoke of residential fires.

DIFFERENTIAL DIAGNOSIS

- **THERMAL INJURY.** Thermal injury to the airway can occur when the patient has inhaled superheated gases. Most of the injury will be limited to the upper airway because the upper airway is very efficient at conditioning the air for the lower airways. Inhalation of steam or hot water vapor may cause a lower airway injury. Thermal injury may appear mild initially but can rapidly progress, causing an upper airway obstruction. Early intubation is recommended. Clues that suggest an upper airway thermal injury include singed nasal hairs, carbonaceous sputum, stridor, a history of a loss of consciousness, a fire in a confined space, and a prolonged exposure.

- **LOCAL CHEMICAL INJURY.** Some of the products of combustion may cause a chemical injury to the airways and lung tissues. It is not common to be able to identify these chemicals, and specific antidotes do not exist. Typical clinical findings can include laryngeal edema or laryngospasm, bronchospasm, noncardiogenic pulmonary edema, arrhythmias, and hypoxia. Symptoms can often have a delayed onset.

- **SYSTEMIC CHEMICAL POISONING.** Two important chemicals that are found in the products of combustion include CO and cyanide. The paramedic must have a high index of suspicion because diagnostic testing of the patient is not usually possible in the field. It is possible to measure environmental CO levels, however.

  o **CO poisoning** will be a clinical diagnosis and should be suspected when the patient has been exposed to smoke and has some of the following signs or symptoms: headache, shortness of breath, tachycardia, tachypnea, altered mental status, seizures, or evidence of cardiac ischemia. The pulse oximeter's reading will indicate the sum of the saturations of both oxyhemo-globin and carboxyhemoglobin. Do not expect to see the "cherry-red" skin coloration—it is an uncommon finding. Most patients with toxic and even lethal levels of CO do not have this skin characteristic.

o **Cyanide poisoning** is even more difficult to determine in the field. Some report the odor of bitter almonds. Cyanide poisons the cellular metabolism of oxygen. The patient will be unable to make use of the oxygen that is available. Anaerobic metabolism will occur, leading to acidosis. The symptoms have a rapid onset. The patient's symptoms will primarily be those of hypoxia—shortness of breath, headache, anxiety, and altered mental status. Tachycardia and hypertension are found initially, but the patient may become hypotensive and bradycardic before suffering cardiac arrest. If the poisoning is mild supplemental oxygen may be all that is needed. In severe poisoning, a cyanide antidote kit should be used.

KEY PHYSICAL EXAMINATION FINDINGS

- ✓ *Initial assessment.* Look for alterations in mental status, respiratory compromise, and hemodynamic instability.

- ✓ *Vital signs.* Careful monitoring of the vital signs is needed.

- ✓ *HEENT.* Examine carefully and note signs of facial burns, singed nasal hairs, carbonaceous sputum, stridor, and anterior neck burns.

- ✓ *Lungs.* Listen to lung sounds for signs of bronchospasm and pulmonary edema. Assess for circumferential burns of the chest.

- ✓ *Extremities.* Assess for burns and other evidence of trauma.

- ✓ *Skin.* Assess for burns. Compute body surface area (BSA).

ELECTROCARDIOGRAM

Evaluate for signs of cardiac ischemia or injury.

GLUCOMETER

Evaluate in patients with an altered mental state.

TREATMENT PLAN

- *Patient assessment.* Perform a rapid and systematic initial assessment, and institute treatment as life-threatening problems are discovered. Prompt transport to the appropriate ED is a key intervention. Frequent reassessment of the patient with smoke inhalation is necessary because of the potential for worsening. Be prepared—the potential for cardiac arrest exists. See chapter 7 regarding specific therapy for the burned patient.

PATIENT WHO IS HEMODYNAMICALLY UNSTABLE

- Administer **O$_2$** and **provide ventilatory support** as needed. Consider early intubation if findings suggest an upper airway injury.

- Place patient in **shock position** if shock is apparent.

- Establish **large-bore IV access with 0.9% NaCL or lactated Ringer's solution** and begin immediate fluid resuscitation. Obtain venous blood specimens for laboratory analysis.

- Consider possibility of cyanide poisoning if no source of hypotension is apparent.

- **Transport expeditiously to the appropriate ED.** Burn units and hyperbaric facilities should be considered.

- Do not needlessly delay transport—expedite transport. Treat associated injuries en route. Ensure patient comfort en route.

PATIENT WHO IS HEMODYNAMICALLY STABLE

- **Administer O$_2$ and provide ventilatory support** as needed. Consider early intubation if findings suggest an upper airway injury.

- Establish **large-bore IV access with 0.9% NaCL or lactated Ringer's solution.** Obtain venous blood specimens for laboratory analysis.

- **Transport expeditiously to the appropriate ED.** Consider transport to burn unit or hyperbaric facility if either of these matches patient needs.

- Do not needlessly delay transport—expedite transport. Treat associated injuries en route. Ensure patient comfort en route.

BIBLIOGRAPHY

Cheeseman, M. M. & H. L. Boozer (2004). Burns and smoke inhalation. In C. K. Stone & R. L. Humphries (Eds.), *Current emergency diagnosis and treatment* (5th ed., pp. 917–929). New York: McGraw-Hill.

Lee-Chong, T. L. (1999, February). Smoke inhalation injury. *Postgraduate Medicine, 105,* 55–62.

NOTES

_____

_____

_____

_____

_____

_____

_____

CHAPTER 41

SPINAL CORD INJURY

Thomas J. Rahilly, Ph.D.

PRESENTATION

Patients with spinal cord injury (SCI) pose a special set of challenges to the prehospital emergency medical services (EMS) provider: They can present with virtually no symptoms to complete paralysis and shock. The patient with obvious signs and symptoms of severe SCI, although in need of immediate immobilization and resuscitation, does not create difficult treatment plan decisions for the paramedic. Such patients must be fully immobilized, receive treatment for shock, and be transported to a Level I trauma center. Recently, however, the treatment of patients with no neurologic deficit, or those with only a mechanism of injury suggesting the possibility of SCI, has created yet another controversy in EMS practice. Recent studies have shown that EMS providers can safely rule out significant SCI if they use a standard evaluation tool. This new strategy is contrary to the old adage that "any trauma patient should be considered spinally injured until proven otherwise." If there are indications that an SCI may have occurred, the patient should be fully immobilized with a cervical collar and long backboard.

IMMEDIATE CONCERNS

❶ **Does the patient require cervical spinal immobilization?**
Two clinical decision rules were recently developed and validated to help reduce the number of patients who require cervical spine x-rays before they can be removed from spinal immobilization devices. These decision rules are being used by some EMS systems to "clinically clear" patients so they do not require cervical spine

immobilization. The rules are described in the physical exam section.

❶ **Is the patient's airway patent and stable?** Patients with a central nervous system (CNS) injury from either head or spinal cord trauma may be unable to protect their airway. Often SCI is associated with facial injuries that cause both bleeding and swelling, leading to airway compromise. All airway interventions must be performed without endangering the cervical spine. Endotracheal intubation may be required, but neutral in-line cervical spine immobilization must be maintained.

❷ **Are there any signs of abnormal respiration?** Patients with an SCI may exhibit signs of inadequate or severely restricted respiratory effort. Depending on the location of the injury, the patient may show signs of unequal or limited excursion of the chest or diaphragmatic breathing. In addition to immobilization and expeditious transport, these patients must receive ventilatory assistance that is coordinated with their own respiratory effort.

❸ **Is the patient hemodynamically stable?** In addition to neurogenic shock, hemodynamic instability in the context of an SCI injury usually means that there may be other, hidden injuries: Look for evidence of internal trauma—intrathoracic, intraabdominal, and intrapelvic. Treat the patient for shock while protecting the spine. Expedite transport to the closest trauma center.

❹ **Is there evidence of an SCI?** During the initial assessment a brief neurologic exam is performed. Spinal precautions should be instituted for patients who are not alert and who have suffered trauma. Alterations in mental status, whether caused by trauma, substance abuse, or dementia, may make the patient unable to accurately report symptoms. The focused history and physical exam may provide additional evidence of a neurologic deficit.

❺ **What is the mechanism of injury?** Direct trauma to the head, neck, or back is the primary cause of SCI.

Although the mechanism is often apparent, the EMS provider must sometimes actively seek a history of trauma. This approach is especially important when evaluating a patient who abuses drugs or alcohol who may have fallen and injured his or her head and cervical spine several days before exhibiting signs and symptoms of the event. Have a high index of suspicion when called to evaluate an elderly patient who may have an SCI. Elderly people have brittle bones, and it take less force to cause a cervical spine injury. The paramedic should carefully evaluate at-risk patients if there is a history or mechanism that indicates the possibility of an SCI. Some believe that SCI can remain silent until something aggravates the injured area, such as displacement of a fracture by movement of a patient who was not immobilized. Even when using out-of-hospital "rule out" SCI protocols, the at-risk patient population deserves special spine care consideration.

IMPORTANT HISTORY

❷ **Has there been a loss of consciousness?** Loss of consciousness requires significant force transmitted to the brain. Patients with a head injury severe enough to have lost consciousness may be at risk of SCI. Patients who have suffered a major trauma leading to loss of consciousness require immobilization of the spine.

❷ **Does the patient have an altered mental status?** It is prudent to assume that any patient with altered consciousness who has suffered trauma has also suffered damage to the cervical spine and spinal cord; subsequent immobilization of the neck and spine must therefore be used. The patient's mental status is the most sensitive indicator of brain function. The range of alteration of consciousness extends from transient and mild symptoms, such as seeing stars, momentary amnesia, restlessness, vomiting, and headache, to profound symptoms, such as focal neurologic deficits, stroke, paralysis, seizures, coma, shock, respiratory arrest, and death.

❼ **Is the patient's neurologic injury improving or worsening?** A patient with a CNS injury, whether to the brain, spinal cord or both, requires constant assessment by the paramedic. The treatment on arrival at the ED may depend on the severity and progression of the injury and requires sequential neurologic assessment. The Glasgow Coma Scale (GCS) should be noted initially and monitored during transport. A loss in the GCS of two or more points is an alarming sign: Expedite transport. A simple way to look at CNS injuries is that they are of three types: those that are improving, those that are stable, and those that are worsening. Those that are worsening may require a more aggressive neurosurgical approach.

❼ **Are there distracting injuries, or is the patient's ability to feel pain impaired?** Often, EMS personnel must rely on the patient's self-reporting of symptoms to discover injury. If there are other significant painful injuries, the patient may not accurately report the pain of a vertebral fracture. Conversely, symptoms of other significant injuries may be blocked by the anesthetic effect of a spinal cord lesion. A patient who has been drinking alcohol or using pain medications or substances of abuse may be too impaired and to report pain. These patients should be treated as if they have a SCI and immobilized.

DIFFERENTIAL DIAGNOSIS

- *CERVICAL, THORACIC, LUMBAR, AND SACRAL SPINE INJURIES.* Injuries of the musculoskeletal portion of the neck and back include fractures, dislocations, and subluxations, as well as injuries to the cervical ligaments, muscles, and tendons. These injuries can exist without SCI. Cervical and lumbrosacral strains are a common sequelae of motor vehicle collisions. Some cervical injuries, particularly bony and ligamentous injuries, may be unstable. The conscious patient typically reports neck pain and possibly stiffness. Posterior midline bony tenderness suggests the possible presence of an injury that would benefit from immobilization.

- **SPINAL CORD INJURIES.**   Although SCIs may be associated with vertebral fractures, or disruption of the spinal ligaments, they may also occur in the absence of bony or ligamentous injury (e.g., where there is a hematoma or vascular compromise). Conversely, vertebral injury, such as fractures or herniated intervertebral discs, can exist without signs of cord injury. SCIs can be classified as complete or partial cord syndromes. Complete spinal cord lesions create a total loss of motor and sensation distal to the site of injury. Three common partial spinal cord lesions exist.

  o In the **central cord syndrome,** the most common type of partial cord lesion, a ligament adjacent to the spine buckles into the cord during hyperflexion, causing a contusion of the central portion of the cord. The findings are usually characterized by weakness in the arms greater than in the legs, with the hands being affected more than the upper arms. This imbalance is due to the more central location of the nerves innervating the upper extremities and hands.

  o The **anterior cord syndrome,** another partial syndrome, is caused by either compression of the anterior spinal cord or compression of the anterior spinal artery that supplies the anterior spinal cord. Paralysis and loss of pain and temperature sensation distal to the injury are evident, but because the posterior aspect of the spinal cord is spared, the ability to sense light, touch, vibration, motion, and position is retained.

  o The **Brown-Sequard syndrome,** or lateral cord syndrome, develops when the lateral half of the spinal cord is transected or injured, often as a result of a knife wound or gunshot wound. Here one finds loss of motor function distal to the injury on the same side of the body and loss of pain and temperature sensation distal to the injury on the other side of the body.

SCIs can cause neurogenic shock. Common findings include quadriplegia, absence of spinal reflexes, and absence of autonomic nervous system reflexes, all leading to poor vasomotor tone. Typical systolic blood pressure is between 80 and 100 mm Hg. The hypotension is accompanied by bradycardia and warm, pink, and dry skin. Thermoregulation is usually impaired secondary to loss of the ability to appropriately vasoconstrict or vasodilate, impaired sweating, and impaired ability to shiver. "Spinal" shock is usually a transient phenomenon, lasting from hours to weeks.

KEY PHYSICAL EXAMINATION FINDINGS

- ✓ *Initial assessment.* Look for compromised airway, difficult breathing, and signs of shock or acute hemorrhage. Consider the mechanism of injury and institute spinal precautions when indicated. If the patient is in shock, look for a hidden injury in addition to suspecting spinal or neurogenic shock.

- ✓ *Vital signs.* Be alert for signs of inadequate respiration: shallow or unequal chest excursion and diaphragmatic breathing.

- ✓ *HEENT.* Look for signs of head injury. If there has been enough force to cause head trauma, also suspect SCI.

- ✓ *Neck.* Stabilize the cervical spine as needed. Examine the cervical spine per cervical spine clearance protocols if authorized by local medical command.

- ✓ *Abdomen/pelvis.* Assess for priapism.

- ✓ *Extremities.* Assess for any gross motor or sensory deficits and warm, pink, and dry skin.

- ✓ *Posterior body.* Carefully palpate the spine for pain, tenderness, and deformity.

🛇 ***Neurologic examination.*** Assess the level of consciousness, record GCS, and perform assessment of motor and
sensory status.

CERVICAL SPINE CLEARANCE PROTOCOLS

Listed below are the two competing protocols for cervical spine clearance. Currently the NEXUS criteria are
more widely used. Controversy exists regarding which of
the two rules performs the best. Decisions regarding the
use of prehospital cervical spine clearance are best left to
local medical direction.

🛇 The **NEXUS** (National Emergency X-Radiology Utilization
Study) **low risk criteria** are as follows:

1. No posterior midline cervical tenderness

2. Normal level of alertness

3. No evidence of intoxication

4. No focal neurologic deficit

5. No distracting injury

If all of the low-risk criteria are present, cervical spine
x-rays are not necessary and the patient therefore does not
require cervical spine immobilization.

🛇 The **Canadian Cervical Spine rule,** a more complex
algorithm, may be used when the adult patient (16 years
of age or older) is alert and stable. The GCS must be 15.

1. The presence of any high risk factor listed below mandates immobilization.

- Age 65 years or older

- Dangerous mechanism

    o Fall greater than 1 meter/5 stairs

    o Axial load to head

o High-speed motor vehicle collision (greater than 62 mph), rollover or ejection, motorized recreational vehicles, bicycle collision

- Numbness or tingling in extremities

2. If there are no high-risk factors, assess for the presence of low-risk factors (listed below) that allow safe assessment of range of motion. If none are present, immobilization is necessary.

o Simple rear-end motor vehicle collisions (exclusions include being pushed into oncoming traffic, being hit by a bus or large truck, rollover, hit by a high-speed vehicle [greater than 62 mph])

o Ambulatory at any time at scene

o No neck pain at scene

o Absence of midline cervical spine tenderness

3. If at least one of the above low-risk factors are present, the patient is asked to actively rotate his or her neck 45 degrees left and right, regardless of pain. If the patient is able to rotate 45 degrees in both directions, cervical spine immobilization is not required. Immobilize the patient if the patient is unable to perform the rotation.

TREATMENT PLAN

- **Patient assessment.** Perform a rapid and systematic initial assessment, and institute treatment as life-threatening problems are discovered. Prompt transport to the appropriate ED, preferably to a Level I trauma center, is a key intervention. A rapid trauma assessment should be performed once the initial assessment and all attendant interventions have been accomplished. Frequent reassessment of the patient with an SCI injury is necessary because of the potential for a rapidly worsening neurologic status. Be prepared—the potential for respiratory insufficiency exists.

- Administer **O₂** and **provide ventilatory support,** including endotracheal intubation, as indicated; protect the cervical spine. **If GCS is 8 or lower, the patient should be intubated**.

- If a mechanism of injury suggests the possibility of SCI, the patient requires spinal immobilization.

- Establish **large-bore IV access** with 0.9% NaCL or lactated Ringer's.

- **Treat for shock.** See chapter 38.

- Consider use of **methylprednisolone, 30 mg/kg IV bolus,** followed by an IV infusion of 5.4 mg/kg per hour. This is a controversial therapy.

- If the patient has an altered mental status, treat for head injury. See chapter 20.

- Treat nonlife-threatening injuries as appropriate (e.g., control bleeding, splint fractures).

- Transport to appropriate ED. Ensure patient comfort en route. Do not needlessly delay patient transport—expedite transport.

BIBLIOGRAPHY

Bledsoe, B. E., R. S. Porter, & R. A. Cherry (Eds). (2003). *Essentials of paramedic care.* Englewood Cliffs, N.J.: Prentice-Hall.

Gabbey, D. (2004). Cervical spine injury. In E. T. Dickinson & A. W. Stern (Eds.), *ALS case studies* (pp. 1068–1097). Upper Saddle River, N.J.: Prentice-Hall.

Hoffman, J. R., Mower, W. R., Wolfson, A. B., Todd, K. H., & Zucker, M. I. (2003). Validity of a set of clinical criteria to rule out injury to the cervical spine in patients with blunt trauma. *New England Journal of Medicine, 353,* 94–99.

National Association of Emergency Medical Technicians. (1999). *Basic and advanced prehospital trauma life support student manual* (4th ed., pp. 186–199). St. Louis, MO: Mosby.

Stiell, I. G., G. A. Wells, K. L. Vandemheen, et al. (2001). The Canadian c-spine rule for radiography in alert and stable trauma patients. *Journal of the American Medical Association, 286,* 1841–1848.

NOTES

_____

_____

_____

_____

_____

_____

_____

_____

_____

_____

_____

_____

_____

_____

_____

_____

CHAPTER 42

SUDDEN INFANT DEATH SYNDROME

Michael A. Nagy, B.S., NREMT-P

PRESENTATION

Sudden infant death syndrome (SIDS) is defined as the sudden death of an apparently healthy infant during the first year of life and without an obvious cause. The death remains unexplained after an autopsy, examination of the infant's and family's medical history, and investigation of the scene and circumstances of death. The SIDS rate has been declining since the 1990s, with an 11% drop seen from the year 2000 to 2001. SIDS remains the third leading cause of death among infants, however, accounting for about 8% of all infant deaths. In 2001, some 2,240 infants died of SIDS.

IMMEDIATE CONCERNS

❶ **Should cardiopulmonary resuscitation (CPR) be performed?** SIDS is a diagnosis of exclusion, and all efforts should be made to resuscitate the patient who presents as pulseless and apneic, especially if the infant is potentially or questionably viable. The paramedic should follow pediatric resuscitation protocols such as pediatric advanced life support (PALS) guidelines. In some cases the patient might meet criteria for pronouncement of death in the field. Medical direction should be obtained regarding whether to initiate or continue resuscitation efforts in these instances. Given the emotional needs of the family, emergency medical services (EMS) personnel should provide rapid transport to a hospital while providing basic life support.

● **What is the emotional state of the family?** If the infant is unable to be resuscitated, the family should be the immediate focus of EMS personnel. Family members may respond to the episode with a gamut of emotions, ranging from anger to shock, denial, self-blame, and grief. Prehospital personnel should expect an unpredictable and often intense display of emotions and remain sensitive to the needs of the family. Offer support and reassurance that everything possible was done for their child. In many areas SIDS support services are available to provide counseling to the family.

IMPORTANT HISTORY

● **Is there a history of apneic events?** The role or previous episodes of apnea have not been clearly linked to SIDS cases. A variety of causes including cardiac, respiratory, central nervous system, and anatomic airway abnormalities are suggested to be risk factors. An apparent life-threatening event (ALTE) is an episode of prolonged apnea (more than 20 seconds) associated with a change in skin color. It is believed that infants who have experienced ALTEs probably have definable pathology and are believed to be at greater risk for cardiac or respiratory arrest.

● **Does the infant have any chronic, congenital, or recent illnesses?** Infants with a history of congenital abnormalities or chronic illness may be predisposed to complicating factors resulting in an ALTE. Recent respiratory illnesses could precipitate severe bronchospasm, hypoxia, or pneumonia. Hypoglycemia or cardiovascular shock in infants may be a result of sepsis.

● **Has there been a recent injury?** Inspection of the surrounding area and recent history may indicate that a traumatic event may have occurred. Appropriate trauma management techniques should be employed in these instances.

❷ When was the infant last seen, and what was the infant doing? Prearrest activity may give a clue as to the cause of the patient's cardiopulmonary arrest. Such events may include aspiration, fall, accidental drug overdose, and poisoning. The infant's sleeping conditions may also be a contributing factor. Hypercarbia resulting from rebreathing carbon dioxide trapped in soft bedding may lead to a lack of arousal from airway obstruction or possible "rebreathing asphyxia." The information gathered can give some indication of the duration of cardiopulmonary arrest and the success of any resuscitation effort.

❷ Was CPR performed by a bystander? As in any arrest situation, this is a necessary piece of information to be gathered. When determining whether CPR was performed, the paramedic should strive to inquire in a way that does not make the family member or guardian feel neglectful if CPR was not promptly instituted.

DIFFERENTIAL DIAGNOSES

- **FOREIGN BODY OBSTRUCTION OR ASPIRATION.** The presence of any airway obstruction requires aggressive clearing of the infant's airway. Techniques such as suctioning, back blows, and chest thrusts may need to be used in clearing the airway.

- **ASPHYXIATION.** Sleeping conditions linked to the increased incidence of SIDS include objects that may entrap gas such as soft bedding, blankets, or soft toys. Accidental smothering can occur from pillows present in the crib. Infants sleeping in a prone position have also been shown to suffer a higher incidence of SIDS. The American Academy of Pediatrics recommend that the infant be placed in a supine position when sleeping to allow good air circulation near the face.

- **HYPOTHERMIA/HYPERTHERMIA.** Because infants have a large body surface area-to-mass ratio, inadequate heating or coverings may result in rapid heat loss. Resumption of a normal cardiac rhythm may be difficult to achieve until adequate rewarming has occurred. Conversely, overheating caused by heavy clothing, overdressing, or high room temperature may cause an increased metabolic rate that leads to life-threatening conditions.

- **SEPSIS.** A major cause of cardiac arrest in previously healthy infants is overwhelming sepsis in the presence of an immature immune system. Meningitis and pneumonia should be considered as primary causes.

- **INGESTION OF TOXINS OR POISONING.** Overdoses of medicines or accidental ingestion of illicit drugs or other substances should be considered. The winter months pose a greater risk for carbon monoxide poisoning.

- **TRAUMA.** The history may include recent instances of trauma or shaking. Such events may lead to subdural hematomas, and the presence of retinal hemorrhages, vomitus in the vicinity of the infant, or bulging fontanelles are some important indicators.

- **ABUSE.** Child abuse may be a possible explanation for the infant found in cardiopulmonary arrest. Be aware of other physical findings such as multiple bruises, abnormal markings, or burns. Such physical findings in conjunction with a vague history, caregiver detachment, and delays in seeking medical treatment for the infant or other curious behavior should be noted and reported as required by local statute. See chapter 12.

KEY PHYSICAL EXAMINATION FINDINGS

- ✅ **Initial assessment.** Assess for airway, breathing, and circulation. Pay particular attention to possible sources of airway obstruction; hypoxia is the most common cause of infant cardiac arrest.

- ✅ **HEENT.** Assess for trauma.

- ✅ **Lungs.** Assess for obstruction and pneumothorax.

- ✅ ***Heart.*** Assess for heart sounds.

- ✅ ***Crib examination.*** Inspect the crib for objects that could cause foreign body airway obstruction or asphyxia, particularly vomitus, buttons, and small toys.

- ✅ ***Environmental assessment.*** Include an assessment of the environment in which the infant was found. Room temperature, electrical hazards, use of space heaters, strange odors, particularly the smell of gas, may provide important information regarding the cause of the arrest.

- ✅ ***Assess effectiveness of CPR efforts.*** Provide BLS care in accordance with current AHA and PALS guidelines.

TREATMENT PLAN

- **Patient assessment.** Assess for airway, breathing, circulation, skin color, and temperature. In some instances, rigor mortis may be present.

- **Initiate BLS.** In some cases, the most appropriate or only option is to institute BLS with rapid transport to a hospital.

- **Establish an airway.** Endotracheal intubation is recommended if a prolonged transport is likely.

- **Establish a route for drug and fluid administration.** IV or IO access is required for medication or fluid administration. If an ET tube has been placed, drugs may be administered by this route according to the requirements for dosages and strengths.

- **Institute advanced life support.** Follow current AHA or PALS guidelines. Local protocols may also provide medical direction to EMS personnel. See chapter 9.

- Consider giving a **fluid bolus** of 20 ml/kg of normal saline solution (0.9% NaCl).

- Consider the administration of 25% **dextrose** at 2 to 4 ml/kg slow IV or IO push.

- Consider persistent hypoxia, acidosis, tension pneumothorax, or cardiac tamponade.

- Ensure **adequate rewarming.**

- **Attend to the emotional needs of the infant's caregivers.** EMS personnel should refrain from being overly optimistic or providing false encouragement. Allow family members to be present during the resuscitation. If resuscitation is not indicated, be supportive and assist them in contacting other family members and mobilizing support. If transported to a hospital, direct the family to a private room or an individual that may provide support resources.

BIBLIOGRAPHY

Centers for Disease Control and Prevention, Division of Vital Statistics. (2001). National vital statistics report, Vol. 52, No. 2. Infant Mortality Statistics from the 2001 Linked Birth/Infant Death Data Set. Washington, D. C.: Author.

Fleisher, G. R. & S. Ludwig (2000). *Textbook of pediatric medicine* (4th ed.). Philadelphia: Lippincott Williams & Wilkins.

Sanders, M. J. (2001). *Paramedic textbook* (Rev. 2nd ed.). St. Louis, MO: Mosby.

NOTES

_____

_____

_____

_____

_____

_____

_____

CHAPTER 43

SYNCOPE

David J. Gross, MPAS, PA-C

PRESENTATION

Syncope is a sudden, transient loss of consciousness with a loss of postural tone. The episode may last from several seconds to several minutes. Syncope may also be accompanied by myoclonic activity normally lasting 30 seconds or less. Longer-lasting myoclonic activity may be due to a seizure. Although most causes of syncope are benign, syncope of a cardiovascular nature is a serious prodromal sympton of sudden death. In athletes, 30% of deaths during exercise have been preceded by a syncopal event.

IMMEDIATE CONCERNS

● **Is the patient hemodynamically stable?** Hemodynamic instability that fails to quickly return to normal after a syncopal episode may indicate a more serious illness. Early monitoring of the electrocardiogram (ECG) as well as performing a history and physical exam will guide early resuscitation efforts.

● **Did the patient suffer any significant injuries resulting from the syncopal episode?** Consider the possibility of central nervous system (CNS) injury as well as orthopedic and soft-tissue injuries resulting from a fall. Protect the cervical spine as indicated.

IMPORTANT HISTORY

● **What was the patient doing immediately before the syncopal episode?** Syncope that occurs in the supine position suggests a cardiac origin. The presence of palpitations or tachycardia suggests syncope of a cardiac origin. Physical or emotional distress, prolonged standing, fatigue, swallowing, micturition, defecation, and severe pain can precede vasovagal syncope. A severe headache before the syncopal episode can occur with a subarachnoid hemorrhage (SAH).

❓ **What were symptoms at the onset of the episode?** The onset of vasovagal syncope is usually gradual. Prodromal symptoms include complaints of nausea, diaphoresis, palpitations, darkening of vision, and a sensation of faintness. Seizures occur suddenly, in any position, asleep or awake.

❓ **Did the patient have seizurelike muscle activity?** It is possible for tonic clonic muscle activity to happen as syncope occurs. The patient with syncope does not have a postictal period. In contrast, the patient with seizures is postictal, often has a history of seizures, and is more likely to have become incontinent. Patients experiencing seizures are also more likely to bite their tongue.

❓ **Is there a serious underlying medical condition?** Syncope can be a symptom of a more serious problem, such as an acute myocardial infarction, pulmonary embolism, abdominal aortic aneurysm (AAA), aortic dissection, cardiac outflow obstruction, pericardial tamponade, pulmonary hypertension, anemia, hypoxemia, or ruptured ectopic pregnancy.

❓ **What medication is the patient taking?** New medications or a change in dosages is a very common cause of syncope in the elderly. Drugs associated with syncope include vasoactive agents such as beta blockers, calcium channel blockers, nitrates, hydralazine, ACE inhibitors, and diuretics. Antihistamines, sedatives-hypnotics, antiemetics, and psychiatric medications have also been associated with syncope, as have illegal drugs.

DIFFERENTIAL DIAGNOSIS

- **VASOVAGAL SYNCOPE.** Vasovagal syncope is the most common and most benign type of syncope. It is also known as simple fainting. The patient develops a relative hypovolemia caused by dilation of blood vessels. There is a prodrome of lightheadedness. The patient is standing or seated when the symptoms begin. Often there is a report of nausea, pallor, and diaphoresis. This type of syncope rapidly corrects without intervention.

- **CARDIAC CAUSES.** Dysrhythmias—either bradycardias or tachycardias—that significantly reduce cardiac output can cause syncope. Valvular or structural heart disease may be responsible as well by decreasing cardiac output or by reducing left ventricular filling. Pericardial tamponade, aortic dissection, pulmonary embolism, and the acute myocardial infarction have also caused syncope.

- **ORTHOSTATIC HYPOTENSION.** The inability to compensate for changes in position can be caused by acute blood loss and dehydration. Patients with a ruptured AAA may present with syncope. Vasovagal syncope is an example of an orthostatic hypotension. Medications that reduce vasoconstriction, such as ACE inhibitors, or cause vasodilation may make the patient prone to hypotension on standing.

- **NEUROGENIC/NEUROLOGIC.** Stroke is a rare cause of syncope. A subarachnoid hemorrhage can cause syncope followed by a severe headache. Carotid sinus syndrome occurs when the carotid sinuses are stimulated by turning the head to the side or when a tight garment is placed around the neck. The paramedic will often have to distinguish between syncope and a seizure.

- **MISCELLANEOUS.** Hypoxia, hypoglycemia, and hyperventilation may cause syncope. Hyperglycemia may indicate possible diabetic ketoacidosis and dehydration in diabetic patients. Psychogenic syncope may occur in patients with a history of marked emotional stress.

KEY PHYSICAL EXAM FINDINGS

- ✔ *Initial assessment.* The patient is usually awake and alert after a brief period of unconsciousness. The airway is usually patent. When something beyond simple fainting has occurred, abnormalities in respiration and circulation may be found. Protect the cervical spine if indicated.

- ✔ *Vital signs.* Assess for orthostatic changes. Be aware that orthostatic vital sign changes may not occur with mild volume loss. An increase in heart rate by 20 despite an unchanging blood pressure is more sensitive than traditional orthostatic changes. Assess for tachycardias, bradycardias, and irregular pulses.

- ✔ *HEENT.* Look for evidence of postsyncope trauma. Assess for tongue biting if seizurelike motor activity was reported.

- ✔ *Neck.* Assess for JVD in tension pneumothorax, pericardial tamponade, and large pulmonary embolisms.

- ✔ *Lungs.* Severe bronchospasm may decrease venous return. Assess for poor airflow and wheezing.

- ✔ *Cardiac.* Assess for muffled heart tones in pericardial tamponade.

- ✔ *Abdomen.* Search for a pulsatile mass when AAA rupture is suspected. Peptic ulcer disease and diverticular bleeding may be a source of hypovolemia.

- ✔ *Extremities.* Look for poor capillary refill. Assess for unequal pulses in aortic dissections.

- ✔ *Neurologic examination.* Postictal symptoms or focal motor findings, such as Todd's paralysis, suggest a seizure.

ELECTROCARDIOGRAM

Monitor the ECG on all patients presenting with syncope. Assess for dysrhythmias or ectopy. Obtain a 12-lead ECG when cardiac ischemia is a possibility.

BLOOD GLUCOSE DETERMINATION

Assess for hypoglycemia and hyperglycemia.

OXYGEN SATURATION

Unexplained hypoxia may indicate pulmonary embolism.

TREATMENT PLANS

- *PATIENT ASSESSMENT.* Assess the need for transport. In cases of vasovagal syncope, the patient may refuse transport. If the history or physical exam suggests another cause of the syncope, recommend further evaluation and transport. The appropriate refusal forms should be documented and signed by the EMS crew and patient. In cases of syncope in the elderly or syncope with an unclear cause in a younger patient, the patient should be transported to the emergency department for evaluation to rule out a serious etiology. If a specific diagnosis is identified (e.g., acute myocardial infarction [chapter 11]), symptomatic bradycardia [chapter 6], or tachycardia [chapter 44], follow the treatment regimens recommended for each disease.

GENERAL TREATMENT GUIDELINES:
PATIENT WHO IS HEMODYNAMICALLY STABLE

- **Administer O₂ and provide ventilatory support** as needed.

- Place the patient in the **shock position** (supine with legs elevated), protecting the cervical spine as needed.

- **Treat nonlife-threatening injuries** as appropriate (e.g., control bleeding, splint fractures).

- Monitor the patient's condition for changes.

- **Transport to the appropriate emergency department (ED).** Ensure patient comfort en route.

GENERAL TREATMENT GUIDELINES:
PATIENT WHO IS HEMODYNAMICALLY UNSTABLE

- **Administer O_2 and provide ventilatory support** as needed.

- Place the patient in the **shock position** (supine with legs elevated), protecting the cervical spine as needed.

- Establish **large-bore IV access with 0.9% NaCl or lactated Ringer's solution.**

- **Treat dysrhythmias, if needed.** See chapters 6 and 44.

- **Begin fluid resuscitation.**

- **Treat nonlife-threatening injuries** as appropriate (e.g., control bleeding, splint fractures, etc.).

- Monitor the patient's condition for changes.

- **Expeditiously transport to the appropriate ED.** Do not needlessly delay patient transport—expedite transport. Ensure patient comfort en route.

BIBLIOGRAPHY

De Lorenzo, R. A. (2002). Syncope. In J. Marx, R. Hockberger, & R. Walls (Eds.), *Rosen's emergency medicine: Concepts and clinical practice* (5th ed., pp. 173–177). St. Louis, MO: Mosby.

Keim, S., & Hocheder, S. (2003). Syncope. In J. J. Schaider, S. R. Hayden, R. Wolfe, R., M. Barkin, & P. Rosen (Eds.), *Rosen & Barkin's 5-minute emergency medicine consult*

(2nd ed., pp. 1092–1093). Philadelphia: Lippincott Williams & Wilkins.

Preblick-Salib, C., A. Jagoda, & L. D. Richardson (Eds.). (1997). Spells, differential diagnosis and management strategies. *Emergency medicine clinics of North America, 15,* 637–647.

NOTES

_____

_____

_____

_____

_____

_____

_____

_____

_____

_____

_____

_____

_____

_____

_____

_____

_____

CHAPTER 44

TACHYCARDIA

Owen T. Traynor, M.D.

PRESENTATION

The adult who has a heart rate in excess of 100 bpm is tachycardic. Tachycardia can be a physiologic response to stress; a compensatory mechanism for acute blood loss or hypoxia; or a sign of pathology, caused by heart disease, drugs, or an unknown mechanism. The clinical presentation of a patient with tachycardia depends on the heart rate, the duration of the tachycardia, the pumping effectiveness of the heart, the cardiovascular status of the patient, and the underlying health of the patient.

IMMEDIATE CONCERNS

❶ **What is the patient's hemodynamic status?** If the patient is hemodynamically unstable, immediate resuscitation is warranted, including oxygen administration, establishment of IV access, possible administration of IV medications, and synchronized cardioversion or defibrillation. If the tachycardia is a response to hypovolemia, fluid resuscitation and treatment for shock are necessary.

IMPORTANT HISTORY

❷ **Is the patient symptomatic?** Tachycardias may lead to inadequate cardiac output resulting in the following common complaints: chest pain, dyspnea, fatigue, syncope, dizziness, or neurologic deficits. Chest pain may be either the result of an acute myocardial infarction (AMI), which may be causing the tachycardia, or the consequence of poor coronary perfusion secondary to the tachycardia. Asymptomatic patients require less aggressive immediate therapy.

❓ Is the patient taking any medication? Many medications, particularly sympathomimetic agents, aminophylline derivatives, thyroid medications, and diuretics (reflex tachycardia secondary to hypovolemia) can cause tachycardias.

❓ Is there a history of hyperthyroidism? Excess thyroid hormones may cause an increased sensitivity to sympathetic nervous system hormones, thereby leading to tachycardias. Signs and symptoms of hyperthyroidism include heat intolerance, increased sweating, weight loss, insomnia, hyperkinetic movements, and tachycardias.

❓ Does the patient have a previous history of heart disease? Patients with valvular heart disease; prosthetic heart valves; cardiomyopathies; or preexcitation syndromes, such as Wolff-Parkinson-White (WPW) syndrome, exhibit an increased incidence of tachycardia.

❓ What events preceded the onset of the tachycardia? Exercise, pain, emotional stress, fatigue, fever, dyspnea, and acute blood loss may cause tachycardias. Nicotine, alcohol, and caffeine may increase heart rate. The use of cocaine and other stimulants may also induce tachycardias.

DIFFERENTIAL DIAGNOSIS

SUPRAVENTRICULAR TACHYCARDIAS (SVT)

- **SINUS TACHYCARDIA.** The sinus node rate is between 100 to 180 bpm, although it can be much faster with even moderate exertion. It is usually characterized by a gradual onset and a gradual recovery. Sinus tachycardia is a response to fever; hypotension; anemia; thyrotoxicosis; anxiety; exercise; pulmonary embolism; AMI; congestive heart failure (CHF); and drugs, such as sympathomimetics, alcohol, caffeine, and nicotine. Therapy should focus on the underlying etiology.

- **ATRIAL FLUTTER.** The atrial rate is between 250 to 350 bpm. With a ventricular rate between 80 to 175 bpm (conduction ratio may be 2:1, 4:1, or least commonly, 3:1). The presence of flutter (F) waves may be noted. Atrial flutter is an unstable rhythm, often spontaneously converting to atrial fibrillation or normal sinus rhythm. Chronic atrial flutter is usually associated with underlying heart disease: mitral and tricuspid valve stenosis, ischemic heart disease, and cardiomyopathies. Paroxysmal atrial flutter, however, can occur in patients without structural heart disease.

- **ATRIAL FIBRILLATION.** This rhythm is characterized by disorganized, chaotic atrial activity, with P waves absent and fibrillation waves present at a rate greater than 350 bpm. Atrial fibrillation is a common arrhythmia, occurring in 1% of adults over 60 years of age. Incidence increases with age. Most patients have underlying heart disease, such as coronary artery disease (CAD), hypertensive heart disease, CHF, or cardiomyopathy. Hyperthyroidism is an important cause of new-onset atrial fibrillation. Patients with atrial fibrillation have an increased risk of embolic events and often take anticoagulants.

- **ATRIAL TACHYCARDIAS.** The atrial rate is greater than 100 bpm but less than 150 bpm, as rates greater than this are usually considered to be paroxysmal supraventricular tachycardia (PSVT); P-wave morphology is different from sinus node P waves in atrial tachycardia. Unlike sinus tachycardia, which has a gradual onset, atrial tachycardia is characterized by a sudden onset, hence paroxysmal. If heart block is present in patients taking digitalis preparations, consider digitalis toxicity.

- **MULTIFOCAL ATRIAL TACHYCARDIA (MAT).** Atrial rates are usually from 100 to 130 bpm. There is a variation in P-wave morphology of at least three etiologies. The rhythm is irregular. This rhythm occurs most commonly in elderly patients with chronic obstructive pulmonary disease (COPD) or CHF; it may degenerate into atrial fibrillation.

- **SICK SINUS SYNDROME.** A sinoatrial (SA) node abnormality that includes persistent spontaneous inappropriate sinus bradycardia, episodes of sinus arrest or sinus exit block, a combination of SA or atrioventricular (AV) node conduction anomalies, or alternating periods of paroxysmal atrial tachycardias with slow atrial and ventricular rhythms. This is also known as the bradycardia-tachycardia syndrome.

- **JUNCTIONAL TACHYCARDIAS.** Junctional tachycardias may result from increased automaticity or, more commonly, a re-entrant phenomenon. They are characterized by a regular rhythm, normal QRS complexes, and P waves that may be absent, precede, or follow the QRS complex. The P waves may be positive, biphasic, or negative in electrocardiogram (ECG) leads where normally positive. Where the P wave is positive, the PR interval is usually less than 0.12 second. Ventricular rates are usually from 130 to 180 bpm.

- **PREEXCITATION SYNDROME.** In preexcitation syndrome, an atrial or ventricular impulse travels not only along the normal conduction system but along an anomalous pathway through the myocardium, resulting in conduction of an impulse earlier than expected. WPW syndrome, in which impulses are conducted along an accessory AV pathway, is the most common type of preexcitation syndrome, with an incidence of 1.5 per 1000 persons. Two key characteristics of WPW syndrome are PR intervals less than 0.12 second during NSR and QRS complexes greater than 0.12 second, with slurred, slowly rising onset of the QRS complex (delta wave) in some ECG leads and usually a normal terminal QRS portion. Rapid ventricular rates are possible when impulses are conducted along the accessory pathway, bypassing the AV node. The most common ventricular rates are 150 to 250 bpm. The tachycardias usually occur with a sudden onset and a sudden termination. Atrial fibrillation is a particularly dangerous rhythm in these patients because very rapid ventricular rates are

SECTION 1

possible. Atrial fibrillation can lead to ventricular fibrillation in WPW patients. The accessory pathways can be mapped and then destroyed using high-frequency radio frequency energy at specialty centers.

VENTRICULAR TACHYCARDIA

Ventricular tachycardia (VT) is defined as three or more consecutive beats of ventricular origin in a row. The QRS complex is usually wide (greater than 0.12 second), and the ST and T waves are usually opposite in direction to the QRS deflection. VT arises distal to the bifurcation of the His bundle, in the conduction system, in the myocardium, or in both locations. The rate is usually from 70 to 250 bpm. VT may be paroxysmal or nonparoxysmal, multiform or mono-form. It may be difficult at times to differentiate between VT and an SVT with aberrant conduction.

NOTE: Ventricular tachycardia is the most common cause of wide-QRS complex tachycardia.

POLYMORPHIC VENTRICULAR TACHYCARDIA

Also known as torsades de pointes, this is a VT vari-ant characterized by a gradual fluctuation in amplitude and axis of the QRS complex. It is generally found in the context of a prolonged QT interval in patients taking type IA antiarrhythmic agents such as procainamide, quinidine, and disopyramide. It also requires different treatment than conventional VT: overdrive transcutaneous pacing, IV mag-nesium sulfate, and possibly IV isoproterenol.

VENTRICULAR TACHYCARDIA VERSUS SUPRAVENTRICULAR TACHYCARDIA WITH ABERRANT CONDUCTION

Although it may be useful to distinguish between su-praventricular and ventricular wide complex tachycardias (WCTs) because their therapeutic modalities differ, it is dif-ficult to do so reliably in the prehospital environment.

FACTORS FAVORING VENTRICULAR TACHYCARDIA

- QRS complexes of morphology similar to premature ventricular contractions (PVCs)

- Tachycardia initiated by a PVC

- Usually unresponsive to vagal maneuvers

- Presence of AV dissociation

- QRS complex greater than 0.14 second

- Presence of fusion beats

- History of CAD

FACTORS FAVORING SUPRAVENTRICULAR TACHYCARDIA WITH ABERRANCY

- Morphology similar to previous baseline rhythm

- Possible slowing or breaking of tachycardia with vagal stimulation

- Responsive to adenosine therapy

- Tachycardia often initiated by a premature atrial contraction (PAC)

KEY PHYSICAL EXAMINATION FINDINGS

The physical examination is geared toward assessing the cardiovascular status of the patient and potential sources of sinus tachycardia.

⊘ ***Initial assessment.*** Look for signs of shock and blood loss.

⊘ ***Vital signs.*** Monitor blood pressure, pulse, respirations, and temperature. Hypotension may be present. Tachypnea may be present, indicating hypoxia. Fever may be present, indicating infection and causing sinus tachycardia.

- ✅ *Lungs.* Listen for the presence of rales, which indicates CHF.

- ✅ *Heart.* Listen for gallops.

- ✅ *Abdomen.* Look for signs of acute abdomen, another etiology for sinus tachycardia.

- ✅ *Extremities.* Assess for pain secondary to injury, which may explain sinus tachycardia.

- ✅ *Mental status.* Assess for signs of altered mental status. Inadequate perfusion can cause an altered mental status.

ELECTROCARDIOGRAM

The ECG is an important diagnostic tool that will help determine therapy.

TREATMENT PLAN

Treatment options begin with the assessment of the patient's stability. Instability is characterized by an altered mental status, chest pain, dyspnea, hypotension, pulmonary edema, CHF, and AMI. The patient's instability must also be related to the patient's tachycardia.

- *Patient assessment.* Provide frequent reassessment because of the potential for a worsening of hemodynamic status and CHF. Cardiac monitoring is necessary. Be prepared—the potential for cardiac arrest exists. Treat for an AMI if the tachycardia is occurring in the context of a myocardial infarction. Transport decisions need to be considered early in the treatment of unstable patients. Early contact with medical control may be helpful.

- *Pharmacologic interventions.* The 2000 AHA ACLS Guidelines recommend using only a single antiarrhythmic agent to treat a patient's arrhythmia. Antiarrhythmic agents are known to be proarrhythmic. The incidence of induced arrhythmias increases dramatically when more than 1 agent is used. New to the AHA guidelines is a warning to choose agents carefully when the patient has a history of CHF or a reduced ejection fraction (below 40%).

STABLE TACHYCARDIAS

The approach to treating stable tachycardias may be divided into four distinct scenarios based on the patient's ECG findings. The four types of tachycardias include (1) atrial fibrillation or atrial flutter, (2) narrow-complex tachycardias (NCTs), (3) stable wide-complex tachycardia (WCT), unknown type, and (4) stable monomorphic VT and/or polymorphic VT.

ATRIAL FIBRILLATION OR ATRIAL FLUTTER

In general, little field treatment needs to be given in cases of atrial fibrillation or flutter other than observation and supportive care. When there is hemodynamic instability or a rapid ventricular response, patients who have been in atrial fibrillation for more than 48 hours are at increased risk of embolic phenomena. When it is not possible to confirm shorter duration of atrial fibrillation, anticoagulation is recommended before attempting to convert the rhythm.

- **Administer O$_2$** and provide ventilatory support as needed.

- **Establish IV access.**

- If the patient has no evidence of impaired heart function, the following agents are recommended for rate control:

  o **Diltiazem, 0.25 mg/kg IV** (not to exceed 20 mg) over 2 minutes. If the patient does not respond adequately, another bolus may be administered in 15 minutes with 0.35 mg/kg IV (not to exceed 25 mg). If this is effective, start diltiazem infusion at 5 to 15 mg/hour.

- o **Verapamil, 2 to 5 mg IV**. Do not use verapamil if the patient has a history of severe bradycardia, is hypotensive, is in CHF, or has acutely received IV beta blockers. Verapamil may be repeated at 5 to 10 mg IV in 15 to 30 minutes if the tachycardia persists.

- o Beta blockers may also be used. The prehospital use of beta blockers for rate control is not common.

- o **Transport to the appropriate ED.** Continue to reassess the patient's ECG and hemodynamic status. Ensure patient comfort en route.

- If the patient has an impaired heart (ejection fraction (EF) below 40% or CHF), the following agents are recommended:

- o **Diltiazem, 0.25 mg/kg IV** (not to exceed 20 mg) over 2 minutes. If the patient does not respond adequately, another bolus may be administered in 15 minutes with 0.35 mg/kg IV (not to exceed 25 mg). If effective, start diltiazem infusion at 5 to 15 mg/hour.

- o **Amiodarone, 150 mg IV** over 10 minutes, followed by an infusion of 1 mg/min for 6 hours, then 0.5 mg/min. Maximum total daily dose is 2.2g. Repeat boluses at 150 mg IV have been used instead of continuous infusions.

- o Digoxin may also be used. The prehospital use of digoxin for rate control is not common.

- o **Transport to the appropriate ED.** Continue to reassess the patient's ECG and hemodynamic status. Ensure patient comfort en route.

- If the patient has evidence of WPW and is in atrial fibrillation or atrial flutter, rate control becomes a risky intervention. Calcium channel blockers and beta blockers can increase conduction down the accessory pathway, resulting in even faster heart rates and ventricular fibrillation. Conversion of the rhythm becomes the primary goal. It is recommended that this be accomplished in the hospital. Recommended agents include the following:

o **Amiodarone, 150 mg IV** over 10 minutes, followed by an infusion of 1 mg/min for 6 hours, then 0.5 mg/min. Maximum total daily dose is 2.2g. Repeat boluses at 150 mg IV have been used instead of continuous infusions.

o **Procainamide, 20 to 30 mg/min IV until effective,** or 17 mg/kg total has been given, or the width of the QRS complex increases by 50%. Do not use if there is evidence of CHF or a history of an ejection fraction below 40%.

o **Flecainide, propafenoner, and sotalol.** The prehospital use of these agents for rate control is not common. These agents should not be used when there is evidence of CHF or a history of an ejection fraction below 40%.

o **Transport to the appropriate ED.** Continue to reassess the patient's ECG and hemodynamic status. Ensure patient comfort en route.

NARROW COMPLEX SUPRAVENTRICULAR TACHYCARDIA (NCT)

It can be difficult at times to distinguish between the various types of supraventricular tachycardias. The 2000 AHA ACLS Guidelines recommend attempting to make a specific diagnosis using a 12-lead ECG, clinical information, vagal maneuvers, and adenosine. Possible findings include paroxysmal SVT, junctional tachycardia, and ectopic or multifocal atrial tachycardia. General treatment guidelines for the treatment of PSVT follow:

* Administer **O₂** and **provide ventilatory support** as needed.

* Establish **IV access with 0.9% NaCl at a KVO rate.**

SECTION 1

- **Perform vagal maneuvers,** such as the Valsalva maneuver, if trained in their proper use. Carotid sinus massage should not be performed in patients with carotid bruits.

- If PSVT persists, administer **adenosine, 6 mg rapid IV bolus.** Adenosine may be repeated at 12 mg IV in 1 to 2 minutes if ineffective. Drug may be repeated a second time at same dosage.

- If the NCT persists, re-evaluate the rhythm. Treat according to the specific arrhythmia treatment plan below.

- *Junctional tachycardia* treatment options include the following:

  o **Amiodarone, 150 mg IV** over 10 minutes, followed by an infusion of 1 mg/min for 6 hours, then 0.5 mg/min. Maximum total daily dose is 2.2 g. Repeat boluses at 150 mg IV have been used instead of continuous infusions.

  o **Diltiazem, 0.25 mg/kg IV** (not to exceed 20 mg) over 2 minutes. If the patient does not respond adequately another bolus in may be administered 15 minutes with 0.35 mg/kg IV (not to exceed 25 mg). If effective, start diltiazem infusion at 5 to 15 mg/hour. AHA guidelines do not recommend calcium channel blockers if there is evidence of impaired heart function.

  o **Verapamil, 2 to 5 mg IV.** Do not use verapamil if the patient has a history of severe bradycardia, is hypotensive, is in CHF, or has acutely received IV beta blockers. Verapamil may be repeated at 5 to 10 mg IV in 15 to 30 minutes if the tachycardia persists. AHA guidelines do not recommend calcium channel blockers if there is evidence of impaired heart function.

  o **DC cardioversion is contraindicated.**

  o **Transport to the appropriate ED.** Continue to reassess the patient's ECG and hemodynamic status. Ensure patient comfort en route.

- *Paroxysmal SVT* treatment options (in priority order) are as follows:

  o **Diltiazem, 0.25 mg/kg IV** (not to exceed 20 mg) over 2 minutes. If patient does not respond adequately, another bolus may be administered in 15 minutes with 0.35 mg/kg IV (not to exceed 25 mg). If effective, start diltiazem infusion at 5 to 15 mg/hour. AHA guidelines do not recommend calcium channel blockers if there is evidence of impaired heart function.

  o **Verapamil, 2 to 5 mg IV.** Do not use verapamil if the patient has a history of severe bradycardia, is hypotensive, is in CHF, or has acutely received IV beta blockers. Verapamil may be repeated at 5 to 10 mg IV in 15 to 30 minutes if the tachycardia persists. AHA guidelines do not recommend calcium channel blockers if there is evidence of impaired heart function.

  o Beta blockers may also be used. The prehospital use of beta blockers for rate control is not common.

  o Digoxin may be considered; however, the prehospital use of digoxin is not common.

  o **Synchronized DC cardioversion** starting at 50 joules. Prehospital pharmacologic treatment of stable SVT is far more common than cardioversion of stable patients.

  o **Procainamide, 20 to 30 mg/min IV until effective.** or 17 mg/kg total has been given, or the width of the QRS complex increases by 50%. Do not use if there is evidence of CHF or a history of an ejection fraction below 40%.

  o **Amiodarone, 150 mg IV** over 10 minutes, followed by an infusion of 1 mg/min for 6 hours, then 0.5 mg/min. Maximum total daily dose is 2.2 g. Repeat boluses at 150 mg IV have been used instead of continuous infusions.

o Sotalol may also be considered. The prehospital use of sotalol is not common.

NOTE: If the patient has CHF or an ejection fraction below 40%, consider amiodarone, digoxin, or diltiazem as preferred treatments. DC cardioversion is not recommended.

o **Transport to the appropriate ED.** Continue to reassess the patient's ECG and hemodynamic status. Ensure patient comfort en route.

- *Ectopic or multifocal atrial tachycardia* treatment options include:

  o **Amiodarone, 150 mg IV** over 10 minutes, followed by an infusion of 1 mg/min for 6 hours, then 0.5 mg/min. Maximum total daily dose is 2.2 g. Repeat boluses at 150 mg IV have been used instead of continuous infusions.

  o **Diltiazem, 0.25 mg/kg IV** over 2 minutes. If patient does not respond adequately, another bolus may be administered in 15 minutes with 0.35 mg/kg IV. If effective, start diltiazem infusion at 5 to 15 mg/hour.

  o **Verapamil, 2 to 5 mg IV.** Do not use verapamil if the patient has a history of severe bradycardia, is hypotensive, is in CHF, or has acutely received IV beta blockers. Verapamil may be repeated at 5 to 10 mg IV in 15 to 30 minutes if the tachycardia persists. Do not use if there is evidence of CHF or an ejection fraction below 40%.

  o **DC cardioversion is contraindicated.**

  NOTE: If the patient has CHF or an ejection fraction below 40%, consider amiodarone or diltiazem as preferred treatments.

  o **Transport to the appropriate ED.** Continue to reassess the patient's ECG and hemodynamic status. Ensure patient comfort en route.

NARROW COMPLEX TACHYCARDIA
(WITH NORMAL OR ELEVATED BP)

• If rhythm persists, **repeat synchronized cardioversion** using the following incremental dosage scheme: 100 J, 200 J, 300 J, 360 J.

• **Transport to appropriate ED.** Continue to reassess the patient's ECG and hemodynamic status. Ensure patient comfort en route.

STABLE WIDE-COMPLEX TACHYCARDIA:
UNKNOWN TYPE

The 2000 AHA ACLS Guidelines recommend making a rapid attempt to diagnose the actual rhythm. Three possible diagnoses are possible: SVT with aberrant conduction, wide complex tachycardia (WCT): unknown type, and Stable VT. "A history of coronary artery disease or structural heart disease makes VT more likely than SVT with aberrancy. A history of SVT with aberrancy, accessory pathways, preexisting bundle branch blocks, or rate-related bundle branch blocks suggests SVT with aberrancy if the current QRS complex matches the aberrantly conducted QRS." It is likely that it will be difficult in the prehospital environment to access prior ECGs for comparison. If the rhythm is determined to be SVT with aberrancy, the patient should be treated as noted in the NCT algorithm. If the rhythm is confirmed to be stable VT, the patient is treated as in the stable VT algorithm.

• Administer O_2 and **provide ventilatory support** as needed.

• Establish IV access with 0.9% NaCl at a KVO rate.

• **Amiodarone, 150 mg IV** over 10 minutes, followed by an infusion of 1 mg/min for 6 hours, then 0.5 mg/min. Maximum total daily dose is 2.2 g. Repeat boluses at 150 mg IV every 10 minutes have been used instead of continuous infusions.

- **Procainamide, 20 to 30 mg/min IV until effective**, or 17 mg/kg total has been given, or the width of the QRS complex increases by 50%. Use with caution if there is evidence of CHF or a history of an ejection fraction below 40%.

- If WCT persists, perform **synchronized cardioversion** as in unstable patients. Consider sedation before cardioversion. Prehospital cardioversion should be avoided if the transport time to the ED is short, unless the patient's hemodynamic status is poor or the patient is symptomatic.

  NOTE: If the patient has CHF or an ejection fraction below 40%, consider DC cardioversion or amiodarone as preferred treatments.

- **Transport to appropriate ED.** Continue to reassess the patient's ECG and hemodynamic status. Ensure patient comfort en route.

STABLE VENTRICULAR TACHYCARDIA

This algorithm has become more complex. The initial determination is to classify the VT as monomorphic or polymorphic. Torsades de pointe is a specific type of polymorphic VT that may be distinguished by a prolonged QT interval. Its treatment differs from other forms of polymorphic VT, and therefore an assessment of QT interval must be made.

- Administer **O₂** and **provide ventilatory support** as needed.

- Establish IV access with 0.9% NaCl at a KVO rate.

- Monomorphic VT treatment options include the following:

  o **Amiodarone, 150 mg IV** over 10 minutes, followed by an infusion of 1 mg/min for 6 hours, then 0.5 mg/min. Maximum total daily dose is 2.2 g. Repeat boluses at 150 mg IV every 10 minutes have been used instead of continuous infusions. This is a preferred agent when there is evidence of impaired heart function.

- o **Lidocaine 1 mg/kg IV,** repeated at 0.5 to 0.75 mg/kg every 5 to 10 minutes, if needed. Maximum total dose is 3 mg/kg. If effective, start infusion at 1 to 4 mg/minute. If there is CHF or a history of an ejection fraction of below 40%, use 0.5 to 0.75 mg/kg IV as the initial bolus. This is a preferred agent when there is evidence of impaired heart function.

- o **Procainamide, 20 to 30 mg/min IV until effective**, or 17 mg/kg total has been given, or the width of the QRS complex increases by 50%. Use with caution if there is evidence of CHF or a history of an ejection fraction below 40%.

- o **Sotalol** may be considered. The prehospital use of sotalol is not common.

- o **Synchronized cardioversion** starting at 100 J. Consider sedation before cardioversion. This is a preferred option when there is evidence of impaired heart function and amiodarone or lidocaine has failed to convert the rhythm.

- o **Transport to the appropriate ED.** Continue to reassess the patient's ECG and hemodynamic status. Ensure patient comfort en route.

- Polymorphic VT with normal QT interval treatment options include the following:

- o **Amiodarone, 150 mg IV** over 10 minutes, followed by an infusion of 1 mg/min for 6 hours, then 0.5 mg/min. Maximum total daily dose is 2.2 g. Repeat boluses at 150 mg IV every 10 minutes have been used instead of continuous infusions. This is a preferred agent when there is evidence of impaired heart function.

- o **Beta blockers** may be used. The prehospital use of beta blockers for this indication is not common.

- o **Lidocaine, 1 mg/kg IV,** repeated at 0.5 to 0.75 mg/kg every 5 to 10 minutes, if needed. Maximum total dose is 3 mg/kg. If effective, start infusion at 1 to 4 mg/minute. If there is CHF or a history of an ejection fraction of below 40%, use 0.5 to 0.75 mg/kg IV as the initial bolus. This is a preferred agent when there is evidence of impaired heart function.

o **Procainamide, 20 to 30 mg/min IV until effective,** or 17 mg/kg total has been given, or the width of the QRS complex increases by 50%. Use with caution if there is evidence of CHF or a history of an ejection fraction below 40%.

o **Sotalol** may be considered. The prehospital use of sotalol is not common.

o **Synchronized cardioversion** starting at 100 J. Consider sedation prior to cardioversion. This is a preferred option when there is evidence of impaired heart function and amiodarone or lidocaine has failed to convert the rhythm.

o **Transport to the appropriate ED.** Continue to reassess the patient's ECG and hemodynamic status. Ensure patient comfort en route.

- Polymorphic VT with prolonged QT (suggests Torsades) interval treatment options include the following:

  o **Magnesium sulfate, 2 to 4 g IV** over 5 minutes.

  o **Overdrive pacing** at 10 to 20 beats above the ventricular rate may entrain the atria. The pacing rate can gradually be decreased to 100 to 120 bpm.

  o **Isoproterenol** 2 to 10 µg/min infusion.

  o **Phenytoin** may be used, although prehospital use of this agent for this indication is not common.

  o **Lidocaine,1 mg/kg IV,** repeated at 0.5 to 0.75 mg/kg every 5 to 10 minutes, if needed. Maximum total dose is 3 mg/kg. If effective, start infusion at 1 to 4 mg/minute. If there is CHF or a history of an ejection fraction of below 40%, use 0.5 to 0.75 mg/kg IV as the initial bolus.

o **Transport to the appropriate ED.** Continue to reassess the patient's ECG and hemodynamic status. Ensure patient comfort en route.

PREEXCITATION SYNDROMES

Patients with WPW who exhibit stable regular narrow complex tachycardias should be treated as indicated for stable PSVT. Adenosine may be administered as the first-line drug, then verapamil (see note). If the tachycardia is an irregular wide complex tachycardia, atrial fibrillation or flutter may be present. Drugs that prolong the refractoriness of the accessory pathway, such as procainamide, must be used to prevent ventricular fibrillation.

NOTE: Verapamil may be dangerous because it may increase the number of impulses conducted down the accessory pathways by prolonging the refractoriness of the AV node, thereby further increasing the heart rate.

UNSTABLE TACHYCARDIAS

- Prepare for immediate synchronized cardioversion if the ventricular rate is greater than 150. Heart rates less than 150 do not usually require immediate cardioversion. A brief trial of antiarrhythmic agents may be tried before cardioversion.

- Administer **O**$_2$ and **provide ventilatory support** as needed.

- Have suction and intubation equipment available.

- Establish **IV access.**

- **Synchronized cardioversion** beginning at 100 J. Consider sedation before cardioversion. Cardioversion may be repeated at 200, 300, and 360 J. Atrial flutter and PSVT patients may respond at 50 J.

- **Transport to appropriate ED.** Transport decisions need to be considered early in the treatment of unstable patients. Continue to reassess the patient and the ECG.

BIBLIOGRAPHY

Brown, K. R. (2003). *Emergency dysrhythmias and ECG injury patterns.* Clifton Park, NY: Delmar Learning.

Votey, S. R., M. Herbert, & J. R. Hoffman (2001). Tachyarrhythmias. In A. Harwood-Nuss, A. B. Wolfson, C. H. Linden, S. M. Shepard, & P. H. Stenklyft (Eds.), *The clinical practice of emergency medicine* (3rd ed., pp. 685–695). Philadelphia: Lippincott Williams & Wilkins.

(2000). Section 5: Pharmacology I: Agents for arrhythmias. *Circulation, 102,* I-112–I-128.

(2000). Section 7D: The tachycardia algorithms. *Circulation, 102,* I-158–I-165.

NOTES

_____

_____

_____

_____

_____

_____

_____

_____

_____

_____

CHAPTER 45

VAGINAL BLEEDING

Jonathan S. Rubens, M.D., FACEP

PRESENTATION

Vaginal bleeding is one of the most common gynecologic complaints in emergency medicine. Patients may present with a variety of signs and symptoms, including those of shock and passage of blood, clots, or tissue from the vagina.

IMMEDIATE CONCERNS

- **What is the patient's hemodynamic status?** Look for and treat if there is evidence of poor perfusion.

- **Is the patient pregnant?** Pregnant patients with vaginal bleeding may have illnesses that risk the life of the patient and the fetus. Consider the possibility of pregnancy; when the patient is of childbearing age and has a uterus and at least one ovary, pregnancy is possible. A missed or delayed menstrual period indicates a possible pregnancy. If the patient has a positive pregnancy test, find out the due date. Symptoms of an early pregnancy include amenorrhea (absent periods), breast tenderness or tingling, nausea and vomiting, and frequent urination.

IMPORTANT HISTORY

- **When was the last normal menstrual period?** Metrorrhagia is defined as noncyclical vaginal bleeding between menstrual periods. Menorrhagia is defined as unusually heavy bleeding associated with an expected menstrual period.

- **Is there pain associated with the bleeding?** Cramping is common in menstruation and spontaneous abortion. Pain is often associated with ectopic pregnancy and abruptions. Painless blood can be seen in a patient with placenta previa.

❷ **What is the amount of bleeding?**   The amount of blood can often be quantified by the number of pads used in a period.

❷ **Is the patient taking any medications?**   Aspirin, warfarin (Coumadin), and nonsteroidal antiinflammatory agents may all contribute to bleeding.

❷ **What is the patient's other medical history?**   Is there any history of malignancy or bleeding tendencies? Women who have undergone embryo transfer techniques and treatment for infertility are at increased risk for ectopic pregnancy.

❷ **Is there a history of trauma?**   Examples include intercourse, sexual assault, or instrumentation (insertion of foreign objects).

DIFFERENTIAL DIAGNOSIS

THE PREGNANT PATIENT

- *ECTOPIC PREGNANCY.*   Any woman of childbearing age with vaginal bleeding should be considered to have an ectopic pregnancy until proven otherwise (with or without pain).

- *HYDATIDIFORM MOLE.*   A hydatidiform mole is an abnormal development of the tissue that forms the placenta. Molar pregnancies occur in approximately 1 out of 1,500 live births. The uterus is usually larger in relation to dates in the pregnancy cycle. Risk is 10 times greater in women older than 45 years of age.

- *SPONTANEOUS ABORTION.*   With spontaneous abortion, termination of pregnancy occurs before the twentieth week of gestation. Approximately 15% to 20% of pregnancies end this way.

- **PLACENTA PREVIA.** A portion of the placenta overlies the cervical os (or opening), usually accompanied by the painless bleeding of bright-red blood.

- **ABRUPTIO PLACENTAE.** Abruptio placentae is the painful separation of the placenta from its implantation site. Bleeding may or may not be present—it is sometimes contained within the uterus.

- **UTERINE RUPTURE.** Uterine rupture is a grave complication that occurs in 1 out of 2000 pregnancies and results in high maternal and fetal mortality.

THE NONPREGNANT PATIENT

- **NORMAL MENSES**.

- **NEOPLASMS.** Neoplasms appear on the uterus, ovaries, or cervix.

- **OVARIAN CYSTS.** Ovarian cysts result in hormonal disruption.

- **ENDOMETRIOSIS.** Endometrial tissue develops outside of the uterus.

- **IUDS** (intrauterine devices).

- **TRAUMA.** Trauma results in disruption of the integrity of the vaginal or cervical anatomy.

- **INFECTION.** A history of vaginal discharge, fever, and dyspareunia (painful intercourse) is usually present.

- Other systemic disease or coagulation disorders may be present.

KEY PHYSICAL EXAMINATION FINDINGS

- ✓ **Initial assessment.** Monitor airway, breathing, and circulation. Look for signs of shock.

- ✓ **Vital signs.** Include orthostatic blood pressures. Remember that pregnant patients may have up to one third greater blood volume and thus may not show signs of shock as early as the nongravid patient.

⊘ ***Abdomen.*** Is a gravid abdomen present? Tenderness, masses, rebound tenderness, and involuntary guarding should all be assessed. Listen for bowel sounds; attempt to gently palpate any uterine contractions.

⊘ ***Genital.*** Inspect the external genitalia for amount of bleeding and the presence of any tissue. Do not perform any internal examination of the vaginal opening in the field.

TREATMENT PLAN

*   Continued vital sign assessment.

GENERAL TREATMENT GUIDELINES:
PATIENT WHO IS HEMODYNAMICALLY UNSTABLE

*   Administer **O₂** and **provide ventilatory support** as needed. Monitor O₂ saturation.

*   Establish **two large-bore IV lines with 0.9% NaCl or LR.**

*   **Position gravid patients on their left side** to avoid inferior vena cavae compression by the uterus and to increase venous return.

*   Monitor ECG.

*   **Transport expeditiously to appropriate ED.** Do not needlessly delay transport—expedite transport. Ensure patient comfort en route.

GENERAL TREATMENT GUIDELINES:
PATIENT WHO IS HEMODYNAMICALLY STABLE

*   **Transport to appropriate ED.** Ensure patient comfort en route.

BIBLIOGRAPHY

Morrison, L. J. & J. M. Spence (2003). Vaginal bleeding in the non-pregnant patient. In J. E. Tintinalli, G. D. Kelen, & J. S. Stapczynski (Eds.), *A comprehensive study guide* (6th ed., pp. 647–653). New York: McGraw Hill.

Valentine C. (2003). Vaginal bleeding. In J. J. Schaider, S. R. Hayden, R. Wolfe, R. M. Barkin, & P. Rosen (Eds.), *Rosen & Barkin's 5-minute emergency medicine consult* (2nd ed., pp. 1184–1185). Philadelphia: Lippincott Williams & Wilkins.

NOTES

_____

_____

_____

_____

_____

_____

_____

_____

_____

_____

_____

_____

_____

_____

SECTION 1

CHAPTER 46

WHEEZING

Deepi Goyal, M.D.
Kurtis A. Judson, M.D.

PRESENTATION

A wheeze is an abnormally high-pitched sound produced by breathing through partially obstructed or narrowed airways. It is more prominent during exhalation and is associated with a prolonged expiratory phase. The wheezing patient may present in many ways. In fact, the patient may not even complain of wheezing. Quite often, the patient may present with complaints of shortness of breath, cough, or chest tightness. Wheezing patients are often apprehensive and distressed. Their shortness of breath may be so severe that they may not be able to speak in complete sentences. Oxygenation may be compromised to the point at which the patient's level of consciousness is decreased. These signs are clues that the patient needs immediate and aggressive therapy. In evaluating the wheezing patient, it is important to remember that asthma and chronic obstructive pulmonary disease (COPD) are not the only causes of wheezing.

IMMEDIATE CONCERNS

❶ **What is the patient's state of oxygenation?** Is the patient cyanotic? Can the patient talk? Patients who are clearly hypoxic may exhibit symptoms such as a decreased level of consciousness and cyanosis. A note of caution: The hypoxic patient may not be cyanotic. Cyanosis occurs when 5 mg% of hemoglobin is unsaturated. Therefore, the severely anemic patient may not be able to produce cyanosis and yet be quite hypoxic. Hypoxic patients need immediate and aggressive therapy, including supplemental oxygen, inhaled bronchodilators, and possibly intubation.

IMPORTANT HISTORY

❷ **Is there a history of wheezing in the past?** Patients who have had episodes of wheezing in the past may know if they have a history of asthma, COPD, or other respiratory disorders. It is important to determine the average duration of prior attacks and the therapy that has been effective in terminating these acute attacks. Furthermore, knowledge of the patient's ventilatory capacity between attacks can help determine the patient's baseline level of functioning, which can help in assessing the patient's response to therapy. For instance, if a patient normally has a poor level of pulmonary function between attacks, the endpoint of therapy will be different from the patient with a normal level of function between attacks. Does the patient have a previous history of intubation?

❷ **Is the patient taking any medications?** Certain medications (e.g., beta blockers) can acutely precipitate asthmatic attacks. Furthermore, the patient's medications, such as metered dose inhalers or cardiac medications, can provide clues to other medical problems and thus help to guide therapy.

❷ **Does the patient have any allergies?** A history of prior allergic reactions may indicate that the patient's symptoms are a manifestation of anaphylaxis.

DIFFERENTIAL DIAGNOSIS

• *CHRONIC OBSTRUCTIVE PULMONARY DISEASE.* Emphysema and chronic bronchitis account for a large percentage of EMS calls for shortness of breath. These patients almost always have a significant tobacco-smoking history. Smoking leads to chronic damage to both the small and large airways, with most of the damage occurring in the large airways. These patients usually have a lowered baseline level of pulmonary function, as opposed to the patient with pure asthma who will return to a normal level of function between asthmatic attacks. Although emphysema and chronic bronchitis are categorized as entirely different entities, there is often a component of both disorders in the patient who presents with wheezing and shortness of breath. These patients often have a history of chronic cough, sputum production, and dyspnea on exertion. The classic appearance of a person with emphysema is the "pink puffer," with rapid, shallow breathing through pursed lips, a thin body habitus with a barrel chest, and the use of accessory muscles of breathing. The classic appearance of a person with bronchitis is the "blue bloater": cyanotic and overweight, with slow, deep, and labored breathing.

- **ASTHMA.** Asthma is characterized by a hypersensitivity of the tracheobronchial tree to a variety of stimuli, leading to bronchoconstriction, inflammation, and increased airway secretions.

- **CONGESTIVE HEART FAILURE.** Congestive heart failure (CHF) is often overlooked as a cause of wheezing, but wheezing may be the only sign of CHF. This diagnosis should be suspected in every middle-aged or older person who complains of wheezing, especially if there is also a history of heart disease.

- **ASPIRATION.** Persistent localized wheezing can suggest the diagnosis of foreign body aspiration, especially in individuals who may not protect their airways well. Foreign body aspiration, however, usually produces an obstruction of the upper airway and therefore is more likely to produce stridor than frank wheezing. Aspiration is more likely in young children and older, debilitated patients who cannot protect their airways.

- **ANAPHYLAXIS.** Wheezing may be a manifestation of anaphylaxis, as histamine release and inflammation lead to narrowing of the airways. Usually, however, other clues are present to indicate an anaphylactic reaction, such as rash, edema, hypotension, and so forth.

- **OTHER CAUSES.** Pneumonia, pulmonary embolism, thoracic cage deformities, tuberculosis, and lung cancer are among the other causes of wheezing. Wheezing, however, is a less common manifestation of these disorders than those mentioned previously.

KEY PHYSICAL EXAMINATION FINDINGS

✓ **Initial assessment.** Form a general impression about the patient; assess the mental status, airway, breathing, circulation, and look for signs of shock or airway compromise. The use of accessory muscles to breathe or the inability to speak in complete sentences secondary to shortness of breath indicates that the patient's respiratory status is in jeopardy.

✓ **Vital signs.** Monitor respirations and pulse. The respiratory rate is usually increased. Tachycardia is often prominent if cardiac output must be increased to compensate for decreased oxygenation.

✓ **Focused history and physical.** Follow the OPQRST-ASPN (Onset, Provocation/Palliation, Quality, Radiation/Region, Severity, Time, Associated Symptoms, Pertinent Negatives) history-taking format, and perform a focused physical exam.

✓ **Peak expiratory flow rate.** Measure peak expiratory flow rate (PEFR). The PEFR provides the only objective measurement of the degree of airway obstruction and can be used to follow the patient's progress. It does depend on the patient's technique and efforts; therefore the patient must be coached in its use and encouraged to give his or her best effort.

✓ **Neck.** Look for distended neck veins as an indicator for CHF or possible pulmonary embolism.

✅ **Chest.**   Listen to the nature and character of the breath sounds. Exercise caution, however, because you may be fooled into a sense of security by a previously noisy chest that becomes quiet. Often this is a sign of impending doom as the patient becomes fatigued and cannot generate enough airflow to create wheezes. This is an indication that the patient is rapidly deteriorating and that steps should be taken immediately to prevent loss of the airway.

✅ **Accessory muscles.**   The use of the neck muscles and chest wall muscles are a sign that the work of breathing is too great for the diaphragm alone. Abdominal breathing is an even later sign, which indicates that the patient is beginning to tire. The energy required to breathe in this manner is great, and once fatigue sets in, the patient will no longer be able to compensate for the extra airway resistance.

✅ **Extremities.**   Check for signs of peripheral edema. Peripheral edema is a sign of heart disease and should make you suspicious that the patient's wheezing may be due to CHF. Failure of the right side of the heart is common in advanced lung disease (cor pulmonale). Clubbing of the fingers is an indication of long-standing hypoxia.

TREATMENT PLAN

- **Patient assessment.**   Reassess the patient frequently for both response to therapy and for signs of further deterioration. The patient may need assisted ventilations with a bag-valve-mask device or even require intubation. The patient who appears fatigued warrants early intervention.

- Administer O_2 either via nasal cannula, face mask, or bag-valve-mask device, depending on the patient's degree of respiratory compromise. A pulse oximeter may be very useful in determining the patient's O_2 saturation.

- Establish **IV access;** it may be necessary for the administration of medications.

- **_Medications._** For the treatment of asthma or COPD, give nebulized beta agonists or nebulized beta agonists and anticholinergics, such as albuterol or albuterol/ipratropium bromide (Atrovent) back to back until the patient's status improves. Steroids are not used often in the field because their benefits take several hours to manifest and may actually worsen some conditions that mimic asthma. If there is evidence of CHF, sublingual nitroglycerin, furosimide (Lasix), and morphine may be indicated. The following agents are most commonly used to treat bronchospasm:

  o **Albuterol, 2.5 to 5 mg in 3 ml 0.9% NaCl via nebulizer or 4 to 8 puffs of a 90 µg per puff MDI with spacer** (pediatric dose: age younger than 12 years, one half of the adult dose (2.5 mg); age older than 12 years, use full adult dosing). Dose may be repeated every 4 hours; however, in cases of severe bronchospasm, it may be given as frequently as back to back.

NOTE: More frequent dosing may result in a greater incidence of side effects.

  o **Ipratropium bromide, 0.5 mg in 3 ml 0.9% NaCl via nebulizer** (pediatric dose: age younger than 12 years, one half of the adult dose (0.25 mg); age older than 12 years, use full adult dosing). Dose giving in conjunction with albuterol for severe episodes of wheezing or respiratory distress.

  o **Epinephrine (1:1000), 0.3 to 0.5 mg SC injection** (pediatric dose: 0.01 mg/kg, not to exceed 0.5 mg per dose). Dose may be repeated every 20 minutes.

- **Transport expeditiously to an appropriate ED.** Do not delay patient transport needlessly—expedite transport. A delay in transport may hinder further diagnostic and therapeutic maneuvers. Ensure patient comfort en route.

SECTION 1

BIBLIOGRAPHY

Cydulka, R. K. & M. A. Kaufman (2001). Asthma. In A. Harwood-Nuss & A. B. Wolfson (Eds.), *The clinical practice of emergency medicine* (3rd ed., pp. 740–746). Philadelphia: Lippincott Williams & Wilkins.

Mandavia, D. P. & R. H. Dailey (2002). Chronic obstructive pulmonary disease. In J. J. Marx, R. S. Hockberger, & R. M. Walls (Eds.), *Rosen's emergency medicine: Concepts and clinical practice* (5th ed., pp. 956–989). St. Louis, MO: Mosby.

Nowak, R. & G. Tokarski (2002). Asthma. In J. J. Marx, R. S. Hockberger, & R. M. Walls (Eds.), *Rosen's emergency medicine: Concepts and clinical practice* (5th ed., pp. 956–989). St. Louis, MO: Mosby.

Stulbarg, M. S. & L. Adams (2000). Dyspnea. In J. F. Murray, & J. A. Nadel, (Eds.), *Murray & Nadel: Textbook of respiratory medicine* (3rd ed., pp. 1247–1289). St. Louis, MO: W. B. Saunders.

NOTES

_____

_____

_____

_____

_____

_____

_____

_____

_____

SECTION 2

SPECIAL TOPICS

CHAPTER 47

ADVANCE DIRECTIVES FOR HEALTH CARE

Thomas J. Rahilly, Ph.D.

PRESENTATION

In the increasingly complex world of medicine, it is becoming more common for individual states to allow their residents to make informed decisions regarding their health care in advance of the need to do so. The need to make such decisions can be the result of a current serious illness or injury with a poor prognosis for recovery. In this case, the individual may assign his or her medical treatment decision-making authority to a trusted person. Advance directives may also be written by those who prefer to have their treatment decisions made by someone they trust, should they suffer a catastrophic illness or injury at some time in the future. For all patients admitted to a hospital, the Federal Patient Self-Determination Act mandates that every patient has the right to sign an advance directive. There is no such statute, however, for out-of-hospital directives.

DO NOT RESUSCITATE ORDER

A Do Not Resuscitate (DNR) order, which requires that resuscitative measures not be instituted when the patient expires, is issued by a physician at the request of the patient or by the patient's legally authorized representative. The DNR order is a written directive that must be signed by the attending physician and, in most states, honored by the EMS providers if they do not have a valid reason to disregard it. A few states have developed standardized DNR forms as well as DNR bracelets. These items must clearly identify the individual patient and must not have exceeded the expiration date if applicable.

DNR orders are not generally considered legal authority for withholding other medical treatment, such as the administration of oxygen and other life-sustaining measures. In the absence of a valid form of documentation indicating that the patient has specifically requested not to be resuscitated, the EMS provider must follow the standard of care as stated in statute or provided by medical control policies through prehospital protocols.

LIVING WILLS

A living will is a legal document that adults in a competent state of mind may use to express their wishes regarding their future health care. The living will can be used to stipulate their desire for certain life-sustaining medical treatments. In many cases, however, the persons who authorize a living will want to make clear their objection to unwanted medical interventions while they still have the capacity for such decisions. The living will is usually intended to apply to situations in which the person would suffer an illness or injury that results in a terminal condition accompanied by a permanent state of unconsciousness. It could also apply to situations in which the person would maintain consciousness, but damage to the brain would be so severe that an expression of wishes regarding treatment cannot be made.

HEALTHCARE PROXY

A healthcare proxy is another mechanism whereby persons are able to decide what health care they will receive during a period in which they are incapacitated. By appointing a healthcare proxy (in writing), a person transfers the authority for informed consent to another person who has the best interests of the patient in mind. Healthcare providers often look to family members for guidance when a person is too sick to make an informed decision about their health. However, family members are not usually permitted to withhold or stop treatment. The line of authority may be complete or specific to a certain treatment that is to be administered or withheld. The healthcare proxy may receive detailed instructions to be followed in the event of a temporary loss of decision-making ability, such as during surgery. Unlike a living will, a healthcare proxy agreement does not require that all of the decisions be made in advance. Unless otherwise specified, the healthcare proxy may interpret the medical circumstances surrounding a particular healthcare situation and make decisions accordingly. In other words, the proxy may make decisions as the patient's condition either improves or deteriorates.

As is the case with most healthcare issues, there is no universal acceptance of the healthcare proxy as a legal document in the prehospital EMS environment. Providers must be familiar with all of the regulations associated with not only advance directives but also each of the medico-legal requirements of their states and local jurisdictions.

SECTION 2

BIBLIOGRAPHY

Bledsoe, B. E., R. S. Porter, & R. A. (Eds.). (2003). *Essentials of paramedic care*. Englewood Cliffs, NJ: Prentice-Hall.

Tintinali, J. E., L. R. Krome, & E. Ruiz (Eds.). (2000). *Emergency medicine: A comprehensive study guide* (5th ed.). New York: McGraw Hill.

NOTES

_____

_____

_____

_____

_____

_____

CHAPTER 48

THE PEDIATRIC APPROACH

Kemedy K. McQuillen, M.D.

Evaluation of pediatric patients can be especially challenging because they differ significantly from adults in emotional development and physiologic function. In addition to being unable to communicate at a level that the adult caregiver can understand, they can be caught in a situation that they find terrifying, thereby limiting communication. What follows are general guidelines to approaching pediatric patients in a way that alleviates their fears while eliciting as much information as possible. Also included are signs and symptoms that are unique to children, which may provide important diagnostic information.

APPROACH

These guidelines apply to children who are aware of their surroundings. Children who are obtunded or rapidly deteriorating should be treated expeditiously to facilitate advanced care at an institution that can properly care for them.

GENERAL GUIDELINES

Remember that fear is often the limiting factor in the examination of children. By keeping them comfortable, you will be able to clarify the situation more rapidly. Watch the child from a distance before approaching: Does the child smile? Does the child play? Whenever possible, allow the child to sit with or next to the parents. Because the child is more likely to talk to the guardian, have the guardian ask the questions. Start simple: what's the child's name; how old is the child; does the child go to school? If the child has a stuffed animal, perform each part of the examination on the toy before you examine the child. Most important, be honest and explain everything before you do it. If something is going to hurt, say so. Offer choices, and make the examination a game: "Do you want me to listen to your front first, or your back first?" Do not ask to do something you have to do. If the child says "no," then you are stuck.

It may also be helpful to allow the child to touch the items you are going to use to examine or treat him or her if it is safe to do so. By permitting a child to hold the stethoscope for a few seconds, you may allay the fear that this is something that will hurt. It is also good practice to warm a cold stethoscope before placing it on the child's body and to listen through the shirt first.

VITAL SIGNS

- Blood pressure is "a big hug on the arm." For kids older than 2 years of age, the normal systolic blood pressure is approximately 90 mm Hg plus 2 times the age in years, with a lower limit of 70 mm Hg plus 2 times the age in years.

- Temperature taking can be done by parents.

- Respiratory rate checks can usually be done visually from a distance.

- Respiratory rate decreases with age:

   o Newborn: 40 breaths per minute

   o 1-year-old: 24 breaths per minute

   o 18-year-old: 18 breaths per minute

- Tachypnea is often the first sign of respiratory distress but can also be present with fever or anxiety.

- Heart rate decreases with age:

   o Infant: 120 to 150 bpm

   o Toddler: 100 to 120 bpm

- o School Age: 90 to 100 bpm

- o Adolescent: 70 to 90 bpm

- In general, heart rate increases in the earliest stages of shock, but in neonates the first response to hypoxia is bradycardia.

- Tachypnea or tachycardia can also result from fever, anxiety, and excitement.

HEENT

- Offer a choice: "Should I look in your mouth or your eyes first?"

- Use keys or a toy (bears are the most popular) to track eye movement.

- Check for neck pain or rigidity with a "tickle on the neck."

- In infants, check the fontanel (soft spot). Is it bulging or sunken?

  - o Bulging fontanels may indicate rising intracranial pressure from various causes, such as head injury, meningitis, or hydrocephalus, or it may be caused by crying.

LUNGS

- Have the child's parent or guardian lift up the child's shirt to watch respirations.

  - o Does the child have retractions (intercostal, sternal, or supraclavicular)?

  - o Does the child have paradoxical movement of the abdomen with respirations?

  - o Is the child using accessory muscles? Sitting forward? Drooling?

- Let the child place the stethoscope on the chest, and listen for everything (heart rate, breath sounds, bowel sounds) wherever it lands.

  o Are breath sounds reduced or unequal?

  o Is there wheezing, stridor, or a prolonged expiratory phase?

  o Is the child grunting?

  o Have the child blow out a penlight to get good expirations.

CARDIAC

- Distract child with a toy or medical instrument, or allow a baby to suck on a pacifier to get a quiet examination.

- Let the child listen to his or her parent's or guardian's heart before you listen to the child's.

- Tickle the feet or hands to evaluate temperature and capillary refill.

- Mucous membranes and nailbeds are good places to check for cyanosis.

  o Acrocyanosis (cyanosis of the hands and or feet) is normal in a newborn, and cutis mamorata (mottling of the legs) is normal in an infant.

ABDOMEN

- Use the stethoscope to push on the abdomen while listening.

- Tell the child that you push on the belly to see if he or she is hungry.

- If the child is ticklish, have him or her place a hand on top of yours and do the pushing (while you do the feeling) to squelch the laughter and allow for a better examination.

NEUROLOGIC EXAMINATION

- Does the child recognize his or her parent or guardian?

  o By 2 months of age, a child should be able to focus on the parent or guardian's face.

- Observe for confusion, lethargy, and agitation, which suggest subacute hypoperfusion.

- Hold or have the parent or guardian hold the child to evaluate muscle tone.

  o Decreased muscle tone, convulsions, or pupillary dilation suggest acute hypoperfusion.

- Watch the child play with the parent or guardian to evaluate strength.

- Check with the parent or guardian to determine the child's baseline movements or gait before assuming the child is ataxic; the child may be just learning to walk or sit.

- Gently tickle the child to evaluate sensation.

- If a parent or guardian says the child is just not right, believe it—this person knows the child best.

SKIN

- Ask the parent or guardian to direct you to any new rashes or discolorations.

These are suggestions. Good common sense and a modicum of patience will carry you through even the most difficult evaluation.

For further information regarding emergent evaluation and treatment of children, contact the American Heart Association for training in pediatric advance life support (PALS) or the American College of Emergency Physicians for its course in advanced pediatric life support (APLS).

CHAPTER 49

CONTINUOUS QUALITY IMPROVEMENT

Thomas J. Rahilly, Ph.D.

Every organization or agency that provides either a product or a service should have a process by which the enterprise seeks to continuously improve its products or services. Businesses realize that in order to grow their base of customers and thrive in a competitive marketplace, the customer must feel that what they are purchasing is necessary to their own existence and growth. They must also believe that their purchase has value when compared with similar commodities. To measure the quality of what it offers, a business will often institute a quality management program. There are many quality management programs with various names from which to choose, but all of them have the same philosophy: Quality can always be improved, but only if everyone in the organization is committed to the program.

Quality management as it relates to EMS organizations is a relatively new endeavor. This is probably a result of the maturation of EMS as a legitimate field of medicine. In its more than 30 years of evolution, EMS has become more professionally managed by individuals who have been educated in the methods of organizational management. In addition, some states now mandate quality improvement programs for EMS services. Regardless of the impetus for improving the quality of service, most organizations that provide EMS realize that a comprehensive quality management program is an essential component of its business plan.

Although there are many models of continuous quality improvement (CQI) from which to choose, perhaps the one most often studied was developed by W. Edwards Deming, a mathematician who began working to revitalize the Japanese economy shortly after the end of World War II. He is universally accepted as the individual most responsible for creating the Japanese economic system, one of the most powerful in the world. His approach was actually quite simple. Deming knew that to survive, an organization needs continuous economic growth, that constant customer satisfaction is essential to economic growth, and growth is only possible if an organization's entire workforce is committed to CQI. Few would argue that Japan's economy could have achieved such dramatic growth without Deming's quality improvement efforts.

Although most of Deming's work was focused on the Japanese manufacturing sector, his "Plan, Do, Check, and Act" (PDCA) cycle of CQI can be applied to almost any organization that seeks to provide its customer with a high-quality product or service while using its resources efficiently to control costs. The PDCA is a never-ending cycle that usually produces substantial initial improvements and then constantly looks for ways to provide "zero defect" service to the customer. While there are those who try to cover up deficiencies or shortcomings, Deming taught the Japanese to believe that "every defect is a treasure." Errors or failures must be seen as a way to improve quality. There is no perfect part of any society. Therefore the search for ways to improve all facets of life should be continuous. Properly implemented, each PDCA cycle will yield benefits to the organization. The yield of one cycle becomes the impetus beginning the next cycle.

Deming developed a process by which the management of an organization could transform its business practices to achieve a high level of quality. He used a 14-point plan to guide the organization along the road to zero defects. This plan can easily be used to promote quality improvement activities within an EMS agency as well.

1. **Create constancy of purpose.** All members of the orga-
    nizations should have a role in defining the highest prior-
    ity of the organization. The community served by an EMS
    organization expects to receive a high level of service at
    the lowest possible cost. Through CQI, the organization
    can achieve maximum efficiency and effectiveness.

2. **Adopt the new philosophy.** CQI is a process that requires
    a contribution from all members of the organization. Pride
    of workmanship must be modeled by the organization's
    leaders and practiced by all employees from recruitment
    to retirement.

3. **Cease dependence on inspection to achieve quality.**
    Periodic inspections as the only means of improvement
    will not achieve quality because they are grounded in the
    assumption that error is likely. By focusing on activities
    that reduce or minimize error, EMS organizations will be
    prepared for inspection by any entity.

4. **Do not purchase on the basis of price tag alone.** The
    lowest bid does not always provide the highest-quality
    item. Purchasers must be accountable for obtaining the
    highest-quality product for the best price. Vendors must
    be considered as partners. They must have their own
    quality management program and be included in the EMS
    organization's CQI efforts.

5. **Constantly improve the system of production and
    service.** Regardless of how well any organization functions,
    that quality of service can always be improved by close coop-
    eration between the suppliers and users of the service.

6. **Institute CQI training on the job.** Every worker must under-
    stand the needs of those served by the organization. CQI is
    not a stand-alone process. It must be viewed as an integral
    part of how the organization strives to meet and improve
    the needs of those who are served on a daily basis.

7. **Institute effective leadership.** Effective leaders are
    knowledgeable about the work of the organization and

SECTION 2

its workers. They create an environment that encourages workers to suggest ways that the service can be improved and quickly implement those ideas that have merit. Effective leaders celebrate successes and find ways to eliminate failures.

8. **Drive out fear.** The identification of an error should not be viewed as poor performance by one or several workers but as an opportunity for improvement by the entire workforce. Workers must feel confident that they will be taken seriously and not be adversely affected by identifying a problem or failure.

9. **Break down barriers between departments.** If the entire organization has unity in purpose, there will be no need for interdepartmental conflict. The synergy of an entire organization seeking ways to improve service and reduce errors will cultivate a culture of CQI.

10. **Eliminate slogans, exhortations, and targets for the workforce for zero defects and new levels of productivity.** Improvement in service performance is brought about by improving work processes.

11. **Eliminate management by numbers and objective.** Substitute leadership. Management by numbers and objectives tends to reward individuals and thereby fractionate the workforce. Developing a team effort to improve processes will yield improved outcomes and higher profits, which will benefit the entire workforce.

12. **Remove barriers to pride of workmanship.** Workers who are proud of their workmanship are the most valuable resource that an EMS organization has. They are most productive when they have a clear understanding of what is expected of them. Management must develop a strong relationship with the workforce and provide it with the infrastructure it needs to accomplish the organization's purpose.

13. **Institute a vigorous program of education and self-improvement.** Lifelong learning must be an organiza-

tional standard for both management and the workforce. Continued growth through education and life experience is essential to the improvement in the quality of the organization as well as each of its members.

14. **Put everybody to work to accomplish the transformation.** CQI is an organization-wide endeavor. The focus must be on the identification of the needs of those who use the service of EMS providers and then developing methods that continuously seek to improve the service delivered. Every aspect of service delivery is included, and every member of the organization has a vital role in ensuring that "every defect is a treasure."

The purpose of every EMS organization must be the provision of the highest quality of patient care at the most economical price possible. To achieve this purpose, there must be management systems in place to ensure that CQI is a part of every worker's daily routine. CQI is the hallmark of an EMS organization that is committed to providing the best possible service to those it serves, with the understanding that even an excellent performance can be improved. The organization's leaders must constantly reinforce the value of quality-driven management by being customercentric. They must also provide the tools and processes by which employees can fulfill the roles they have been asked to perform. Workers must be confident that the organizational culture promotes the identification of weak performance and rewards suggestions to improve processes. Workers perform best when they know that they have a vested interest in the organization's mission. A quality improvement program improves not only the delivery of service but self-improvement for the workforce as well.

BIBLIOGRAPHY

Polsky, S. (1992). *Continuous quality improvement in EMS.* Dallas, TX: American College of Emergency Physicians.

United States Department of Transportation. (1999). *A Leadership Guide to Quality Improvement.* Retrieved September 30, 2004 at http://www.nhtsa.dot.gov/people/injury/ems/leaderguide/index.html.

NOTES

_____

_____

_____

_____

_____

_____

_____

_____

_____

_____

_____

_____

_____

_____

_____

_____

_____

_____

_____

CHAPTER 50

EXPOSURE TO INFECTIOUS DISEASES

Thomas J. Rahilly, Ph.D.

Exposure to disease has always been a hazard to humans. A number of devastating diseases over the course of time have been carefully recorded by historians. There are several diseases, both airborne and bloodborne, that may be included in the worst ever contracted by man. Hepatitis B virus, human immunodeficiency virus (HIV), and tuberculosis are serious threats to the health of the general population and especially that of healthcare workers.

Prehospital emergency medical service (EMS) providers are especially susceptible to acquiring a disease through occupational exposure. The prehospital area is more dangerous than other healthcare work environments because the worker has little, if any, control over the setting in which the health care is delivered. EMS workers often find themselves in unfamiliar surroundings that were never meant to be places where health care was delivered. Motor vehicle and industrial accident sites, as well as the homes, offices, and even the streets where people experience events that lead to the need for emergency medical assistance, all pose a danger for the emergency medical technician. Unlike other areas where emergency medical care takes place, such as the emergency departments of hospitals, there is usually limited or no control of environmental conditions such as light, temperature, and the engineering controls that may reduce the potential exposure to communicable disease.

Having read the previous paragraph, you may feel that the acquisition of a communicable disease is only a matter of time. This, however, is not true. By implementing a comprehensive infection control program, EMS and first-responder agencies can greatly improve the chances that their employees (including volunteers) can remain safe in the workplace. The establishment of an effective health maintenance system, the development of an objective-based training program, and the routine use of appropriate personal protective equipment can provide a high level of protection for the EMS worker. Although the potential for infection will always be present, the risk of becoming occupationally exposed to a communicable disease can be minimized.

Governmental agencies such as the Occupational Safety and Health Administration (OSHA) and state departments of labor require employers in the healthcare industry to develop and maintain an exposure control plan for the protection of its employees. Most of these agencies—including OSHA—specify a plan that protects against bloodborne pathogens. The components of an effective plan, however, provide protection from all pathogens. At a minimum, such a plan should include policies for the following:

- Health maintenance

- Personal protective equipment

- Incident operations and recovery

- Postexposure

- Equipment disinfection and storage

To prevent the spread of infection in the prehospital field, EMS providers must develop a proactive attitude. The procedures needed to reduce the risk of acquiring an infectious disease are known as body substance isolation (BSI). Those who practice BSI consider the blood, body fluids, and tissues of all patients to be infectious. BSI requires those emergency service personnel who have the potential to come in contact with a patient to place a barrier between themselves and the potentially infectious materials found at every emergency medical incident. By using barrier protection, or personal protective equipment, the responders isolate their skin and mucous membranes from contact with the potentially infectious materials. The only exceptions to the use of barrier protection are when the use of personal protective equipment interferes with the proper delivery of health care or when such equipment poses a significant risk to the personal safety of the responder or a coworker. These cases are considered extraordinary situations, and the decision not to use personal protection rests solely with the emergency service providers, not their employers.

At a minimum, BSI requires the use of disposable gloves. They should be donned before any patient contact, worn until all patient care and cleanup activities are complete, and disposed of according to the response agency's written policy. There must also be written policies that indicate when masks, protective eyewear, gowns, and other forms of personal protection must be worn. Training programs that inform emergency providers about the use of these devices must be included in the agency's exposure control plan.

All emergency service providers are at risk for acquiring an infectious disease while providing health care. They may, however, provide a high degree of personal protection by maintaining their health, practicing BSI, and ensuring that their patient-care equipment and transport vehicles are kept free from potentially infectious materials.

BIBLIOGRAPHY

National Fire Protection Association. (2000). *NFPA 1581: Standard on Fire Department Infection Control Program.* Quincy, MA: Author.

U.S. Fire Administration. (1992, September). *Infection control for emergency response personnel: The supervisor's role.* Emmitsburg, MD: Author.

West, K. (Ed.). (2001). *Infectious disease handbook for emergency care personnel* (3rd ed.). Cincinnati, OH: American Conference of Governmental and Industrial Hygienists.

NOTES

_____

_____

_____

_____

_____

_____

_____

_____

_____

_____

_____

_____

_____

_____

_____

_____

_____

_____

_____

_____

CHAPTER 51

THE FIRE SCENE

Thomas J. Rahilly, Ph.D.

In many communities, the fire department is also the provider of emergency medical services (EMS). This means that when responding to a fire call, the ambulance personnel are under the direct control of the chief fire officer and are fully integrated into the department's response plan. The ambulance usually accompanies the fire apparatus. Firefighter or emergency medical technicians (EMTs), or other fire-medic personnel, perform specific tasks on the fire scene that are delineated in the fire department's standard operating procedures. Not all emergency medical services, however, are provided by the fire service. In fact, there are a great many areas where the provider of EMS may serve a region that is protected by several different fire departments. Because a chance exists that there may either be an injured person at the fire scene as a result of the fire or that one of the firefighters could be injured during the firefighting operation, ambulances are generally dispatched to the scene of a fire. It is therefore imperative that EMS responders know exactly what their responsibilities are at the scene of a fire.

For the most part, the fire service has been the leader in a move to establish a system whereby the scene of an emergency is managed in a coordinated manner. The incident command system (ICS), when properly implemented, assigns areas of responsibility according to the task being performed. These responsibilities are assigned to sectors with an officer in charge who reports to a single incident commander. The desired effect of this system is to reduce the amount of freelancing by the various agencies that may become involved during a fire or other multiagency response. ICS provides more efficient use of resources, reduces personal risk, and improves on-scene communication.

All EMS responders, whether fire or third service, must report to the incident commander on arrival at the scene of a fire or other emergency where the chief fire officer has been placed in charge. In communities where there is an integrated approach to emergency management, each response organization understands its specific responsibility within the system. The ICS identifies EMS as a separate sector, and an officer, preferably from EMS, will be assigned as the sector commander. Under this system all emergency medical providers must report to the sector commander on arrival at the emergency scene. From this point, personnel can be assigned to activities in the order of highest priority. There may be a need for the treatment of fire victims and firefighters, or EMS responders may be needed to staff the rehabilitation sector, where emergency workers are evaluated and monitored for any negative physiologic effects resulting from the operation.

In the event that a community has not implemented an emergency incident management system or if the ambulance arrives before the fire department, EMS personnel should not undertake firefighting operations on their own. This includes entering structures that are on fire or those that appear to be emitting smoke. Untrained or poorly equipped persons who attempt to gain entry to a building that is on fire not only risk personal injury to themselves but also place an added burden on firefighters who now must consider them to be potential victims. This may actually delay the rescue of the building's occupants. Additionally, the EMS responders will be needed to treat any victims who are rescued from the building. If they become injured themselves, they only add to the problem at hand.

It is not uncommon for an ambulance to come to a structure that is on fire or arrive before the firefighters. The EMS responder's first action must be to notify the fire department. Do not rely on reports at the scene that the fire department has already been called. Advise the EMS dispatcher to make a separate notification. The EMS responder's next action should be to alert the occupants of the building from a position of personal safety. The use of the ambulance public address system and siren are a particularly effective means of accomplishing this. Once again, without the proper training and personal protective equipment, EMS personnel should not enter a burning building.

BIBLIOGRAPHY

Delmar Publishing. (2000). Firefighter's Handbook: Essentials of firefighting and emergency response. Albany, NY: Thomson Delmar Learning.

National Fire Protection Association. (2002). *NFPA 1500: Standard for fire fighter health and safety*. Batterymarch Park, MA: Author.

NOTES

_____

_____

_____

_____

_____

_____

_____

_____

_____

_____

_____

_____

SECTION 2

CHAPTER 52

THE HAZARDOUS MATERIALS INCIDENT

Thomas J. Rahilly, Ph.D.

Every day millions of pounds of hazardous materials are produced, transported, stored, and used worldwide to support modern technology. Considering the number of industries that are using substances that are potentially harmful to humans and the environment, there are surprisingly few accidents. But they do occur and will continue to place workers and the public in danger. As is the case in just about every other emergency incident, an emergency medical services (EMS) response will be necessary either to help mitigate the problem or provide support services to those who must confine and control the situation.

When called to the scene of a hazardous materials (HAZMAT) incident, EMS workers must take a more conservative approach to the operation than they would at another type of incident. The dangers to the responders are great, and many of these dangers are not obvious. Hazardous material incidents should not be considered routine because the use of day-to-day procedures can result in longer exposure for the victims and contamination of ambulance and emergency department personnel and equipment. The Occupational Safety and Health Administration (OSHA) requires all emergency service personnel who respond to emergencies as first responders to complete a hazardous materials awareness training course. This course is the first step in recognizing the inherent dangers associated with responses to hazardous materials incidents. It does not, however, prepare the emergency worker to mitigate the problem or to treat victims associated with these emergencies.

THE INCIDENT COMMAND SYSTEM

Any emergency response organization that may be called to the scene of a hazardous materials incident should have an operational plan that has been developed in cooperation with the other agencies that will also be on the scene. The use of the incident command system (ICS) will help to ensure a coordinated approach to a situation that is as dangerous to the responders as it is to the victims. Responding EMS units should report to the incident commander and follow the directions of the command post.

An effective hazardous materials operation managed by ICS will have zones established to identify the areas that pose a danger to victims of the incident as well as to the emergency responders. The "hot zone" is the area that actually contains the material that has caused the event. Depending on the material involved and the atmospheric conditions present or expected, this zone will vary in size. No responders may enter this area unless they are expressly ordered to do so by the command post, and then, only if they are currently certified to work there. Activity in the hot zone requires special equipment and training. Independent actions by unauthorized persons may result in injury or death and will usually endanger the safety of the other emergency responders.

The "warm zone" is the area immediately surrounding the hot zone. This is where such activities as patient and hazardous materials technician decontamination is accomplished. Once again, if responders are not adequately trained and protected, entry to this zone is restricted. Perimeter identification and control are essential to ensure that unwary responders do not inadvertently enter a dangerous area of the incident.

The "cold zone" is established well beyond the area of potential danger. It is here that all of the support functions, such as the provision of EMS, occur. The "cold zone"

SECTION 2

contains the command post, EMS sector, and staging areas for additional resources. Incoming EMS units should receive direction from the command post before their arrival whenever possible. Preplanning and multiagency training drills help prevent the confusion associated with multiagency emergency response when these agencies do not normally work with each other on a day-to-day basis.

THE EMERGENCY MEDICAL SERVICES SECTOR

The EMS, or medical, sector of the ICS has several important functions. Depending on the other resources available, these functions may include medical surveillance of the hazardous materials response team, the decontamination of victims, and treatment and transport of victims to an appropriate medical facility. Rarely will EMS providers be part of the hazardous materials team, which is responsible for rescuing victims or controlling the release of the material. A well-designed hazardous materials plan will assign the following responsibilities to the EMS sector:

- *Medical surveillance of the hazardous materials team.* Members of the hazardous materials team are frequently placed under severe physical stress as a result of the effects of the personal protection equipment that must be used to protect them from the hazardous materials present. EMS personnel should be present to establish baseline vital signs of the team before the commencement of their operations. All members of the team should be monitored after the completion of their duties to ensure that they have not been adversely affected by either the stress of the incident or the hazardous materials themselves. Complete documentation is essential for the protection of the team's future health benefits.

- *Decontamination of patients.* Although many hazardous materials response teams are trained and equipped to handle this task, there may be a need in certain jurisdictions for the EMS sector to assume this responsibility. When developing the overall response plan, the emergency management staff must determine which agency will be given the resources and training to properly perform patient decontamination. Some hazardous materials plans identify decontamination as a separate sector. Regardless of which agency or organization is charged with the responsibility of decontaminating patients exposed to hazardous substances, proper training and equipment are necessary if the decontamination process is to be successful. During decontamination, victims should be decontaminated in the "warm zone."

- ***Treatment of patients.*** After patients have been decontaminated, they must receive a thorough evaluation and treatment according to the presenting problem, with consideration given to the substance involved. Before any patient contact, EMS personnel should don the appropriate personal protective equipment. Use extreme caution during patient care because incomplete decontamination may result in personal injury to the caregiver.

Because most chemical emergencies adversely affect the respiratory system of those victims who were exposed, basic life support is a priority. Immediate attention must be given to protecting the airway, with ventilatory assistance as appropriate. Information about the treatment of specific injuries from substances identified by the hazardous materials technicians may be found in the U.S. Department of Transportation's *Hazardous Materials Response Guidebook*. This reference is updated periodically and often contains the method for neutralizing the substance. All EMS vehicles should have a copy of this guidebook, which is available from the U.S. Government Printing Office.

Whenever possible, labels used to identify the material should be brought to the emergency department to assist the physician in treating the patient. If material safety data sheets (MSDS) are available, copies of these documents will also be useful in the evaluation and treatment of the patient. Because all entities that use or store hazardous materials must disclose their use to the agency responsible for hazardous materials, it might prove helpful to provide the medical facility with copies of the disclosure documents before an emergency.

- **Transport of patients.** After treatment and packaging of the patients is complete, they should be transported to the closest appropriate medical facility. Before placing patients who have been exposed to hazardous materials in the ambulance, it may be necessary to remove nonessential equipment and supplies to keep them from potential contamination. In addition, it may be prudent to drape the inside of the patient compartment with a plastic sheet to help protect the interior of the ambulance. Seal off the opening to the driver's compartment as well if there is such an opening.

Because not all medical facilities are staffed with appropriately trained personnel or are equipped to handle victims of a hazardous materials incident, preplanning is essential to a successful outcome for the victims. Medical facilities identified as prepared and willing to receive patients exposed to hazardous materials must be included in the planning process and involved in training drills to increase the likelihood that they will maintain a high level of readiness. Notification from the command post will help the medical facility prepare itself and its personnel for the arrival of a patient that may pose a danger to the other people in the facility.

The nature of emergency response is becoming more complex and, if not adequately planned, may be cause for injury or death to those called on to control the incident. EMS providers must be prepared to assume their role in the overall response to hazardous materials incidents. Training, personal protective equipment, and, most of all, self-discipline are the fundamental components of a plan that will help to ensure that the rescuers will not become victims themselves.

BIBLIOGRAPHY

Stutz, D. R. & S. Ulin. (1997). *Hazardous materials injuries: A handbook for pre-hospital care*. Greenbelt, MD: Bradford Communication.

Varela, J. (Ed.). (1996). *Hazardous materials: Handbook for emergency responders*. New York: Joseph Wiley & Sons.

NOTES

_____

_____

_____

_____

_____

_____

_____

_____

_____

_____

_____

_____

_____

_____

_____

_____

CHAPTER 53

INTERPRETING THE 12-LEAD ELECTROCARDIOGRAM

Gary Goodman, M.D.

The electrocardiogram (ECG) is a representation of the electrical events of the heart over time. It must be interpreted in the context of the clinical picture of the patient. The traditional prehospital use of the ECG was for rhythm analysis. Advancements in the care of the ischemic heart have led to a need for earlier diagnosis and treatment. It is hoped that the addition of the 12-lead ECG to the prehospital armamentarium will reduce the morbidity and mortality rates associated with acute coronary syndromes. This chapter serves as a brief review of 12-lead electrocardiography for paramedics.

In the 12-lead configuration, nine additional leads are added. The 12-lead configuration consists of three sets of leads:

- Three bipolar leads: I, II, and III

- Three augmented limb unipolar leads: aVR (augmented Voltage Right arm), aVL (augmented Voltage Left arm), and a VF (augmented Voltage Foot)

- Six precordial (chest) leads: V_1, V_2, V_3, V_4, V_5, and V_6, which spread from the sternum laterally across the precordium from the right sternal border to the left midaxillary line.

To best understand the differences between each lead set, it is easiest to visualize the view of the heart as though one was looking from the direction of the positive electrode. Thus in the bipolar leads (I, II, and III), the heart is viewed from the left shoulder, left hip, and right shoulder, respectively. The depolarization of the myocardium will display a positive inflection as the heart depolarizes from the direction of the right shoulder to the left hip as seen in lead II.

The three bipolar leads and the three augmented leads combined display the six intersecting limb leads of the standard ECG and lie in a flat "frontal" plane across a patient's chest. The 6 chest leads cut the body into top and bottom halves displaying the "horizontal" plane. Again, each lead is always a positive lead—therefore V_1 is the most negative deflection because the heart lies in the mediastinum tilted downward and to left hip. Moving further left across the precordium to V_6, the leads become increasingly more positive.

The best source of orientation for proper lead placement is the sternum. Begin by placing each limb lead at each extremity or "truncally" at each shoulder and hip. Once the limb leads are applied, begin applying the V leads: V_1 is placed at the right sternal border, fourth intercostal space. Continue across the chest to the left sternal border, fourth intercostal space for V_2. Leads V_3 through V_6 will then create a small half-circle ending in the anterior axillary line. In patients with excessive breast tissue, it is acceptable to place the precordial leads under the breast because placing them on the breast will cause the *a* tracing to be perceived as that of low voltage, commonly seen in some medical diagnoses, or that of pericardial effusion. Care should be taken to place the electrodes in their standard locations to facilitate valid comparisons between the current tracing and past tracings.

By convention, the ECG machine is calibrated so that a 1 mV (1 millivolt) signal deflects the stylus 10 mm. Low voltage tracings may be found in patients with chronic obstructive pulmonary disease (COPD) or those with pericardial effusions. High-voltage tracings are common in patients with left ventricular hypertrophy. The gain may be adjusted so that these tracings are more easily evaluated. ECG paper speed is set at 25 mm per minute. The speed may be increased to 50 mm/minute to increase the space between complexes when the patient is tachycardic to facilitate evaluation of atrial complexes.

SECTION 2

A systematic, stepwise approach to 12-lead ECG interpretation is recommended. Be sure to evaluate the following ECG features:

- Rate
- Rhythm (regularity of atrial and ventricular rhythm)
- Axis
- Ventricular or atrial hypertrophy
- Area of injury and/or ischemia (ST segment elevation or depression, inverted T waves, right bundle branch block (RBBB) or left bundle branch block (LBBB), and Q waves)
- Specific electrolyte abnormalities (peaked T waves, decreased or increased QT segments, PR intervals, etc.)
- Miscellaneous waves (delta, Osborne waves, etc.)

EMS providers should be expert at recognizing the abnormalities that require EMS interventions, affect transport decisions, or indicate a potential for a worsening clinical situation. These include the following:

- Rhythm disturbances
- Ischemia and infarction
- Hyperkalemia
- Tricyclic antidepressant (TCA) overdose

Rate does not usually require calculation from the ECG tracing because most ECG machines calculate the rate and display it digitally. However, rate can be determined using standard ECG recording paper. On a standard ECG recording, each 1-second interval consists of 5 large ECG boxes, or 25 small (1-mm) ECG boxes. Using a "300-box" counting method, the number of large ECG boxes separating two consecutive R waves are counted and then divided by 300. This equation is only accurate if the rhythm is regular, with R-R intervals that are constant. This method is not useful for irregular rhythms, such as atrial fibrillation. If the rhythm is not regular, one can closely approximate the rate by using the "six-second method," whereby one counts the amount of R-R intervals in a 6-second interval and multiplies that amount by 10. Finally, another popular method used is the "300, 150, 100, 75, 60, 50" method. To calculate the ventricular rate, start by counting dark lines from any R wave. If the next R wave falls on the fourth dark line, the rate is equal to 75 beats per minute. It should be noted that this is the number of electrical impulses produced by the heart.

To identify the inherent cardiac rhythm, follow these steps: (1) Evaluate the atrial and ventricular rates, (2) evaluate the P wave configuration in lead II, (3) establish the number of P waves in relation to the number of QRS complex (1:1; 2:1; 3:1, etc.), and (4) establish the configuration of the QRS complex. Table 53-1 identifies 15 inherent rhythms distinguishable from each other by four independent criteria: rate, P wave, P : QRS ratio, and QRS complex. Each inherent rhythm possesses only one of the four criteria. Exceptions may exist where different ECG abnormalities might appear identical (i.e., supraventricular tachycardia with aberrancy versus ventricular tachycardia).

Although it is not of critical concern in the prehospital arena, the axis of the heart can be determined simply by using the QRS complex in leads I and AVF; as this may help distinguish one rhythm or block from others. See Table 53-1 for clarification.

Of major interest to most EMS providers is the concept of the acute coronary syndrome. The current American Heart Association guidelines recommend a 12-lead ECG within the first 10 minutes as part of the immediate assessment of patients who are suspected of having cardiac ischemia. This ECG is used to triage the patient into one of three groups:

1. ST-segment elevation myocardial infarction (MI) (STEMI). These ECGs have ST segment elevation or presumably new LBBB. This finding strongly suggests injury.

2. High-risk unstable angina/non-ST-segment elevation MI. These ECGs have ST depression or dynamic T-wave inversion. This finding strongly suggests ischemia.

3. Intermediate/low-risk unstable angina. These ECGs do not have suspicious changes in ST segments or T-waves. They are considered nondiagnostic ECGs.

The location of ischemia or infarction can be determined by looking for the following abnormalities:

- Inferior region—leads II, III, and aVF.
- Septal region—leads V_1 and V_2
- Anterior region—leads V_3 and V_4
- Lateral region—leads I, aVL, V_5, and V_6
- Posterior region—indirectly through evaluation of V_1 and V_2

The triage schema listed above does not include an assessment of the Q-wave. A Q-wave may be a normal finding in some leads, such as III or V_1, or a pathologic finding. A significant Q wave is defined as one greater than 0.04 seconds (1 mm) in duration or exceeding 25% of the total QRS complex. Although found in some acute MIs, the Q-wave may also indicate a prior MI.

The interpretation of 12-lead ECGs seems daunting at first. In time, the diligent paramedic will become expert. Although the modern 12-lead ECG machine provides a computer-generated interpretation, the paramedic should perform his or her own analysis. It is not uncommon for the computer-generated interpretation to be wrong. Consultation with medical direction may be helpful when the paramedic's interpretation differs from the computer-generated interpretation.

The 12-lead ECG is one of the newest diagnostic tests used in the emergency medical services. It has great potential to improve the care of patients suffering an acute coronary syndrome, especially when healthcare systems are able to act rapidly on information that was previously available only after the patient arrived at the hospital.

Table 53-1. Characteristics of Selected Cardiac Arrhythmias

Rhythm	Atrial Rate	Ventricular Rate	P Wave in Lead 11	P to QRS Ratio	QRS Morphology
Sinus bradycardia	< 60	Equal	Upright	1 to 1	Normal width
Normal sinus rhythm	60–100	Equal	Upright	1 to 1	Normal width
Sinus tachycardia	> 100	Equal	Upright	1 to 1	Normal width
Atrial tachycardia	120–150	Equal	Usually upright	1 to 1	Normal width
Atrial flutter	250–350	60–120*	Upright and spiked	4 or more:1	Normal width
Atrial fibrilliation	> 350	60–120*	Upright and irregular	Indeterminable	Normal width
Nodal rhythm†	40–60	Equal	Missing/ downward	1 to 1 (if present)	Normal width
Accelerated nodal rhythm	60–100	Equal	Missing/ downward	1 to 1 (if present)	Normal width
Nodal tachycardia	> 100	Equal	Missing/ downward	1 to 1 (if present)	Normal width
Ventricular rhythm†	xxx	< 50	Missing	xxx	Wide/aberrant
Accelerated ventricular rhythm	xxx	50–1000	Missing	xxx	Wide/aberrant
Ventricular tachycardia	xxx	100–200	Missing	xxx	Wide/aberrant
Ventricular flutter	xxx	200–300	Missing	xxx	Wide/aberrant
Ventricular fibrilliation	xxx	150–300	Missing	xxx	Wide/aberrant
Torsades de Pointes	xxx	250–350	Missing	xxx	Wide/aberrant

*These values are approximate and show that a varying ventricular response is not unusual. In the case of atrial flutter, a fixed ventricular response is most frequent. In the case of atrial fibrillation, on the other hand, a varying ventricular response is both classic and a hallmark sign.

†These are the truly inherent rhythms occurring within the specialized conductive system of the heart. Atrial and ventricular rhythms such as tachycardia, flutter, and fibrillation are not "true" rhythms because they occur outside the normal conductive system.

According to Dubin, "Each QRS complex gradually increases and then decreases resembling that of a series of end to end spindle shapes 3."

SECTION 2

BIBLIOGRAPHY

Brown, K. R. (2003). *Emergency dysrhythmias & ECG injury patterns.* Clifton Park, NY: Thomson Delmar Learning.

CHAPTER 54

MULTIPLE CASUALTY INCIDENTS

John Fitzwilliam, B.S., B.A., EMT-CC

Statistics show that the experience of most advanced emergency medical technicians (EMTs) with multicasualty incidents (MCIs) are limited to motor vehicle accidents involving fewer than a dozen persons. Most paramedics spend their entire career without ever confronting a mass casualty disaster situation. Nevertheless, all paramedics and EMTs should be highly skilled in handling MCIs because of the potential for great loss of life. There are numerous definitions of an MCI. As a practical matter, we should understand that when the number of patients exceed the number of rescuers, we must go into an MCI operations mode. Leadership, triage, rapid scene control, and intelligent resource utilization are the key elements to effective management of these situations.

INCIDENT COMMAND SYSTEM

Under the incident command system (ICS), one person, the incident commander (IC), is responsible for the overall management of the MCI. The IC delegates job assignments (sectorization) to the treatment sector, extrication (rescue) sector, staging sector, triage sector, supply sector, or any other sectors needed at a particular operation. Note that here a sector is a function, not necessarily a geographic location. The sector officer is the supervisor for that particular function. On-scene communications between sectors should occur primarily through sector officers, not through providers. This allows command personnel to see the big picture, and use their resources more efficiently. Personnel assigned to a specific task report to only one supervisor. ICS greatly improves efficiency and supervision. Its scope can be narrowed or expanded as needed for each MCI. Using ICS routinely is good training. Vests of different colors should be used to identify sector officers whenever possible.

EARLY ON-SCENE OPERATIONS

The first ambulance on the scene becomes the initial medical aid station, supply pool, and communications center. Do not let this ambulance drive off with the first victim because you will be stranded without any resources in the middle of chaos. The personnel arriving first will be the medical sector officers, who will be relieved by officers who arrive later. The initial responsibilities of the first responders include the following:

- Confirming the location

- Assessing scene safety

- Sizing up the scene

- Establishing communications

- Performing triage

- Designating a staging area and a central patient collection area

- Implementing the ICS

- Implementing the local MCI plan

TRIAGE

Triage is the sorting of patients into categories based on the severity of their injuries and their potential for survival. The most medically experienced person should do the triaging. Most systems sort patients into three groups:

- Critical (RED)—those who need immediate care or transportation

- Serious (YELLOW)—those who are in urgent need of care but can wait up to 1 hour

- Delayed (GREEN)—those who do not require urgent care and can wait more than 1 hour. Deceased patients or those not expected to survive are often included in this last group.

Triage is an ongoing process, because patient conditions can change. Emergency medical personnel must try to do the most good for the most victims. A popular triage system is called "START" (simple triage and rapid treatment).

- On arrival at an MCI, tell anyone who can walk to move to a designated area. This method immediately places those who do not require urgent care in a "delayed" category until further triage can take place.

- Go to those patients left behind. Check their ventilation. If no ventilations are present, position airway once. If no ventilation can be discerned, this patient is dead.

- If ventilation is present at rates greater than 30 breaths per minute, this patient is an immediate priority.

- If rate is less than 30 breaths per minute, assess capillary refill. If capillary refill exceeds 2 seconds, this patient is an immediate priority.

- If capillary refill is less than 2 seconds (normal), proceed to assess mental status. If patient can follow simple commands, this patient is a delayed priority.

- If this patient cannot follow simple commands, this patient is categorized as an immediate priority.

- While triaging patients, do not start treatment. The only exceptions would be to attempt to open the airway once or put a pressure bandage on patients who have severe bleeding. Cardiopulmonary resuscitation (CPR) is not started during field triage.

The first arriving EMT or paramedic starts triage, not treatment. The use of triage tags is strongly recommended to provide an at-a-glance assessment of the patient's triage category, to speed documentation of medical care, and to track the condition and disposition of each patient at the scene.

STAGING AREA

The staging area should have good access and exit routes. Have police control traffic as soon as possible. Drivers should stay with ambulances if possible. The staging area should be away from the actual incident but near enough for rapid response.

CENTRAL PATIENT COLLECTION POINT

The central patient collection point (often called the *medical aid station* or *treatment sector*) is a location where all triaged patients are taken for continuing care and to await disposition. It should be located close enough to the incident site to offer rapid care, yet far enough to offer protection from fire, smoke, explosion, hazardous material run-off, toxic fumes, leaking fire hose lines, vehicle exhaust, and so forth. It should be an area that is more than large enough to handle the anticipated number of casualties. Consider uphill and upwind positioning, or place a fire engine between you and the threat. It is generally better to establish only one treatment area.

The most efficient means of moving patients is via backboards. Use nonEMS-trained personnel for patient transfer roles as much as possible. Use of a central patient collection point permits maximum utilization of rescuers and resources on hand. These EMS providers can function as a team and rapidly gain scene control. Whenever possible, personnel trained in advanced life support (ALS) should perform ALS tasks; they should not be litter carriers or drivers.

SECTION 2

The use of physicians at an MCI site is controversial. Many believe that doctors should stay at the hospital where they are more useful. Others say that on-scene physicians are valuable for making difficult triage decisions or performing advanced procedures on trapped victims.

Contact your Medical Control Communications Center (MEDCOM) early to allow local hospitals sufficient time to implement their MCI plans and be ready for the delivery of patients. MEDCOM contact with the scene, other than patient-specific on-line medical direction, should be through the medical sector commander only. Have MEDCOM determine individual hospital capabilities.

Do not overload the nearest hospital. Doing so only moves the disaster from the field to the hospital. The patient's needs and the system's capabilities will determine transport priorities and dispositions. Individual ambulances should not use the radio to contact MEDCOM during an MCI except for on-line medical direction.

ON-SCENE COMMUNICATIONS

Effectively managing communications at an MCI can be challenging. The radio communications system can easily be overwhelmed. The best on-scene communication is face to face. Do not hesitate to use messengers. The IC should have access to a portable radio from each agency at the MCI (if not, consider parking a fire chief's car, police car, ambulance, and so forth together for coordinated radio coverage). Use plain English, not radio codes. Interjurisdictional operations make the use of codes confusing and, at times, dangerous. An MCI is not the time to experience mistaken messages.

Prevent open microphones by placing the microphone in its proper holder. Some people drop the microphone on a car seat or inadvertently depress the "push to talk" switch. One open microphone causes enormous frustration at the MCI. Proper radio procedure and frequency coordination is critical. Try to establish separate channels for administration, scene-to-hospital contact, and so forth.

There should be no unnecessary transmissions; talk only when you have something important to say. In rural areas, consider involving amateur radio (ham) clubs in providing state-of-the-art communications assistance. Encourage radio interoperability among all units and agencies.

TERRORISM CONSIDERATIONS

• Ask yourself whether this MCI could actually be a terrorist attack.

• An explosion or fire could hide a secondary explosive device aimed at emergency service crews.

• Are the victims exhibiting signs and symptoms of respiratory distress or seizure disorder? If so, consider biochemical weapons. Call HAZMAT immediately. Do not enter such a scene without proper equipment and training.

• Do not let the rescuers congregate closely, creating one big target.

• Do not get tunnel vision. Be alert for suspicious persons trying to enter the scene. Watch for people who are dressed inappropriately for the climate. Remember that a bulky coat worn in the summer can conceal a bomb.

• Ambulances and emergency vehicles have been used in the past by terrorists to get explosives into secured areas. If you do not recognize the vehicle's markings or the driver's uniform, summon authorities to investigate immediately.

HINTS FOR INCREASED EFFECTIVENESS

• Use red, yellow, or green plastic tarps, flags, or tape to indicate the treatment area.

• Have stocked disaster boxes available for rapid transport to scene. These can also be colored coded to indicate ALS or basic life support (BLS) supplies.

• Have a stockpile of backboards for MCIs. Take a 4 × 8 piece of 3/4-inch plywood. You can make two 2 × 6-foot boards and one 2 × 4-foot board (child) from each piece. You can have three boards if you make them 16 inches wide. Keep 25 or more at various locations with cravats.

- Have available some portable oxygen manifolds, a box of nonrebreather masks, and a large oxygen tank to treat the many patients requiring oxygen.

- Use worksheets to write everything down.

- Bring extra pencils, triage tags, writing paper, grease pencils, and portable radio batteries.

- Make colored sector officer vests widely available at any hour.

- Remove injured or emotionally distraught EMS providers and rescue workers from the scene immediately. The other EMS providers will not remain focused on their tasks if a fellow worker is suffering. It is also better for scene morale and control to remove injured children and hysterical persons as soon as possible. Also remove relatives of EMS crews for the same reason.

- Have plans to protect patients from inclement weather. You might be able to move patients indoors to schools, shopping malls, barns, airplane hangars, or other structures. You can also bring shelter to the scene in the form of school buses, moving vans, or tractor trailer trucks.

- Plan for situations in which there are not sufficient ambulances available. Consider transporting via school bus. Place the wooden backboards over the seat tops, and secure them in place with cravats. Assign several EMTs or paramedics to remain on board with standard portable ambulance equipment and proceed to the hospital with a police escort.

- Make arrangements to supply local maps to incoming units. Keep a resource book and the local Yellow Pages phone directory on hand to use as needed. If all else fails, make sure that you have change for a phone call.

In conclusion, remember the six Ts of MCI Operation.

- **Take charge**

- **Triage**

- **Treat**

- **Transport**

- **Terminate (field and hospital emergency operation)**

- **Talk** (critical incident stress debriefings)

When people are accustomed to following a procedure, that procedure becomes a habit. Emergency medicine personnel must develop good habits to successfully handle MCIs.

BIBLIOGRAPHY

Briggs, S. M. & K. H. Brinsfield. (Eds.) (2003). *Advanced disaster medical response for providers*. Boston: Harvard Medical International Trauma and Disaster Institute.

Christen, H. & P. M. Maniscalo. (1998). *The EMS incident management system: Operations for mass casualty and high impact incidents*. Englewood Cliffs, NJ: Prentice-Hall.

NOTES

_____

_____

_____

_____

_____

_____

_____

CHAPTER 55

PSYCHIATRIC EMERGENCIES

Owen T. Traynor, M.D.

The American Psychiatric Association defines a psychiatric emergency as a "situation that includes an acute disturbance in thought, behavior, mood, or social relationship" requiring an immediate intervention. Paramedics often see patients with depression and anxiety disorders, aggressive or violent behavior, hallucinations, delusions, and personality changes. Paramedics also see patients with psychiatric disorders for other reasons, such as acute medical and traumatic illnesses and substance abuse.

The unusual behavior exhibited by some patients experiencing a psychiatric emergency may distract the paramedic from looking for medical causes of abnormal behavior and comorbid medical problems. Some studies of both inpatient and outpatient psychiatric services indicate that between 5% and 30% of patients have undiagnosed medical problems.

Paramedics must develop strategies for dealing with patients who present with psychiatric emergencies. The priority must be the safety of the patient, bystanders, and EMS workers. Second, the paramedic must consider the medical problems that may have caused the psychiatric emergency. Next, the paramedic must provide safe transportation, if needed, for the patient. The paramedic must also be prepared to safely restrain the patient, if indicated.

Patients who are severely depressed, anxious, agitated, confused, or psychotic pose the greatest threat to safety. Paramedics must perform a risk assessment for suicide in all patients with a psychiatric emergency. Consider the following risk factors:

- Alcohol or substance abuse

- A history of physical or sexual abuse

- A positive family history of a suicide attempt

- A previous suicide attempt

- A prior psychiatric diagnosis such as depression, anxiety or panic disorders, schizophrenia, and personality disorders

- A history of chronic severe medical illnesses

- Poor social support

- Access to weapons

- A well-developed suicide plan, including a strong intent and the means available to complete the plan

In addition to assessing the risk of suicide, the paramedic must assess for the possibility of violent behavior. Unfortunately, there are no reliable predictors of violent behavior. However, those who have behaved violently in the past are at high risk for further violence. Male gender and alcohol or substance abuse are also associated with violent behavior. Violent behavior is often preceded by aggressive language and threats of violence. Often the patient appears to be anxious, speaking in a loud voice and pacing. A preemptive strategy usually provides the most safety. Review the dispatch data carefully. Request police assistance when the dispatch data indicates a potential for danger. The 911 caller and other bystanders may provide useful information, such as the nature of the patient's behavior, the presence of weapons or hostages, and the location of the patient. Find out about entrances and exits to the patient's location. Keep at a safe distance if your safety is in jeopardy. Once the scene has been secured or the initial data indicate that it is safe, approach cautiously. Some recommend considering violent behavior as a continuum, from mild agitation to explosive physical violence.

Be ready to adapt as the patient's behavior moves along the continuum. Some choices of action may be to change the environment (e.g., moving to a quieter area with ready access to an exit). Ensure that the patient is not between you and the exit. Have adequate police backup present to demonstrate a show of force. Ensure that no weapons are available to the patient. Be direct and empathetic during your medical interview. You may need to set limits on what constitutes acceptable behavior. Ensure the patient's safety, and respect his or her personal space. If the behavior continues to escalate, offer medications to help the patient remain calm. Medications that may be helpful include haloperidol and benzodiazepines such as diazepam and lorazepam.

If violent behavior appears imminent and sufficient personnel are present, cease negotiations and physically restrain the patient. Only those specially trained and skilled in the safe use of restraints should apply the restraints. Always use the least restrictive and most effective means of control. Retreat when there is not sufficient personnel to restrain the patient.

All physically or chemically restrained patients must be carefully monitored to prevent accidental injury and death. Never hog-tie or restrain a patient in a prone position. The supine position with the head elevated or a lateral recumbent position are considered the safest positions.

Seek potential medical causes of abnormal behavior or an altered mental status. Possible medical causes include hypoxia, hypoglycemia, hypovolemia, substance abuse, head injury, hypertensive encephalopathy, renal and hepatic failure, seizure disorder, and CNS infection. Refer to chapter 4 for further details. Obtain a thorough medical and psychiatric history, including the use of prescription and nonprescription drugs. Many psychiatric patients who suffer an acute relapse have been noncompliant with their medication regimen. Ask directly about a history of substance abuse.

Paramedics should be familiar with the following psychiatric disorders:

- **Depressive disorders.** Typical features include a persistent sad or dysphoric mood with sleep disturbances, fatigue or low energy, problems with concentration, poor appetite, and loss of interest in usual activities. These patients are at increased risk of suicide.

- **Manic syndromes.** Typical features include a persistent elevated, expansive, or irritable mood causing decreased function, grandiose behavior, pressured speech, decreased need for sleep, racing thoughts, flight of ideas, and excessive involvement with pleasurable activities with a high potential for serious consequences.

- **Anxiety syndromes.** Typical features include anxiety, fearfulness and feelings of panic, chest pain, shortness of breath and palpitations, avoidance behavior, ritualistic counting or checking, rumination, obsessive thoughts, restlessness, and depression.

- **Psychotic disorders.** Typical features include abnormal thought content or processes, delusions and hallucinations, disorganized speech, flattened affect, and inability to maintain goal-directed behavior. Delusions are fixed abnormal beliefs. Common delusions include paranoia, religious preoccupation, and delusions of grandeur. Hallucinations are false sensory perceptions. Auditory and visual hallucinations are the most common, although any sense may be involved.

Paramedics can provide excellent care for patients with psychiatric illness by following the guidelines below.

- Ensure the safety of the patient, bystanders, and emergency workers.

- Demonstrate respect, compassion, and empathy for the patient.

SECTION 2

- Protect the patient's privacy.

- Seek out medical diagnoses for abnormal behavior.

BIBLIOGRAPHY

Milner, K. K., T. Florence, & R. L. Glick (1999). Mood and anxiety syndromes In emergency psychiatry. *Psychiatric Clinics of North America 22,* 755–777.

Sanders, K. (2003). Depression. In J. J. Schaider, S. R. Hayden, R. Wolfe, R. M. Barkin, & P. Rosen (Eds.), *Rosen & Barkin's 5-minute emergency medicine consult* (2nd ed., pp. 304–305). Philadelphia: Lippincott Williams & Wilkins.

Traynor, O. T. (2004). Violent psychiatric patient. In E. T. Dickinson & A. W. Stern (Eds.), *ASL case studies in emergency care* (pp. 265–270). Upper Saddle River, NJ: Pearson Education.

Vissers, R. J. (2003). Psychosis, acute. In J. J. Schaider, S. R. Hayden, R. Wolfe, R. M. Barkin, & P. Rosen (Eds.), *Rosen & Barkin's 5-minute emergency medicine consult* (2nd ed., pp. 912–913). Philadelphia: Lippincott Williams & Wilkins.

Williams, E. R. & S. M. Shepard (2000). Medical clearance of psychiatric patients. *Emergency Medicine Clinics of North America 18,* 185–198.

NOTES

_____

_____

_____

_____

_____

CHAPTER 56

RESPONSE TO ACTS OF TERRORISM

Thomas J. Rahilly, Ph.D.

INTRODUCTION

Since the events of September 11, 2001, many emergency responders have taken the threat of terrorism more seriously than in past years. The magnitude of 9/11 has shown that the entire United States is vulnerable to an attack by terrorists. The Department of Homeland Security is spending billions of dollars to prevent future attacks by terrorists on both the U.S. and its interests around the world. An equal amount is being spent to educate and equip the emergency response organizations and their responders, who will be called upon after an act of terrorism. Planning, training, and organizing a coordinated response provide the only real chance for a successful outcome to an attack by terrorists. Although generally considered to be mass casualty incidents (MCIs), acts of terrorism contain elements that make them dramatically different "ordinary" MCIs, not the least of which is the possibility of secondary explosions or releases of toxic and infectious agents targeting the emergency responders.

As the threat of terrorism increases, EMS responders must continually prepare for a situation in which a weapon of mass destruction (WMD) will be used. Over the course of history, WMDs have been employed many times. For the most part, however, they have been a component of the wartime military strategy of one sovereign nation against another. Today, however, rogue terrorist groups around the world are attempting to either create or purchase agents and weapons delivery systems that would cause widespread death, injury, and destruction. Although these groups do not have large military forces, they do have the desire to unleash an offensive attack against their enemies of the type and scope required to effect political and cultural change, change that historically has required a potent military structure. Without a powerful military to launch a consistent campaign against its foes, terrorists must strike with as much force as they can on a more limited basis; WMDs provide this devastating potential.

WEAPONS OF MASS DESTRUCTION

A WMD can be any device that uses radioactive material, chemical and biological agents, or explosive and incendiary forces that intentionally kill, injure, and disrupt the normal activity of a community and its infrastructure. Although technically a hazardous materials (HAZMAT) incident, WMD attacks have the potential to be hundreds of times more deadly than most HAZMAT events. Although the vast majority of governments and entities that have radioactive materials in their inventories maintain them under tight control, many of the chemical and biological agents used to make WMDs are relatively easy to obtain. Recipes for the manufacture and instructions for use of WMDs are as close as the Internet. Some of the most toxic agents known to man can be created in a modestly configured laboratory in the average American home. Although a nuclear strike would be the most highly desirable event for a terrorist, an attack using a chemical or biological agent is more probable. Historically, however, the use of explosives and incendiary devices are the most prominent method employed by terrorists.

ACTIONS BY RESPONDERS

The actions of emergency responders are mostly defensive during the initial response to a terrorist event, especially if a WMD was used. The first action of all responders must be to protect themselves from exposure to the agent deployed by the terrorists. Proper on-scene procedures and the early implementation of an incident command system (ICS) can save many lives. Every EMS system should have an emergency preparedness plan that includes response to a WMD event. Because more than 10% of the victims of some terrorists events in the United States and abroad are rescue personnel, it is essential that EMS responders position themselves in a location that is free from the effects of the agent or device deployed by the terrorists. They should also be aware of the potential for secondary events that target the emergency responders. A WMD event combines all of the elements of an MCI incident and a HAZMAT event. Unless specifically trained in tactical operations and equipped to do so, EMS responders should not rush to the scene and arbitrarily begin treating victims. Upon arrival at the scene, EMS personnel should either establish or report to the medical sector of the ICS. In most cases, the EMS sector should be positioned in the "cold zone," and EMTs and paramedics should treat only victims that have been decontaminated.

SECTION 2

AGENTS AND DISSEMINATION

One of the most important considerations for creating a plan of action in response to a terrorist event is the identification of the agent used and the method by which it was disseminated. In the case of an explosive or incendiary device, identification is not as complicated as when a chemical or biological agent is deployed, although a "dirty" bomb, one that contains radiological material, may not be recognized as such until specialized detection equipment is available. The release of a chemical agent will have an immediate impact on the community, whereas most biological attacks will take time to become apparent, depending on the incubation time of the pathogen. Although patients exposed to each of these types of agents may require care that is specific to the agent used, they will all require basic life support (BLS) and transport to a medical facility capable of providing definitive care. The following is a brief description of the clinical presentation and type of care that patients exposed to a WMD may require. More information is contained in Appendix K.

Explosive and incendiary devices. Treatment for casualties of an explosive or incendiary device without an associated WMD agent depends on the destructive power of the device and the proximity of the patient when it detonated. Burns and other traumatic injuries associated with blast overpressure, such as falls and flying debris, require a thorough assessment of the patient. The most life-threatening injuries from the pressure wave of a powerful explosive will be to the respiratory system. Pneumothorax, pulmonary contusions, edema, and bleeding can each result in death if not detected and treated promptly. Hollow organ and tympanic injury are frequently reported after explosions and require supportive care and treatment for shock (see Chapter 38).

Chemical agents. Use of a chemical agent will likely be suggested by the presence of a large number of people complaining of respiratory, neurologic, gastrointestinal, and dermatologic signs and symptoms. The class of agent used will determine the patients' clinical presentation. Although knowing exactly which chemical agent or agents were released would be helpful, appropriate treatment can be provided on the basis of the clinical appearance of the patients. Nerve agents, vesicants, blood agents (cyanides), choking agents, and riot control agents all have characteristics that are unique enough to allow the astute EMS provider to identify the agent type. Specific treatment modalities beyond those of BLS must be initiated before scientific analysis of the agent if most of the severely exposed patients are to survive. Protocols that define resuscitative efforts and the use of antidotes must be in place before response to a terrorist attack involving the release of a chemical agent.

Biological agents. Unlike explosive and chemical agents events, biological agent release is somewhat more passive. The effective release of a biological organism by a terrorist will not be evident to the medical community until the disease-causing agent has incubated in its human hosts. Such an attack will probably not be detected until a significant number of confirmed cases have been reported to public health officials or until EMS dispatch centers notice a clustering of signs and symptoms from those calling for an EMS response. In most cases, an epidemiologist will be required to determine whether the outbreak of a certain disease is naturally occurring or the work of a terrorist. However, some diseases, such as smallpox, do not require a great deal of research before being identified as the work of a terrorist. EMS responders will provide supportive care and transport to a facility capable of caring for the patient. Self-protection by EMS personnel should be the primary concern.

Radiological agents. Injuries to victims surviving a nuclear explosion include blast injuries, thermal burns, and radiation exposure. Some individuals have one, two, or all three of these types of injury. Patients must be decontaminated before transport to the treatment area for their own protection as well as that of the emergency medical providers. Radiation monitoring equipment should be available and operated by responders trained in its use. As with conventional explosives, the most devastating blast injuries will be to the respiratory system; these will require airway control and ventilatory support. Trauma to the ears and abdomen is also to be expected. Care for thermal injuries is the same as for any burn patient. Prehospital care for severe noncontact radiation exposure is limited to supportive care and transport to a medical facility. Many radiation exposure victims do not show any immediate signs or symptoms of exposure, but they still may have experienced severe internal injury. Because the damage caused by radiation exposure is at the cellular level, little definitive care can be provided for these patients. Those who come in direct contact with nuclear material exhibit severe burns within hours of contact. Eye damage is possible for those who were looking in the direction of the detonation as it happened.

SUMMARY

National experts have predicted that we should prepare for terrorist attacks that are expected to occur over the next 10 years. Emergency medical response to a terrorist event, in which WMDs are frequently used, must be coordinated with the other agencies involved through the ICS. Unless properly trained and in appropriate personal protective equipment, EMS providers should be directed to the treatment area, which should be upwind and uphill in the cold zone. Patient care protocols for chemical, biological, and radiological agents should be developed and emergency preparedness drills conducted. It is essential that EMS providers practice personal protection at all times to keep from becoming a victim of the event.

BIBLIOGRAPHY

Centers for Disease Control and Prevention. (May 26, 2004). The Public Health Emergency Preparedness-and Response page. Retrieved September 30, 2004 at http://www.bt.cdc.gof/Agent/AgentlistChem.asp.

DeLorenzo, R. A. & R. S. Porter (2000). *Weapons of mass destruction: Emergency care.* Englewood Cliffs, NJ: Prentice-Hall.

Mistovich, J. J., B. Q. Hafen, & K. J. Karren (2004). *Pre-hospital emergency care,* Englewood Cliffs, NJ: Prentice-Hall.

The United States Army Medical Research Institute of Chemical Defense. The Textbook of Military Medicine: Medical Aspects of Chemical and Biological Warfare page. Retrieved March 24, 2004, at http://ccc.apgea.army.mil/products/handbooks/books.htm.

SECTION 3

PROCEDURES

CHAPTER 57

CAPNOGRAPHY AND CAPNOMETRY

Michael Cassara, D.O., FACEP

For several years, EMS providers have been using color-imetric end-tidal carbon dioxide (CO_2) detectors to confirm proper placement of endotracheal tubes. These single-use devices can provide a simple indication of the presence of CO_2 in exhaled gases. The more sophisticated and expensive devices used by anesthesiologists are now becoming available for field use. These technologies are being adopted to prevent unrecognized esophageal intubations.

Although *capnography* and *capnometry* have been used interchangeably, more precise definitions are needed. The capnometer is a device that provides a numeric measurement of the CO_2 in expired gas. The capnograph can provide a real-time graph of the level of CO_2 as well as a numeric value. It is possible for some devices to measure tissue CO_2, but we will consider only devices that measure exhaled CO_2.

CO_2, produced by cells during normal aerobic respiration, plays a key role in our acid base balance. CO_2 may be found in three forms in the body: bound to hemoglobin (carbaminohemoglobin), dissolved in water, or as part of the bicarbonate ion (HCO_3^-). Its bicarbonate form represents the greatest store of CO_2.

$$CO_2 + H_2O \leftrightarrow H_2CO_3 \leftrightarrow H^+ + HCO_3^-$$

The equation above indicates that CO_2 can move freely, combining with water to form carbonic acid, a weak acid, and then dissociating into bicarbonate ion.

CO_2 does not normally reach high levels in tissues during periods of normal ventilation and perfusion. It accumulates in tissues during periods of hypoperfusion (i.e., hypovolemic shock, hemorrhagic shock, sepsis). CO_2 does not routinely accumulate in the air contained within the stomach, esophagus, or the intestines.

The presence of CO_2 in exhaled gas usually indicates that the patient is still alive, with perfusion to the lungs.

COLORIMETRIC CAPNOMETRY

The most common method of capnometry used in the field is colorimetric end-tidal capnometry. Disposable color-imetric devices have a pH-sensitive paper encased within a chamber. The device is placed on the advanced airway device between the patient and the source of ventilation. The initial state of the indicator is purple. When exposed to CO_2, the detector changes color. Higher concentrations of CO_2 cause a change from purple to tan to yellow. These devices can last up to 20 minutes (if kept dry) and provide a visual feedback with each breath. These devices can give a false negative reading (no color change when the endotracheal tube is in the trachea) when the patient has absent or poor perfusion, such as during cardiac arrest or profound shock. False positive color changes (when the endotracheal tube is in the esophagus) may occur when the patient has recently ingested a carbonated beverage.

END-TIDAL CAPNOMETRY

The most widely used method of capnometry in criti-cal care medicine and in the operating room is quantitative capnometry. Quantitative capnometry is performed through various techniques of spectrographic analysis. The most common clinically used technique is infrared spectroscopy. CO_2 absorbs a specific wavelength of infrared light. Mea-suring the amount of the specific infrared light wavelength absorbed in a chamber of end-tidal air, when compared with known controls, provides an accurate determination.

There are two major types of quantitative capno-meters: mainstream and sidestream. The mainstream units analyze the gas within the ventilation circuit. Sidestream devices analyze the gas outside the ventilation circuit. The advantages and disadvantages of each method of sampling are listed in Table 57-1. The results can be displayed as either a numeric value, a continuous graph (capnography), or both. The results are expressed most commonly in millimeters of mercury (mmHg). The normal values for quantitative capnometry is 37 mmHg. Under normal conditions, a small gradient (below 6 mmHg) exists between the arterial CO_2 and the end-tidal CO_2.

Table 57-1: Mainstream Versus Sidestream Quantitative Capnometry

Mainstream	
Advantages	**Disadvantages**
1. Gas analysis is instantaneous.	1. It places added stress on ventilation tubing.
2. Capnograph may be generated.	2. It creates additional dead space.
3. It may be combined with pulse oximetry in same unit display.	3. It is limited to use with intubated patients.
4. Some newer units are portable or battery powered.	4. It may cause burns because of heat generation.
	5. Older units are bulky and are not portable.

Sidestream	
1. It may be used on nonintubated patients.	1. Tube may become obstructed with water vapor or secretions (requires special filters).
2. Capnograph may be generated.	2. It affords slower analysis than mainstream units.
3. It may be combined with pulse oximetry in same unit display.	3. It is inaccurate in patients with high ventilatory rates with small tidal volumes (e.g., neonates); it results in underestimation of CO_2).
4. Older units are more portable than mainstream units from the same area.	

INDICATIONS FOR CAPNOMETRY

- Initial and continued evaluation of respiratory status, including initial and continuous verification of endotracheal or tracheal tube placement, is necessary.

- Proper assessment requires early detection of the following:

  o Equipment failure (e.g., endotracheal tube obstructed by mucous secretions).

  o Acute changes in respiratory conditions (e.g., asthma, pulmonary embolism).

  o Acute changes in patient metabolism and homeostasis (e.g., malignant hyperthermia, hypotension, and other low perfusion states).

- Cardiopulmonary resuscitation efforts must be assessed. Higher levels of CO_2 indicate more effective compressions. Better compressions indicate better perfusion. Better perfusion may result in better outcomes. Studies have shown that patients in both asphyxial and primary cardiac arrest with initial end-tidal CO_2 levels greater than 10 mmHg had a better chance for return of spontaneous circulation.

- Shock resuscitation (e.g., from hypovolemia, hemorrhagic shock, sepsis) is necessary. Sublingual capnometry has been reported as beneficial in distinguishing between compensated versus decompensated shock, in assessing patient response to and the effectiveness of treatment modalities in shock scenarios, and in accurately predicting patient survival. Capnometry may represent an as-yet-unrealized advance in the treatment of shock.

SUMMARY

• The use of capnometry should be considered the standard of care for the objective initial assessment of endotracheal tube placement.

• Capnometry should be used whenever endotracheal or tracheal tube dislodgment is part of the differential diagnosis for an acute change in a patient's condition.

• Practitioners should recognize and understand the limitations of qualitative colorimetric capnography when compared with methods of quantitative capnometry in the continuous assessment and management of patients receiving noninvasive or invasive support of ventilation.

• Capnometry may be a useful adjunct in the assessment and resuscitation of patients in cardiopulmonary arrest and in various forms of shock.

BIBLIOGRAPHY

Baker, W. E., R. Lanoix, D. L. Field, & J. R. Hedges (1998). Noninvasive assessment and support of oxygenation and ventilation. In J. R. Roberts & J. R. Hedges (Eds.), *Clinical procedures in emergency medicine* (3rd ed., pp. 90–96). Philadelphia: W.B. Saunders.

Bhende, M. S. & D. C. LaCovey. (2001). End-tidal carbon dioxide monitoring in the prehospital setting. *Prehospital Emergency Care 5,* 208–213.

Biedler, A. E., W. Wilhelm, S. Kreuer, et al. (2003). Accuracy of portable quantitative capnometers and capnographs under prehospital conditions. *American Journal of Emergency Medicine 21,* 520–524.

Kobler, A., B. Schubert, P. Bertanlanffy, et al. (2004). Capnography in non-tracheally intubated emergency patients as an additional tool in pulse oximetry for pre-hospital monitoring of respiration. *Anesthesia and Analgesia 28,* 206–210.

NOTES

_____

_____

_____

_____

_____

_____

_____

_____

_____

_____

_____

_____

_____

_____

_____

_____

_____

_____

_____

CHAPTER 58

CARDIOVERSION AND DEFIBRILLATION

Thomas J. Rahilly, Ph.D.

NOTE: Use body substance isolation whenever the possibility exists of contact with blood or any body fluids. This precaution should include gloves, eye protection, masks, and other protective barriers as necessary.

CARDIOVERSION

INDICATIONS

CARDIOVERSION is indicated for patients with supraventricular tachycardias with signs and symptoms of decompensation. Cardioversion is also indicated for patients with ventricular tachycardia who have a pulse and signs and symptoms of decompensation.

CONTRAINDICATIONS

Patients with permanent (implanted) pacemakers may suffer loss of pacemaker action from the electrical shock of a defibrillator. Placement of the paddles or pads should be at least 1 inch from the device.

EQUIPMENT

The following equipment is required: a defibrillator and monitor with synchronized cardioversion capabilities, defibrillator pads or a conductive medium, and a sedative.

PROCEDURE

1. Sedate the patient if indicated according to local protocol.

2. Turn on the defibrillator and activate the synchronizer mode.

3. Ensure that the synchronizer is marking the R wave of the patient's ECG. The R wave must be at least 1 to 3 cm high for cardioversion, depending on the unit being used. Adjust the gain as necessary.

4. Place conductive medium on the paddles (gel) or on the patient (saline pads or defibrillator pads), or use hands-free electrode pads.

5. Turn on the recorder.

6. Charge the paddles to the appropriate energy level.

7. Advise all present to stand away from the patient and to avoid contact with the patient.

8. Place paddles on the patient's chest in the proper locations, and apply firm pressure.

9. Begin audible warning of cardioversion ("I'm clear; you're clear; everyone is clear"). During the warning, check to ensure that no one is in contact with the patient.

10. Make a final confirmation of the dysrhythmia requiring cardioversion.

11. Shout "clear" and make a visual check to ensure that there is no contact with the patient.

12. Simultaneously press both discharge buttons until the defibrillator discharges on the next R wave.

13. Check the patient's pulse and ECG.

DEFIBRILLATION

INDICATIONS

DEFIBRILLATION is indicated for patients with ventricular fibrillation or pulseless ventricular tachycardia.

CONTRAINDICATIONS

There are no contraindications in the presence of a pulseless patient. Place the paddles or pads at least 1 inch from an implanted defibrillator.

EQUIPMENT

The following equipment is required: defibrillator and monitor and defibrillator pads or conductive medium.

PROCEDURE

1. Turn on the defibrillator power.

2. Place the conductive medium (gel) on the paddles or on the patient (saline pads or defibrillator pads), or use hands-free electrode pads.

3. Charge the paddles to the appropriate energy level.

4. Advise all present to stand away from the patient and to avoid contact with the patient.

5. Place paddles on the patient's chest in the proper locations, and apply firm pressure.

6. Begin audible warnings of defibrillation ("I'm clear; you're clear; everyone is clear"). During countdown, check to ensure that no one is in contact with the patient.

7. Make a final confirmation of ventricular fibrillation.

8. Shout "clear" and make a visual check to ensure that there is no contact with the patient.

9. Simultaneously press both discharge buttons until the defibrillator discharges.

10. Check for evidence of successful defibrillation.

BIBLIOGRAPHY

Bledsoe, B. E., R. S. Porter, & R. A. Cherry (Eds.). (2003). *Essentials of paramedic care.* Englewood Cliffs, NJ: Prentice-Hall.

Roberts, J. R. & J. R. Hedges (Eds.). (2004). *Clinical procedures in emergency medicine* (4th ed.). Philadelphia: W.B. Saunders.

NOTES

_____

_____

_____

_____

_____

_____

_____

_____

_____

_____

_____

_____

_____

_____

_____

_____

_____

CHAPTER 59

CENTRAL VENOUS CATHETERIZATION VIA THE SUBCLAVIAN VEIN

Wanda Millard, M.D.

NOTE: This procedure should be performed only when indicated and authorized by the local medical control physician. Use body substance isolation whenever the possibility exists of contact with blood or any body fluids. Use gloves, eye protection, masks, and other barriers as necessary.

INDICATIONS

CENTRAL VENOUS CATHETERIZATION is indicated in the following situations:

- The patient requires high-flow infusion of fluids or blood (when the patient is in hypovolemic shock).

- Peripheral access is limited because of burns; trauma; plaster casts; or chemically sclerosed, thrombosed, or inadequate peripheral veins.

- Access is necessary during cardiac arrest. The supraclavicular route is recommended for access during cardiopulmonary resuscitation (CPR) because it minimizes interference with compressions and airway management.

- Preparation for passage of Swan-Ganz catheter or transvenous pacemaker is necessary.

CONTRAINDICATIONS

Central venous catheterization is contraindicated in the following situations:

- Local anatomy or landmarks are distorted (use the opposite side instead).

- Chest wall is deformed.

- The patient is extremely overweight or underweight.

- Superior vena cava injury is suspected.

- Subclavian vessel injury is suspected (use the opposite side instead).

- Pneumothorax is evident (cannulate same side so as to avoid creation of bilateral pneumothoraces).

- The patient has a bleeding disorder or is undergoing anti-coagulation therapy.

- The patient is combative.

EQUIPMENT

The following equipment is necessary: sterile swabs or sponges; sterile drapes; introducer needle (usually 18-gauge   walled needle); catheter or sheath introducer; IV tubing and solution; antibiotic ointment; antiseptic solution; 1% lidocaine solution; 5-ml nonLuer-lok syringe; vessel dilator; silk sutures; gauze pads; sterile gloves; 25-gauge, 1.5-inch needle with 3-ml Luer-lok syringe; guidewire; No. 11 scalpel; suture scissors; cloth tape.

Selection of the type of needle and catheter set depends on the indication for the procedure. Hypovolemic shock is an indication for high-flow infusion. Although the placement of peripheral large-bore catheters is preferred, the aforementioned indications may preclude the use of the peripheral route. In such cases, the paramedic may elect to place a large-bore (8.5 French [Fr]) catheter in the subclavian vein. In cases that do not require high-flow infusion, the paramedic may opt to place a smaller device, such as a 16-gauge, 20-cm catheter.

PROCEDURE

Both the infraclavicular and supraclavicular approaches to the subclavian vein require the Seldinger or guidewire technique. The Seldinger technique has many positive aspects. Significant trauma to adjacent structures is less likely because of the smaller introducer needle. This technique is also excellent for placement of large-bore introducers for high-volume infusion.

The infraclavicular approach is more widely used. The anatomic landmarks are consistent and are generally rapidly located. The right subclavian vein is usually chosen owing to anatomic considerations, but the aforementioned indications and contraindications must be considered.

1. Explain the procedure to the awake patient during preparation.

2. Place the patient in the supine position with the head in a neutral position and arms at the patient's side. Placing the patient in the Trendelenburg position (10 to 15 degrees) helps to decrease the risk of air embolism.

3. The area of needle entry is prepared with an appropriate antiseptic solution and should include the anterior part of the neck, supraclavicular fossa, and the anterior part of the chest to 3 cm across the midline and just above the nipple. Once the area is prepared, sterile gloves should be worn for the remainder of the procedure. If time permits, the area may be draped.

4. The area of needle entry should be just inferior to the junction of the middle third and medial third of the clavicle (costoclavicular junction). This area may be infiltrated with 1% lidocaine using the 3-ml syringe and the 25-gauge needle.

5. The forefinger is placed in the suprasternal notch and the thumb is placed at the costoclavicular junction for points of reference.

6. The nonLuer-lok syringe with the introducer needle attached is inserted, bevel down, immediately inferior to the clavicle at the costoclavicular junction, while the syringe is gently aspirated. The needle should be kept nearly flush with the skin and directed behind the clavicle toward the sternal notch.

7. Return of dark venous blood signals penetration of the vein at a depth of 3 to 4 cm. If the blood is bright red, the artery has been penetrated. In such a case, the needle should be removed, and, if possible, pressure should be applied in the area of puncture.

8. Remove the syringe, stabilize the needle, and cover the hub of the needle with a finger. To prevent air embolism, this should be performed while the breathing patient exhales or while the mechanically ventilated patient inhales.

9. Thread the guidewire through the needle and into the vein. The wire should thread easily and should never be forced. If the wire must be removed, the needle and wire should be removed together to prevent shearing off the wire.

10. Always remove the needle while holding the wire either above or below the needle to avoid losing the wire in the central circulation.

11. Make a small incision in the skin with the scalpel at the site of the wire.

12. Advance the dilator and catheter with a twisting motion into the vein after placing the dilator and catheter assembly on the guidewire. The wire must be visible through the back of the device before entering the vein or the wire may get lost in the central circulation.

13. Remove the dilator and wire. Cover the catheter with a finger until the intravenous tubing can be attached.

14. If placing a small catheter, rather than the 8.5 Fr introducer, thread the dilator over the wire and insert into the vein.

Remove the dilator and thread the catheter over the wire until the tip is approximately 2 cm below the sternal angle. This distance may be determined by placing the catheter along the chest wall before insertion.

15. Secure the catheter to the skin with the silk suture if time permits.

The supraclavicular approach is reportedly easier for the less experienced EMS provider, and it does not interfere with the performance of CPR. Also, some studies have shown that there are fewer complications with this approach as compared with the infraclavicular approach. Of the several methods described in the literature, the following was chosen for its simplicity:

1. Explain the procedure to the awake patient during preparation.

2. Place the patient in the supine position with the head in a neutral position and arms at the patient's side. Placing the patient in the Trendelenburg position (10 to 15 degrees) helps to decrease the risk of air embolism. Turning the patient's head to the opposite side may help identify landmarks.

3. The area of needle entry is prepared with an appropriate antiseptic solution and should include the anterior part of the neck, supraclavicular fossa, and the anterior part of the chest to 3 cm across the midline and just above the nipple. Once the area is prepared, sterile gloves should be worn for the remainder of the procedure. If time permits, the area may be draped.

4. With the patient in the neutral position, place a finger on the most anterior part of the shoulder. Draw an imaginary line medially until it intersects the clavicle. The site of needle entry is just posterior to the clavicle. This area may be infiltrated with 1% lidocaine using the 3-ml syringe and the 25-gauge needle.

5. Keeping the needle parallel to the surface of the stretcher, advance toward the ipsilateral sternoclavicular joint while gently aspirating. The bevel should be directed medially.

6. The nonLuer-lok syringe with the introducer needle attached is inserted, bevel down, immediately inferior to the clavicle at the costoclavicular junction, while the syringe is gently aspirated. The needle should be kept nearly flush with the skin and directed behind the clavicle toward the sternal notch.

7. Return of dark venous blood signals penetration of the vein. If the blood is bright red, the artery has been penetrated. In such a case, the needle should be removed, and, if possible, pressure should be applied in the area of puncture.

8. Remove the syringe, stabilize the needle, and cover the hub of the needle with a finger. To prevent air embolism, this should be performed while the breathing patient exhales or while the mechanically ventilated patient inhales.

9. Thread the guidewire through the needle and into the vein until at least one quarter of the wire is in the vein. The wire should thread easily and should never be forced. If the wire must be removed, the needle and wire should be removed together to prevent shearing off the wire.

10. Always remove the needle while holding the wire either above or below the needle. This is to avoid losing the wire in the central circulation.

11. Make a small incision in the skin with the scalpel at the site of the wire.

12. Advance the dilator and catheter with a twisting motion into the vein after placing the dilator and catheter assembly on the guidewire. The wire must be visible through the back of the device before entering the vein or the wire may get lost in the central circulation.

13. Remove the dilator and wire. Cover the catheter with a finger until the intravenous tubing can be attached.

14. If placing a smaller catheter, rather than the 8.5 Fr introducer, thread the dilator over the wire and insert into the vein. Remove the dilator and thread the catheter over the wire until the tip is approximately 2 cm below the sternal angle. This distance may be determined by placing the catheter along the chest wall before insertion.

15. Secure the catheter to the skin with the silk suture if time permits.

COMPLICATIONS

The following complications are possible:

- Pneumothorax, hemothorax, hydrothorax

- Hemomediastinum

- Tracheal perforation

- Artery puncture, arteriovenous fistula

- Air embolism

- Hematoma at puncture site

- Infection leading to cellulitis and sepsis

- Phrenic nerve and brachial plexus injury

NOTE: Unsuccessful attempts should be reported to the ED staff members so that they may monitor the patient for complications.

BIBLIOGRAPHY

Doren, D. C. & J. G. Younger (1999). Central venous catheterization and central venous monitoring. In J. R. Roberts & J. R. Hedges (Eds.), *Clinical procedures in emergency medicine* (3rd ed., pp. 367–372). Philadelphia: W.B. Saunders.

SECTION 3

Sacchetti, A. D. (1999). Guide-wire (Seldinger) technique for catheter insertion. In J. R. Roberts & J. R. Hedges (Eds.), *Clinical procedures in emergency medicine* (3rd ed., pp. 334–341). Philadelphia: W.B. Saunders.

Sztajnkrycer, M. D. (2001). Subclavian central venous access. In P. Rosen, et al. (Eds.), *Atlas of emergency procedures* (pp. 78–81). St. Louis, MO: Mosby.

NOTES

_____

_____

_____

_____

_____

_____

_____

_____

_____

_____

_____

_____

_____

_____

_____

_____

CHAPTER 60

CRICOTHYROTOMY

Daniel S. Miller, EMT-P

NOTE: Use body substance isolation (BSI) whenever the possibility of contact with blood or any bodily fluids exists. Use gloves, eye protection, masks, and other protective barriers as necessary. When sharp instruments are used (e.g., needles or cricothyrotomy equipment), a container must be available for the safe disposal of the equipment.

Cricothyrotomy is defined as the placement of a cuffed tracheostomy tube or endotracheal tube through a surgical opening in the cricothyroid membrane.

NEEDLE CRICOTHYROTOMY

INDICATIONS

The primary indication for **NEEDLE CRICOTHYROTOMY** is to establish and secure an airway after oral or nasal intubation attempts have failed and definitive airway management is needed. A secondary indication is when oral and nasal intubation is not feasible or possible.

CONTRAINDICATIONS

There are no absolute contraindications in an emergency situation. Relative contraindications include the following:

- Anatomic anomaly

- Crush injury to larynx

- Tracheal transection

- Preexisting abnormalities in the area of the cricothyroid membrane (e.g., trauma, tumor, subglottic stenosis)

- Anticoagulation therapy

- Lack of operator expertise

EQUIPMENT

The following equipment is necessary: aseptic solutions (povidone-iodine or alcohol), commercially prepared cricothyrotomy kit or a 14- to 16-gauge over-the-needle IV catheter and transtracheal jet ventilator, 5- to 10-cc syringe, tape, sterile dressings, 3 cc of sterile saline or water (optional), bag-valve-mask device. NOTE: Needle cricothyrotomy requires the use of a device capable of delivering 50 psi.

PROCEDURES

1. Establish need for procedure (i.e., because other attempts to secure airway have failed or are inappropriate).

2. Prepare equipment for procedure, with necessary oxygen delivery devices ready for use.

3. Prepare the patient by applying povidone-iodine or alcohol to the general area of insertion.

4. For traumatic presentations, place the patient in a neutral position, providing cervical stabilization. A hyperextended position is preferred for patients who have not experienced trauma.

5. Identify the cricothyroid membrane.

6. Stabilize the cricoid and thyroid cartilage with the nondominant hand.

7. Insert the needle with a syringe attached through the midline of the cricothyroid membrane at a slight angle toward the feet.

8. Withdraw the syringe plunger until air is freely withdrawn.

9. Advance the catheter an additional 1 cm (1/2 inch).

10. While holding the needle steady, advance catheter off the needle to hub. Safely dispose of needle.

11. Attach jet ventilator, assess for chest rise, and auscultate lung sounds. Note: The use of a bag-valve-mask device or automatic ventilator will not produce sufficient pressures to adequately ventilate through a needle cricothyrotomy. Patients under the age of 5 years may be ventilated with a bag-valve-mask device.

12. Secure catheter.

13. Ventilate once every 5 seconds (every 3 seconds in pediatric patients younger than 8 years of age), and frequently assess lung sounds and ventilatory status.

NOTE: With commercially prepared cricothyrotomy kits, induction of larger catheters or dilators (up to 4 mm I.D.) will allow ventilation to be accomplished by bag-valve-mask device, mouth, or automatic ventilator. Although use of these devices is similar to the procedure listed above, personnel should be properly trained in the use of any device or kit selected for use.

SURGICAL CRICOTHYROTOMY

INDICATIONS

The primary indication for **SURGICAL CRICOTHYROTOMY** is to establish and secure an airway after oral or nasal intubation attempts have failed and definitive airway management is needed. A secondary indication is when oral and nasal intubation is not feasible or possible.

CONTRAINDICATIONS

The only absolute contraindication in an emergency situation is in patients younger than 12 years of age. Relative contraindications include the following:

• Anatomical anomaly

• Crush injury to larynx

• Tracheal transection

- Preexisting laryngeal abnormalities (e.g., trauma, tumor, subglottic stenosis)

- Anticoagulation therapy

- Lack of operator expertise

EQUIPMENT

The following equipment is necessary: aseptic solutions (povidone-iodine or alcohol), commercially prepared cricothyrotomy kit or an endotracheal tube (No. 6), scalpel, 5- to 10-cc syringe, tape, sterile dressings, bag-valve-mask device, suction unit, Magill forceps.

1. Establish need for procedure (i.e., other attempts to secure airway have failed or are inappropriate).

2. Prepare equipment for procedure, with necessary oxygen delivery devices and suction unit ready for use.

3. Prepare the patient by applying povidone-iodine or alcohol to the general area of incision.

4. For traumatic presentations, place the patient in a neutral position, providing cervical stabilization. A hyperextended position is preferred for patients who have not experienced trauma.

5. Identify the cricothyroid membrane.

6. At the level of the cricothyroid membrane, make a 2- to 3-cm (approximately 1-inch) midline vertical incision through the skin and subcutaneous tissue, exposing the cricothyroid membrane.

7. Make a 1-cm (approximately 1/2-inch) horizontal stabbing incision through the cricothyroid membrane.

8. Using Magill forceps to maintain the opening, insert an endotracheal tube (usually a No. 6 endotracheal tube will suffice) or a commercially prepared cricothyrotomy kit tube. NOTE: The handle side of the scalpel may be inserted into the incision of the cricothyroid membrane to

maintain the opening, should Magill forceps not be readily available.

9. Inflate endotracheal tube cuff.

10. Attach a bag-valve-mask device, ventilate, assess for chest rise, and auscultate.

11. Confirmation of endotracheal tube placement should also be confirmed by the use of an end-tidal CO_2 detector.

12. Secure the tube.

13. Ventilate once every 5 seconds and frequently assess lung sounds and ventilatory status.

COMPLICATIONS

The following complications are possible:

- Surrounding tissue injury and hemorrhage

- Subcutaneous emphysema

- Barotrauma (i.e., tension pneumothorax)

- Airway obstruction (from surrounding tissue hemorrhage and edema)

- Hypoventilation and hypoxia

- Perforation of posterior tracheal wall, esophageal cannulation

- Infection

SECTION 3

BIBLIOGRAPHY

American Heart Association. (2003). Airway, airway adjuncts, oxygenation, and ventilation. In *Advanced cardiac life support: Principles and practice*. South Deerfield, MA: Channing Bete.

North Carolina College of Emergency Physicians. (2002). Standard procedure skill. Airway surgical cricothyrotomy page. Retrieved September 30, 2004, at http://www.nccep.org/

content/ems/standards/EditableNCCEPProceduresand
Policies.pdf.

Walls, R., R. C. Luten, M. F. Murphy, & R. E. Schneider (Eds.).
(2000). *The manual of emergency airway management.*
Philadelphia: Lippincott Williams & Wilkins.

NOTES

_____

_____

_____

_____

_____

_____

_____

_____

_____

_____

_____

_____

_____

_____

_____

_____

_____

_____

CHAPTER 61

ENDOTRACHEAL INTUBATION AND EXTUBATION

Owen T. Traynor, M.D.

NOTE: Use body substance isolation (BSI) whenever contact with blood or body fluids is possible. This precaution should include gloves, eye protection, masks, and other barriers as necessary. When sharp instruments are used (e.g., needles), a container must be available for their safe disposal.

OROTRACHEAL INTUBATION

INDICATIONS

OROTRACHEAL INTUBATION is indicated whenever there is a need to secure the airway of a patient who has lost or is at risk of losing airway control. Patients who would benefit from the insertion of an endotracheal tube include those who have experienced cardiac or respiratory arrest, coma, or ventilatory or respiratory failure.

NOTE: Endotracheal intubation may be performed in the patient who has experienced multiple trauma if cervical spine stabilization is maintained by a second EMS provider.

CONTRAINDICATIONS

If the endotracheal intubation procedure will compromise cervical spine control or precipitate laryngospasm, it is contraindicated.

EQUIPMENT

The following equipment is required: laryngoscope handle and blade, endotracheal tube, 10-ml syringe, malleable stylet, water-soluble lubricant (e.g., K-Y jelly), suction device and equipment, Magill forceps, bag-valve-mask (BVM) device, oxygen source, end-tidal CO_2 detector or esophageal detector device, pulse oximeter, tape, commercial ET tube holder.

PROCEDURE

1. Confirm the order to intubate or proceed on standing order.

2. Determine the correct size needed for the tube, and assemble and check the equipment, including inflation and deflation of the ET tube cuff. Lubricate tip of ET tube.

3. Hyperventilate or preoxygenate the patient for at least 30 seconds before attempting to insert the endotracheal tube.

4. If cervical spine precautions are not indicated, place the patient in the "sniffing" position, and remove the oropharyngeal airway. If cervical spine precautions are indicated, an assistant must continue to stabilize the cervical spine throughout this procedure.

5. Hold the laryngoscope in the left hand and insert it into the patient's mouth without causing trauma.

6. Maneuver the laryngoscope to visualize the vocal cords (do not use the teeth or gums as a fulcrum).

7. While maintaining direct visualization of the vocal cords, insert the ET tube into the trachea.

8. Remove the laryngoscope blade from the patient's mouth and the stylet from the ET tube, taking care to manually stabilize the tube in place.

9. Ventilate the patient no later than 30 seconds from the time of the last ventilation.

10. Note the rise and fall of the chest.

11. Instruct another EMS provider to continue ventilations using a BVM device.

12. Auscultate the chest and abdomen to ensure correct placement of the ET tube.

13. Check tube placement with an end-tidal CO_2 monitor or esophageal detector device.

14. Inflate the cuff with the minimum volume of air needed to seal the tube.

15. Auscultate the chest and abdomen to ensure correct placement of the ET tube.

16. Insert an oropharyngeal airway and secure the ET tube in place with tape or a commercial holder.

NASOTRACHEAL INTUBATION

INDICATIONS

NASOTRACHEAL INTUBATION is indicated whenever there is a need for control of the airway and orotracheal intubation is not feasible, owing to spontaneous respirations, clenched teeth, intact gag reflex, facial trauma, and so forth.

CONTRAINDICATIONS

Patients with a known bleeding disorder, severe facial trauma, or basilar skull fracture should not be intubated by the nasotracheal method.

EQUIPMENT

The following equipment is required: Endotracheal tubes (7.0, 7.5, and 8.0 mm for adults), 10-ml syringe, water-soluble lubricant, anesthetic agent (lidocaine jelly), oxymetazoline spray (Afrin) or 0.25% phenylephrine (Neo-Synephrine), suction device and equipment, Magill forceps, BVM device, oxygen source, end-tidal CO_2 detector or esophageal detector device, pulse oximeter, tape or a commercial holder.

PROCEDURE

1. Confirm the order to intubate or proceed on standing order.

2. Determine the correct size needed for the tube, and assemble and check the equipment, including inflation and deflation of the ET tube cuff. Lubricate the ET tube with viscous lidocaine.

3. Apply intranasal oxymetazoline spray or 0.25% phenylephrine to vasoconstrict vessels in nasal passages to decrease bleeding.

4. Gently insert the tip of the ET tube into the nare and push (do not jab) until the tip is at the tracheal opening (breathing sounds will be loudest). If sounds diminish, indicating entry into the esophagus, pull back slightly until sounds increase. Be prepared to use suction on the patient.

5. Listen at the open end of the ET tube for the sound of inspiration, and gently insert the tube into the trachea.

6. Connect a BVM device to the ET tube and ventilate the patient.

7. Note the rise and fall of the chest.

8. Instruct another EMS provider to continue ventilations using a BVM device.

9. Auscultate the chest and abdomen to ensure correct placement of the ET tube. If the tube has entered the esophagus, withdraw to the nasopharynx and attempt to place the tube in the trachea again.

10. Check tube placement with end-tidal CO_2 monitor.

11. Inflate the cuff with the minimum volume of air needed to seal the tube.

12. Auscultate the chest and abdomen to ensure correct placement of the ET tube.

13. Confirm tube placement with an end-tidal CO_2 detector or an esophageal detector device.

14. Secure the ET tube in place with tape or a commercial holder.

EXTUBATION

INDICATIONS

EXTUBATION is indicated any time the patient regains control of the airway and exhibits nontolerance (e.g., gagging) of the ET tube.

CONTRAINDICATIONS

There are no contraindications for extubation, but you should be prepared to suction the airway if the patient vomits.

EQUIPMENT

The following equipment is necessary: suction device and equipment, bandage, and scissors.

PROCEDURE

1. Turn on and test the suction unit.

2. Turn the patient's head to the side. If the patient is immobilized to a spine board, turn the entire body.

3. Remove the oral airway and the device securing the tube.

4. Deflate the distal cuff.

5. Remove ET tube on inspiration.

6. Suction as needed.

7. Reassess the airway.

SECTION 3

FOREIGN BODY REMOVAL

INDICATIONS

FOREIGN BODY REMOVAL is indicated whenever there is a history of airway obstruction, and basic life support techniques to clear the airway have failed.

CONTRAINDICATIONS

There are no contraindications if the airway remains obstructed.

EQUIPMENT

The following equipment is necessary: laryngoscope handle and blade, Magill forceps, suction device and equipment, BVM device, oxygen source.

PROCEDURE

1. Confirm obstruction and reattempt basic life support procedures.

2. Position the patient's head and neck in a sniffing position.

3. Insert a laryngoscope and visualize glottic opening.

4. Identify obstruction. NOTE: If no foreign body is visible, intubate the patient. If the patient still cannot be ventilated, consider passing the ET tube distally into the right mainstem bronchus. This may push the foreign body into the right bronchus and allow ventilation of the left lung after the ET tube is withdrawn to its normal location. DO NOT force the ET tube distally.

5. Insert Magill forceps and position at the obstructing object.

6. Grasp obstruction and remove, using caution not to cause trauma.

7. Remove the laryngoscope.

8. Reassess and position the airway.

9. Attempt ventilation.

BIBLIOGRAPHY

Clinton, J. E. & J. W. McGill (1998). Basic airway management and decision-making. In J. R. Roberts & J. R. Hedges (Eds.), *Clinical procedures in emergency medicine* (3rd ed., pp. 1–15). Philadelphia: W.B. Saunders.

McGill, J. W. & J. E. Clinton (1998). Basic tracheal intubation. In J. R. Roberts & J. R. Hedges (Eds.), *Clinical procedures in emergency medicine* (3rd ed., pp. 15–34). Philadelphia: W.B. Saunders.

Walls, R., R. C. Luten, M. F. Murphy, & R. E. Schneider (Eds.). (2000). *The manual of emergency airway management.* Philadelphia: Lippincott Williams & Wilkins.

NOTES

_____

_____

_____

_____

_____

_____

_____

_____

_____

_____

SECTION 3

CHAPTER 62

ESOPHAGEAL TRACHEAL COMBITUBE

Myron J. Rickens, EMT-P

NOTE: Use body substance isolation whenever contact with blood or any body fluids is possible. This should include gloves, eye protection, masks, and other protective barriers as necessary. When sharp instruments are used (e.g., needles), a container must be available for their safe disposal.

INDICATIONS

The esophageal tracheal combitube (ETC) may be used for control of the airway when it is not feasible to insert an endotracheal tube, such as with patients who are trapped in unusual positions, patients who have experienced trauma and in whom head and neck movement is contraindicated, morbidly obese patients with difficult airways, patients with massive bleeding or regurgitation that prevents visualization of the cords, or patients in coma or respiratory arrest for whom endotracheal intubation attempts have failed.

CONTRAINDICATIONS

ETC is contraindicated in the following situations:

- Patient has intact gag reflexes.

- Patient's height is under 5 feet (under 4 feet if the combitube SA is available).

- A known esophageal pathology is present.

- A caustic substance has been ingested.

- The central airway is obstructed.

EQUIPMENT

The following equipment is necessary:

- ETC (patients 5 feet or taller)

- ETC SA (patients between 4 and 5 1/2 feet)

- Water-soluble lubricant, oxygen, bag-valve-mask device, and suction unit

PROCEDURE

1. Complete basic manual and adjunctive maneuvers, and provide supplemental oxygen and ventilatory support with a bag-valve-mask device and hyperventilation.

2. Prepare and check the equipment.

3. Place the patient's head in neutral position. Stabilize the cervical spine if cervical injury is possible.

4. Insert the ETC gently in a curved, downward movement at the midline through the oropharynx, using a tongue-jaw-lift maneuver, and advance it past the hypopharynx to the depth indicated by the markings on the tube. The black rings on the tube should be between the patient's teeth. Use of a laryngoscope will make insertion successful in many cases when insertion is difficult.

5. The ETC pharyngeal cuff (blue pilot balloon) should be inflated with 100 ml of air and the distal cuff (white pilot balloon) inflated with 10 to 15 ml of air.

   The ETC SA pharyngeal cuff (blue pilot balloon) should be inflated with 85 ml of air and the distal cuff (white pilot balloon) inflated with 10 to 12 ml of air.

6. Ventilate through the longer blue proximal port with a bag-valve-mask device connected to 100% oxygen while auscultating over the chest and stomach. If you hear bilateral breath sounds over the chest and no sounds over the stomach, continue ventilating. Use multiple confirmation

SECTION 3

techniques (auscultate, use CO_2 detector, and monitor clinical improvement).

7. If you hear sounds over the stomach and no breath sounds over the chest, change ports and ventilate through the clear connector. Confirm breath sounds over the chest with no gastric sounds; continue ventilating with 100% oxygen. Use multiple confirmation techniques (auscultate, use CO_2 detector, and monitor clinical improvement).

8. Secure the tube and continue ventilating with 100% oxygen. It is good practice to mark with a piece of tape the unused port so that it is not mistakenly used during resuscitation.

9. Frequently reassess the airway and adequacy of ventilation.

TRICKS OF THE TRADE

1. The Lipp maneuver, curving or bending the ETC between the balloons, is useful for blind insertion. After performing this maneuver, the tip of the ETC must be directed along the tongue with a soft and rapid movement parallel to the patient's chest into the hypopharynx. This movement is in contrast to the insertion of the laryngeal mask airway along the hard palate. During insertion, the tongue should be pressed out of the way with the help of the deeply inserted thumb.

2. When advancing the ETC is difficult, rotate the tube to the left so that the tip passes more easily around the epiglottis or the glottic structures.

3. Hyperextension of the cervical spine could make insertion difficult.

4. Use of the laryngoscope is strongly recommended when insertion is difficult. Keep in mind that the inability to pass the ETC has been cited as the number-one reason for unsuccessful placement.

5. In a few cases, ventilation does not work in both the blue connector and the clear connector. The reason may be that the oropharyngeal balloon is inserted too deeply. Deflate the pharyngeal cuff (blue pilot balloon) and withdraw the ETC out of the patient's mouth approximately 2 to 3 cm. Reinflate pharyngeal cuff (blue pilot balloon) and repeat the confirmation steps.

COMPLICATIONS

The following complications are possible: perforation of the vallecula, perilaryngeal structures, and esophagus.

BIBLIOGRAPHY

Agro, F., M. Frass, J. L. Benumof, & P. Kraft (2002, June). Current status of the combitube: A review of the literature. *Journal of Clinical Anesthesia 14*, 307–314.

Bledsoe, B. E., R. S. Porter, & R. A. Cherry (2000). *Paramedic care: Principles and practice.* Upper Saddle River, NJ: Brady Prentice Hall Health.

Calkins, T. R., M. I. Langdorf, K. T. Miller, T. A. Bey, & M. A. Hill, (2002). Comparison of the combitube and endotracheal tube in the out-of-hospital setting. *Annals of Emergency Medicine 40*, S6.

Combitube homepage. Retrieved on December 2, 2003, at http://www.akh-wien.ac.at/Combitube/.

Della Puppa, A., G. Pittoni, & M. Frass (2002, August). Tracheal esophageal combitube: A useful airway for morbidly obese patients who cannot intubate or ventilate. *The Acta Anaesthesiologica Foundation 46,* 911–913.

Urtubia, R. N. (2002, March). "Tricks of the trade" with the esophageal-tracheal combitube. *The Acta Anaesthesiologica Foundation 46,* 340.

SECTION 3

CHAPTER 63

INTRAOSSEOUS INFUSION

Patrick R. Coonan, R.N., Ed.D.,
CEN, EMT-CC

Owen T. Traynor, M.D.

NOTE: Use body substance isolation whenever the possibility exists of contact with blood or any body fluids. This precaution should include gloves, eye protection, masks, and other protective barriers as necessary. When sharp instruments are used (e.g., needles), a container must be available for their safe disposal.

INDICATIONS

INTRAOSSEOUS INFUSION (IO) should be used with critically ill or injured patients when there is a need for venous access and

- Attempts at IV access have failed

- There is no evident peripheral venous access

CONTRAINDICATIONS

Intraosseous infusion should not be attempted if

- There was a previous IO attempt in the same tibia

- There is a fracture above the intended site

- Infected or burned skin is evident at the insertion site

EQUIPMENT

The following equipment is necessary: IV fluid, microdrip, or burette solution administration set; two 15-gauge

IO or bone marrow needles; povidone-iodine (Betadine) swabs; antibiotic ointment; 10-ml syringe; injectable sterile saline solution; arm board; sterile dressings (4" × 4"); 2-inch cling tape; F.A.S.T.1 kit or B.I.G. kit.

PROCEDURE: PEDIATRIC PATIENTS

1. Assemble and prepare all necessary equipment.

2. Locate the insertion site on the flat surface of the tibia, approximately 1 to 3 cm below the tibial tuberosity.

3. Prepare the site with povidone-iodine. Keep the site aseptic throughout the procedure.

4. Insert the IO needle at a 60-degree angle from the leg, and aim **away** from the knee. This method will prevent accidental damage to the knee.

5. Apply firm, steady pressure with a twisting motion to reduce the chances of fracturing the tibia.

6. Continue to twist and apply firm pressure until you feel a sudden decrease in resistance. This sudden "pop" means you have entered the marrow space.

7. Remove the stylet and attach the syringe. Correct position is assumed if 5 to 10 ml of fluid can be infused without resistance or subcutaneous infiltration or if bone marrow can be freely aspirated by drawing back on the syringe plunger.

8. Infuse fluids or medications as needed.

9. Secure the IO needle. Apply antibiotic ointment around the site and stabilize the IO needle as you would any impaled object using tape, bulky dressings, and cling tape. The needle should be freestanding because it is being supported by the patient's bone, but it requires added stabilization to prevent accidental removal.

PROCEDURE: ADULT PATIENTS

F.A.S.T.1

1. Assemble and prepare all necessary equipment.

2. Locate the site at the manubrium of the sternum.

3. Use aseptic technique to prepare the insertion site with the iodine prep pad followed by the alcohol prep pads provided.

4. Remove the top half of the backing of the target patch.

5. Place the target patch on the manubrium by aligning the locating notch with the sternal notch, and ensure that the patch's target zone is in the midline.

6. Remove the remaining backing on the target patch, and secure the patch to the patient.

7. Remove the protective cap from the introducer.

8. Place the bone probe needles within the target zone of the target patch.

9. Hold the introducer perpendicular to the skin, and apply constant firm pressure until the mechanism releases.

10. Expose the infusion tube by withdrawing the introducer.

11. Safely dispose of the introducer using a sharps container.

12. Connect the infusion tube to the right-angle connector on the target patch.

13. Verify placement by aspirating with a syringe from the straight connector on the target patch.

14. Connect IV administration set to the straight connector.

15. Infuse fluids or medications as needed.

16. Place the protector dome over the target patch, and press down to engage the Velcro fastener. The infusion tubing

and the right-angle connector should be contained within the protector dome.

17. Attach the remover package to the patient for transport.

BONE INJECTION GUN (B.I.G.)

1. Assemble and prepare all necessary equipment.

2. Choose the desired depth of penetration (2.5 cm) on the scale by unscrewing the sleeve from the cylindrical housing.

3. Locate the site 1 to 2 cm medially and 1 cm proximally to the tibial tuberosity.

4. Prepare the site with povidone-iodine. Keep the site aseptic throughout the procedure.

5. Position the B.I.G. at the injection site, and release the safety latch.

6. Trigger the B.I.G. by squeezing the trigger mechanism.

7. Disconnect the B.I.G. barrel from the needle, pull out the trocar, and stabilize the cannula.

8. Safely discard the B.I.G. using a sharps container.

9. Verify placement by aspirating with a syringe from the straight connector on the target patch.

10. Connect IV administration set to the straight connector.

11. Infuse fluids or medications as needed.

12. Secure the B.I.G. Apply antibiotic ointment around the site, and stabilize the B.I.G. as you would any impaled object.

COMPLICATIONS

The following complications are possible:

- Swelling of soft tissues resulting in compartment syndrome

SECTION 3

- Injury to the growth plate

- Fracture of the tibia

- Local bleeding

- Injection into the knee joint

- Periostitis

- Embolism of clots or bone marrow

- Fat embolism (rare)

- Osteomyelitis (rare)

BIBLIOGRAPHY

Stanley, R. (2004). Intraosseous infusion. In J. R. Roberts & J. R. Hedges (Eds.), *Clinical procedures in emergency medicine* (4th ed., pp. 475–485). Philadelphia: W.B. Saunders.

Pyng Medical Corp. The F.A.S.T.1 Adult Intraosseous Infusion System page. Retrieved September 30, 2004, at http://www.pyng.com/pym/products/product.htm.

WaisMed Medical Products. The Bone Injection Gun page. Retrieved September 30, 2004, at http://www.waismed.com.

NOTES

_____

_____

_____

_____

_____

_____

_____

_____

CHAPTER 64

LARYNGEAL MASK AIRWAY INSERTION

Lawrence Sherman, EMT-CC

Laryngeal mask airway (LMA) insertion should be performed only when indicated and authorized by local medical control.

NOTE: Use body substance isolation whenever the possibility exists of contact with blood or any body fluids. This precaution should include gloves, eye protection, masks, and other protective barriers as necessary. Although insertion of the LMA takes time, a patient should not remain unventilated for more than 30 seconds.

INDICATIONS

LMA is indicated as an alternative to direct endotracheal intubation in respiratory or cardiorespiratory arrest. Use LMA if endotracheal intubation is not possible or after two unsuccessful attempts to intubate.

CONTRAINDICATIONS

LMA is contraindicated in the following situations:

- The patient has an intact gag reflex.

- The patient is conscious.

- The patient has a known esophageal disease (e.g., cancer, varices).

- The patient has ingested a caustic substance (e.g., acid, lye).

- The patient has ingested a petroleum product (e.g., Vaseline).

EQUIPMENT

The following equipment is necessary: LMA, 50-cc syringe, water-soluble lubricant, adhesive tape, oropharyngeal airway (OPA), pulse oximeter, BVM with supplemental oxygen source, suction equipment.

PROCEDURE

1. Place the patient in the supine position, and extend the head while flexing the neck ("sniffing position"); if cervical spine trauma is suspected, stabilize the cervical spine in a neutral position.

2. Open the airway, and suction the mouth and oropharynx if necessary.

3. Insert an OPA and adequately ventilate patient using BVM device, confirming air entry bilaterally, and ruling out foreign body airway obstruction.

4. Select the correct size LMA for the patient.

5. Check the integrity of the cuff on the mask of the LMA.

6. Lubricate the distal end of the LMA.

7. Hyperventilate the patient with a BVM device and supplemental oxygen before attempting to insert the LMA.

8. Position the LMA for insertion with the mask facing down (note that the mask of the LMA is at the distal end of the device and is inserted into the oropharynx).

9. While maintaining the head in the "sniffing position," remove the OPA and then grasp the mandible and tongue between the thumb and fingers of one hand.

10. Using the index finger of the other hand, advance the LMA along the hard palate until you feel resistance.

11. Stabilize the LMA with the first hand as you remove your index finger.

12. The LMA is properly positioned when the black line on the LMA faces upward and is in line with the middle of the patient's nose.

13. Inflate the inflatable part of the mask on the LMA with the appropriate amount of air for the size of the device (No. 3: 20 cc, No. 4: 30 cc, No. 5: 40 cc).

14. Confirm LMA placement by auscultating for bilateral breath sounds, absent gastric sounds. Use secondary confirmation devices, such as an esophageal detector device or capnography, to confirm its correct placement.

15. Reinsert the oropharyngeal airway (or other bite block), and secure the LMA.

NOTE: The LMA does not enter the trachea; proper placement of the LMA is at the level of the trachea, just adjacent to it.

COMPLICATIONS

The following complications are possible:

- Vomiting during insertion

- Airway obstruction (if not placed properly)

- Inadequate ventilation

- Aspiration

BIBLIOGRAPHY

Bledsoe, B. E., R. S. Porter, & R. A. Cherry (Eds.). (2003). *Essentials of paramedic care* (1st ed., pp. 547–549). Upper Saddle River, NJ: Prentice-Hall.

Mistovich, J. J., B. Q. Hafen, & K. J. Karren (2004). *Prehospital emergency care*. Englewood Cliffs, NJ: Prentice-Hall.

SECTION 3

CHAPTER 65

MEDICATION ADMINISTRATION

Thomas J. Rahilly, Ph.D.

NOTE: Use body substance isolation whenever the possibility exists of contact with blood or any body fluids. This precaution should include gloves, eye protection, masks, and other protective barriers as necessary. When sharp instruments are used (e.g., needles), container must be available for their safe disposal.

INTRAVENOUS BOLUS ADMINISTRATION

INDICATIONS

INTRAVENOUS BOLUS ADMINISTRATION is indicated in any situation that requires the rapid administration of a medication.

CONTRAINDICATIONS

There are no contraindications if the IV is functioning properly.

EQUIPMENT

The following equipment is necessary: medication, syringe with needle or prefilled syringe, alcohol-prepared pads, sharp-instrument container.

PROCEDURE

1. Confirm order, including medication, dosage, and route.

2. Explain the procedure to the patient, and confirm that the patient is not known to be allergic to the medication.

3. Assemble the necessary medication and equipment.

4. Select the correct medication, and inspect it for expiration date, discoloration, and particulate matter.

5. Fill syringe with medication or assemble the prefilled syringe.

6. Expel air and excess medication from the syringe (only the ordered dosage should remain in the syringe).

7. Select the medication administration port closest to the cannula, and cleanse the port with an alcohol pad.

8. Pinch the IV tubing above the medication administration port to close it. Closing the drip-rate control valve is also acceptable.

9. Insert the needle into the port and inject the correct amount of medication. If the patient is in cardiac arrest, medications should be followed by a 20-ml flush and the extremity elevated to speed medication delivery to the central circulation.

10. Remove the needle and syringe, and dispose of it safely.

11. Flush the IV line by opening the drip-rate control valve.

12. Readjust the drip rate.

INTRAVENOUS INFUSION (PIGGYBACK)

INDICATIONS

INTRAVENOUS INFUSION, or piggyback administration is indicated in any situation that requires the immediate administration of a second IV fluid or titrated infusion of a specific medication.

CONTRAINDICATIONS

There are no contraindications if the primary IV is functioning properly.

SECTION 3

EQUIPMENT

The following equipment is necessary: appropriate IV fluid, medication, secondary administration set, needle, syringe with needle or prefilled syringe, alcohol pads, tape, and sharp-instrument container.

PROCEDURE

1. Confirm order, including medication, dosage, and route.

2. Explain the procedure to the patient, and confirm that the patient has no known allergies to the medication.

3. Assemble the necessary medication and equipment, including the secondary IV setup.

4. Select the correct medication, and inspect it for expiration date, discoloration, and particulate matter.

5. Calculate the required amount of medication, and fill the syringe or assemble the prefilled syringe.

6. Expel air and excess medication from the syringe (only the ordered dosage should remain in the syringe).

7. Cleanse the medication port of the secondary IV bag with an alcohol pad, inject the medication into the port, and gently shake the bag to mix the medication and solution.

8. Label the IV bag with the medication, amount injected, medication concentration, the time and date, and your initials.

9. Attach a sterile needle to the administration set, cleanse the injection port closest to the patient with an alcohol pad, and insert the needle up to the hub.

10. Close the primary IV control valve, and open the secondary IV control valve to the desired drip rate.

11. Secure the secondary needle to the primary set with tape.

INTRAMUSCULAR INJECTION

INDICATIONS

INTRAMUSCULAR INJECTION is indicated for administration of medications that require a slow rate of absorption.

CONTRAINDICATIONS

Intramuscular injection is contraindicated for hypotensive patients.

EQUIPMENT

The following equipment is necessary: medication; syringe; 21- to 23-gauge needle, 3/8- to 1-inch long; alcohol or betadine prep pads.

PROCEDURE

1. Confirm order, including medication, dosage, and route.

2. Explain the procedure to the patient, and confirm that the patient has no known allergies to the medication.

3. Assemble the necessary medication and equipment.

4. Select the correct medication, and inspect it for discoloration, particulate matter, and expiration date.

5. Select the proper size syringe and needle.

6. Fill syringe with medication as appropriate.

7. Expel air and excess medication from the syringe (only the ordered dosage should remain in the syringe).

8. Locate the deltoid area, and prepare the injection site with an alcohol preparation using a concentric motion.

9. Stretch the skin taut around the injection site, and insert the needle at a 90-degree angle.

10. Aspirate for blood; if blood appears, withdraw the needle and select another site.

SECTION 3

11. Inject full dosage of medication with a slow, steady push of the syringe.

12. Withdraw needle at the same entry angle.

13. Properly dispose of needle and syringe.

14. Massage the injection site with an alcohol pad.

SUBCUTANEOUS INJECTION

INDICATIONS

SUBCUTANEOUS INJECTION is indicated for the administration of medications requiring injection into the fatty subcutaneous tissue, such as those for allergic or anaphylactic reactions.

CONTRAINDICATIONS

Patients with inadequate perfusion should not receive medication by the subcutaneous route.

EQUIPMENT

The following equipment is necessary: medication; 1- to 3-ml tuberculin syringe; 24- to 26-gauge, 3/8- to 1-inch needle; alcohol prep pads; sharp-instrument container.

PROCEDURE

1. Confirm order, including medication, dosage, and route.

2. Explain the procedure to the patient, and confirm that the patient has no known allergies to the medication.

3. Assemble the necessary medication and equipment.

4. Select the correct medication, and inspect it for expiration date, discoloration, and particulate matter.

5. Select the proper size syringe and needle.

6. Fill syringe with medication as appropriate.

7. Expel air and excess medication from the syringe (only the ordered dosage should remain in the syringe).

8. Locate the deltoid area, and prepare the injection site with an alcohol or betadine pad using a concentric motion.

9. Pinch the skin away from the underlying tissue, and insert the needle at a 45-degree angle.

10. Aspirate for blood; if blood appears, withdraw the needle and select another site.

11. Inject the full dosage of medication with a slow, steady push of the syringe.

12. Withdraw needle at same entry angle.

13. Properly dispose of needle and syringe.

14. Massage the injection site with an alcohol pad.

ENDOTRACHEAL TUBE ADMINISTRATION

INDICATIONS

Endotracheal tube (ET) administration is indicated in any situation that requires the rapid administration of certain medications when no IV access is available and an ET tube is in place.

CONTRAINDICATIONS

There are no contraindications, although the medications administered by this route include only the "LEAN" drugs: lidocaine, epinephrine, atropine, naloxone (Narcan).

EQUIPMENT

The following equipment is necessary: medication, syringe without needle or prefilled syringe, injectable normal saline, sharp-instrument container.

PROCEDURE

1. Confirm order, including medication, dosage, and route.

SECTION 3

2. If possible, confirm that the patient has no known allergic reaction to the medication.

3. Assemble the necessary medication and equipment.

4. Select the correct medication, and inspect it for expiration date, discoloration, and particulate matter.

5. Prepare the medication aseptically, and expel air and excess medication from the syringe (only the ordered dosage should remain in the syringe). Drugs administered through the ET tube are usually 2 to 2.5 times the recommended dose. In addition, the drug should be diluted in or flushed by 10 ml of normal saline or sterile water.

6. Hyperventilate the patient.

7. Stop ventilations, and remove the ventilating device from the ET tube.

8. Stop CPR (if in progress), and quickly spray the medication down the ET tube. NOTE: Remove the needle from the syringe before administration.

9. Reconnect the ventilating device to the ET tube and hyperventilate the patient.

10. Resume CPR after the medication has been nebulized (several brisk ventilations).

11. Properly dispose of needle and syringe.

BIBLIOGRAPHY

Bledsoe, B. E., R. S. Porter, & R. A. Cherry (Eds.). (1994). *Essentials of paramedic care* (2nd ed.). Englewood Cliffs, NJ: Prentice-Hall.

Kozier, B., et al. (2000). *Fundamentals of nursing* (6th ed.). Upper Saddle River, NJ: Prentice-Hall.

CHAPTER 66

NEEDLE CHEST DECOMPRESSION

Owen T. Traynor, M.D.

Needle chest decompression should be performed only when indicated and authorized by local medical control.

NOTE: Use body substance isolation whenever the possibility exists of contact with blood or any body fluids. This precaution should include gloves, eye protection, masks, and other protective barriers as necessary. When sharp instruments are used (e.g., needles), a sharp-instrument container must be available for their safe disposal.

INDICATIONS

NEEDLE CHEST DECOMPRESSION is indicated for patients with a life-threatening tension pneumothorax.

CONTRAINDICATIONS

There are no contraindications when this procedure is used in the treatment of a tension pneumothorax.

EQUIPMENT

The following equipment is necessary: povidone-iodine solution, sterile gauze sponges, 14- to 16-gauge over-the-needle IV catheters, 1-inch adhesive tape, flutter-type valve.

PROCEDURE

1. Assess the patient's respiratory status and breath sounds.

2. Administer high-flow oxygen and ventilate as necessary.

3. Explain the procedure to the awake patient, without delaying the procedure.

4. Place the patient in a supine position, with the head of the stretcher elevated 30 degrees, if cervical spine precautions are not necessary.

5. Locate the second intercostal space at the midclavicular line on the side of the tension pneumothorax.

6. Rapidly prepare the site using the povidone-iodine solution, if time permits.

7. Insert a 14- to 16-gauge over-the-needle catheter into the second intercostal space at the midclavicular line by passing just superior to the third rib. By doing so, you will avoid puncturing the neurovascular bundle found inferior to the rib.

8. Advance the needle until the parietal pleura is punctured. A rush of escaping air will occur as the chest is decompressed.

9. Advance the catheter over the needle and remove the needle. Safely dispose of the needle.

10. Attach a flutter device (Penrose drain) to the hub of the catheter.

11. Secure the catheter to the chest wall using adhesive tape.

12. Be sure to frequently reassess the patient's respiratory status and breath sounds. Maintain high-concentration oxygen therapy.

COMPLICATIONS

The following complications are possible:

- Pneumothorax
- Hemorrhage
- Pleural infection

- Local hematoma

- Skin infection

BIBLIOGRAPHY

Ross, D. S. (1998). Thoracentesis. In J. R. Roberts & J. R. Hedges (Eds.), *Clinical procedures in emergency medicine* (3rd ed., pp. 130–136). Philadelphia: W.B.Saunders.

NOTES

_____

_____

_____

_____

_____

_____

_____

_____

_____

_____

_____

_____

_____

_____

_____

_____

CHAPTER 67

PERIPHERAL INTRAVENOUS INSERTION

Owen T. Traynor, M.D.

NOTE: Use body substance isolation whenever the possibility exists of contact with blood or any body fluids. This precaution should include gloves, eye protection, masks, and other protective barriers as necessary. When sharp instruments are used (e.g., needles), a container must be available for their safe disposal.

INDICATIONS

An intravenous (IV) line should be placed whenever the need for the administration of IV fluids or medications exists or potentially exists.

CONTRAINDICATIONS

There are no contraindications in emergency situations; however, IV insertion should not significantly delay the transport of a critically ill or injured patient to the ED.

EQUIPMENT

The following equipment is necessary: appropriate IV fluid or saline lock, administration set and catheters, alcohol or povidone iodine (Betadine) preparations, venous constricting band (VCB), blood tubes and collection equipment, sterile dressings (4" × 4" squares), armboard, tape or commercial site cover.

PROCEDURE

1. Inform the patient about the procedure, and obtain the patient's consent.

2. Assemble and ready the equipment.

3. Select the proper fluid, and inspect it for expiration date, contaminants, and leaks.

4. Select the appropriate administration set, unroll tubing, and position and close the drip-rate control valve.

5. Remove the protective cover, and insert the administration set into the fluid bag port using an aseptic technique.

6. Open the control valve, squeeze the drip chamber, and fill one half of the chamber with fluid.

7. With the fluid flowing, bleed all of the air from the IV tubing.

8. Close the control valve, and inspect for air bubbles in the IV tubing.

9. Place a VCB and palpate a radial pulse.

10. Select a suitable vein.

11. Prep the IV site with Betadine and alcohol (use concentric circles).

12. Stabilize the vein distal to the IV site.

13. Aseptically puncture the skin with the catheter (bevel up), enter the vein (from the top or side), and obtain a flash-back.

14. Release the VCB.

15. Remove the needle aseptically, draw blood if necessary, and then connect the IV tubing or saline lock to the catheter.

16. Dispose of the needle safely.

17. Open the drip control valve or flush the saline lock, and note the free flow of fluid.

18. If IV fluid is used, adjust flow rate to the appropriate rate as directed by medication control physician or protocol.

19. Inspect the surrounding tissue for infiltration of fluid.

20. Secure the catheter and IV tubing or saline lock using tape or commercial site cover.

BIBLIOGRAPHY

Hambrick, E. L. & G. C . Benjamin (1998). Peripheral intravenous access. In J. R. Roberts & J. R. Hedges (Eds.), *Clinical procedures in emergency medicine* (3rd ed., pp. 322–338). Philadelphia: W.B. Saunders.

NOTES

_____

_____

_____

_____

_____

_____

_____

_____

_____

_____

_____

_____

_____

_____

CHAPTER 68

PHARYNGOTRACHEAL LUMEN AIRWAY (PtL®) INSERTION

Lawrence Sherman, EMT-CC

Pharyngotracheal lumen airway (PtL®) insertion should be performed only when indicated and authorized by local medical control.

NOTE: Use body substance isolation whenever the possibility exists of contact with blood or any body fluids. This precaution should include gloves, eye protection, masks, and other protective barriers as necessary. Defibrillation should not be delayed to insert PtL®. Although insertion of the PtL® takes time, a patient should not remain unventilated for more than 30 seconds.

INDICATIONS

PtL® is indicated as an alternative to direct endotracheal intubation in respiratory or cardiorespiratory arrest. Use PtL® if endotracheal intubation is not possible or after two unsuccessful attempts to intubate.

CONTRAINDICATIONS

PtL® is contraindicated in the following situations:

- The patient is conscious or semiconscious with a gag reflex.

- The patient is younger than 14 years.

- The patient is less than 5 feet tall.

- The patient has ingested a caustic substance (e.g., acid, lye).

- The patient has ingested a petroleum product (e.g., gasoline).

- The patient has a known esophageal disease (e.g., cancer, varices).

EQUIPMENT

The following equipment is necessary: PtL®, water-soluble lubricant, oropharyngeal airway (OPA), BVM device with supplemental oxygen source, pulse oximeter, suction equipment.

PROCEDURE

1. Place patient in supine position, and hyperextend the neck; if cervical spine trauma is suspected, stabilize the cervical spine in a neutral position.

2. Open the airway, and suction the mouth and oropharynx if necessary.

3. Insert an OPA and adequately ventilate patient using BVM device, confirming air entry bilaterally and ruling out foreign body airway obstruction.

4. Test the integrity of both cuffs of the PtL® by inflating with a BVM device through the No. 1 inflation valve.

5. Hyperventilate the patient with a BVM device and supplemental oxygen before attempting to insert the PtL®.

6. Lubricate the tip of the PtL® with water-soluble lubricant.

7. While maintaining cervical positioning, remove the OPA and then grasp the mandible and tongue between the thumb and fingers of one hand.

8. Insert tube **gently** with the other hand in midline of the pharynx, making sure that the curve of the tube follows the natural curvature of the palate and pharynx. Advance the PtL® until the teeth strap/bite-block flange touches the patient's teeth.

NOTE: A rescuer might encounter modest resistance when making the 90-degree turn with the PtL® at the posterior pharynx. Do not use excessive force to advance the tube; if the tube does not advance, withdraw the PtL® and attempt insertion again.

9. Secure the retaining strap around the patient's head.

10. Inflate both cuffs simultaneously with a BVM device into the No. 1 inflation valve. Inflation is complete when moderate resistance to the airflow from the BVM device is encountered.

11. Ventilate immediately through the No. 2 short green tube.

    a. Observe for chest rise with each ventilation.

    b. Auscultate bilaterally for the presence of breath sounds.

    c. Auscultate the abdomen for the absence of gurgling.

    d. If all signs of adequate ventilation are present, continue to ventilate the patient according to appropriate local protocols.

    e. Perform secondary confirmation of correct placement using the esophageal detector device or other exhaled CO_2 detector.

    f. If signs of adequate ventilation are absent, remove the stylet from the No. 3 long clear tube, and ventilate through that tube.

    g. Assess for signs of adequate ventilation.

    h. If all signs of adequate ventilation are present, continue to ventilate.

    i. Perform secondary confirmation of correct placement using the esophageal detector device or other exhaled CO_2 detector.

      j. If all signs of adequate ventilation are absent, remove the airway and hyperventilate directly with the BVM device for 2 minutes.

12. If the patient begins gagging or regains consciousness, the PtL® must be removed.

      a. Have working suction ready.

      b. If not contraindicated, roll patient into recovery position (left laterally recumbent).

      c. Open white cap on No. 1 tube to deflate both cuffs.

      d. Remove tube and suction as necessary.

COMPLICATIONS

The following complications are possible:

- Vomiting during insertion
- Inadequate ventilation
- Soft-tissue trauma
- Migration of the pharyngeal balloon

BIBLIOGRAPHY

Bledsoe, B. E., R. S. Porter, & R. A. Cherry (Eds.). (2003). *Essentials of paramedic care.* Englewood Cliffs, NJ: Prentice-Hall.

Mistovich, J. J., B. Q. Hafen, & K. J. Karren (2004). *Prehospital emergency care.* Englewood Cliffs, NJ: Prentice-Hall.

NOTES

_____

_____

_____

_____

CHAPTER 69

PULSE OXIMETRY

Robert L. Kerner, R.N., J.D., CEN

Pulse oximetry became a standard EMS tool in the mid 1990s. The devices are easy to use, noninvasive, and cost effective. The devices are not foolproof, however, and the practitioner must be aware of the limitations.

GAS TRANSPORT

Oxygen (O_2) is transported primarily bound to hemoglobin as oxyhemoglobin, with only 2% of the O_2 dissolved in plasma. The amount of O_2 present is measured as the partial pressure of O_2 (p_{O_2}). As the p_{O_2} increases, the saturation of hemoglobin also increases. The relationship, however, is nonlinear. In other words, doubling the p_{O_2} will not necessarily lead to twice the hemoglobin saturation. This can be seen on the oxygen dissociation curve depicted in Figure 69-1. The S-shaped curve demonstrates the relationship between percent hemoglobin saturation and p_{O_2}.

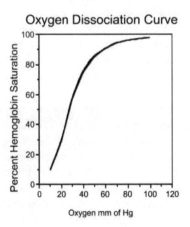

Oxygen Dissociation Curve

Notice that between a p_{O_2} of 60 to 100 mm Hg, the curve is relatively flat. An increase in p_{O_2} in this range will produce only a small increase in hemoglobin saturation. At the steep portion of the curve, between p_{O_2} of 0 to 60 mm Hg, a small change in the p_{O_2} will yield a significant change in the hemoglobin saturation. The significance of this concept is that a small decrease in p_{O_2} can lead to a tremendous decrease in hemoglobin desaturation.

Other factors affect hemoglobin saturation and must be taken into account when using the pulse oximeter. An increase in p_{CO_2} will decrease the affinity of hemoglobin for oxygen, causing an increased oxygen-hemoglobin dissociation at the tissue level, thereby shifting the curve to the right. A shift in the curve to the right means that the hemoglobin will bind less avidly to the oxygen, resulting in increased oxygen delivery to the tissues. An increase in acidity or an increase in temperature also shifts the curve to the right.

The presence of carbon monoxide will also affect hemoglobin-oxygen saturation. Carbon monoxide's affinity for hemoglobin is 240 times greater than that of oxygen, and a relatively small amount of carbon monoxide can bind with a much greater amount of hemoglobin. This phenomenon may lead to serious oxygen deprivation. The presence of carboxyhemoglobin shifts the oxygen dissociation curve to the left, resulting in oxygen that is strongly bound to hemoglobin. This means decreased oxygen delivery to the tissues.

PULSE OXIMETER

The pulse oximeter is a noninvasive method of measuring the oxygen saturation of arterial blood. Although many models of pulse oximeters are now available, all work according to the same basic principle. A probe is applied to the patient, and a beam of light is passed through the tissues to a photodetector on the other half of the probe. The photodetector senses the amount of light absorbed by the oxyhemoglobin molecules in the arterial blood as it passes through the tissues beneath the probe. This information is transmitted to the processing unit of the oximeter, and the percentage of oxygen saturation is displayed. Most pulse oximeters also provide a reading of the patient's pulse rate as well as alarm features such as low saturation or high pulse rate.

The probe-patient interface is perhaps the weakest link in the system. Probes come in many sizes, including adult, pediatric, and neonatal models. Of these, some models have multiple-use probes, such as finger clips, whereas others have single-use probes, such as a tape-type probe. In general, the probe should be applied snugly to a clean, dry surface to allow an accurate reading. Common areas for probe placement include the fingers, toes, nose, and foot. In most cases, nail polish should be removed from fingers or toes before probe placement because colored polish may interfere with the probe. The probe must then be plugged into the oximeter unit directly or to a connecting cable. Check the operation manual to see which types of probes are recommended for the particular machine being used. A probe that is not applied properly will give inaccurate information.

Clinical use of pulse oximetry is increasing. The fact that it is noninvasive means that prehospital care providers can perform an important diagnostic test with no patient discomfort involved. Even small children are able to tolerate this procedure when it is presented in a calm, nonthreatening manner. When the technique is applied properly, the results are reliable. Prehospital EMS providers can be quickly taught to use the oximeter, and it is perhaps one of the easiest biomedical devices to apply and use.

The pulse oximeter is not without a few drawbacks that must be taken into account each time the device is used. The device must sense a pulse in order to calculate the oxygen saturation. States of decreased cardiac output, such as low heart rate, decreased blood pressure, tachycardia, and cardiovascular collapse, will greatly limit the probe's ability to sense the pulse. Likewise, vasoconstrictive states such as shock or hypothermia will have a similar effect. A tourniquet or automated blood pressure cuff proximal to the probe will also interfere with oximetry for the same reasons. Excessive patient movement may cause artifacts to appear, and carbon monoxide poisoning has actually been shown to cause high saturation readings.

Remember that the pulse oximeter measures only arterial oxygen saturation. It does not measure the actual Po_2, nor does it measure the p_{CO_2} or the pH. It also does not assess ventilation. A patient with chronic obstructive pulmonary disease who has a hypoxic drive may have an excellent p_{O_2} when given 100% oxygen but will soon hypoventilate and have dangerously high carbon dioxide levels while maintaining the excellent p_{O_2}.

TROUBLESHOOTING

When the patient's chief complaint, physical examination, and pulse oximeter measurements do not correlate, you must troubleshoot the situation. Does the patient appear sicker than the pulse oximeter reading or vice versa? Always base your interventions on the total evaluation of the patient; treat the patient, not the device. Gather more data if necessary.

Check the mechanical aspects of the machine. Is it plugged in, and does it have sufficient power to operate? Is the probe on properly? Is there any indication that the machine is sensing a pulse? Is the pulse being occluded by a blood pressure cuff? Is the probe placed in such a way that is not being perfused adequately? Has someone accidentally disconnected the cable?

Reassess your patient. Is the patient hypothermic, in shock, or seizing? Could the patient be compensating for an occult problem such as pneumonia? Could the patient be anemic? The possibility exists that if the hemoglobin level is low and if all hemoglobin molecules are bound to oxygen, then the oxygen saturation will be 100%. Yet the patient is still hypoxic because of his or her reduced oxygen-carrying capacity. Is it possible that the patient has carbon monoxide poisoning?

IMPLICATIONS FOR FIELD USE

A pulse oximeter can provide you with important information about the oxygen saturation of patients in respiratory distress. This information was not previously available to the paramedic. Oxygen saturation is only part of the picture. The assessment of the ventilatory status remains one of clinical judgment.

NOTE: Never use the pulse oximeter as a tool to withhold oxygen from a patient in respiratory distress.

BIBLIOGRAPHY

Fluck, R. (2003). Does ambient light affect the accuracy of pulse oximetry? *Respiratory Care 48,* 677–680.

Hartert, T. (1999). Use of pulse oximetry to recognize severity of airflow obstruction in obstructive airway disease. *Chest 115,* 475–481.

NOTES

_____

_____

_____

_____

_____

_____

_____

_____

SECTION 3

CHAPTER 70

RAPID SEQUENCE INTUBATION

Henry E. Wang, M.D.

NOTE: Rapid sequence intubation (RSI) represents one of the most controversial topics in EMS today. Published success rates have varied from 84% to greater than 95%. In addition, several recent studies have questioned the success of prehospital intubation. We originally intended to publish a brief procedure-oriented chapter but quickly realized a more comprehensive chapter would be needed to do justice to this topic. It is our hope that future research will reveal the truth about prehospital RSI.—The editors

RSI is the use of an intravenous paralytic agent to facilitate rapid endotracheal intubation (ETI). A paralytic (neuromuscular blocking) agent is a drug that causes temporary paralysis of all muscles, including those that control respiration. Sensory and autonomic function, however, are preserved. Because paralytics are not sedatives, a powerful sedative or induction agent is usually given with the paralytic so that the patient is not awake during the procedure. The primary purpose of RSI is to enable rapid ETI in the face of a combative or inadequately relaxed patient. However, a secondary purpose of RSI is to control the physiologic response to intubation. The process of intubation is stressful and can cause increases in heart rate, blood pressure, and intracranial pressure; and it is believed that these increases can potentially be harmful to a critically ill patient. It is believed that RSI can help to facilitate intubation while minimizing physiologic response to intubation. Giving a sedative only is **not** RSI. Giving a sedative only is "sedation-facilitated" or "sedation-only intubation." **Do not confuse these terms with RSI.** RSI is not the same as "sedation-only intubation."

INDICATIONS

RSI is indicated for patients who require rapid endotracheal intubation but who have intact protective airway reflexes. Protective airway reflexes include biting, clenching, gagging, and general combativeness. Although there are many opinions about the patient conditions that require RSI, no scientifically based rules for using this technique have been established yet.

CONTRAINDICATIONS

RSI is contraindicated in the following situations:

- **Patients with relative contraindications to selected RSI drugs.** For example, if succinylcholine is used, suspected hyperkalemia is a relative contraindication.

- **Potentially difficult airway anatomy.** Certain anatomic features are believed to make ETI difficult (e.g., morbid obesity, short neck, small mouth, large tongue). RSI is relatively contraindicated in these cases because if intubation is unsuccessful after paralytic administration, ventilation by BVM device may be impossible.

- **Patient entrapment or unstable or dangerous environment.** RSI requires full access to the patient's airway and constant physiologic monitoring, which is impossible to accomplish when the patient is entrapped or located in an unstable or dangerous environment.

- **Absence of qualified personnel or necessary equipment.** Only qualified personnel should perform RSI. RSI should be performed only when all necessary equipment is available.

- **Use of RSI as a punitive measure or to control a combative patient.** RSI should never be used to punish a patient. However, it may be necessary to use RSI to facilitate control of an uncooperative patient in order to ensure the rescuer's safety.

SECTION 3

EQUIPMENT

The following equipment is necessary: IV access, monitoring equipment (continuous pulse-oximetry and ECG), standard intubation equipment (e.g., laryngoscope, blades, endotracheal tubes), RSI drugs (noted in following section), endotracheal tube confirmation devices (esophageal detector device, end-tidal CO_2 detector or capnometer, or waveform end-tidal capnometry), and rescue airway devices and plan (at least two of the following should be readily available: BVM device with oral or nasal airway, laryngeal mask airway [LMA], combitube, cricothyroidotomy).

RSI DRUGS

The selection of specific RSI drugs is determined by local protocol. The following list summarizes the most commonly used agents, with key features and a brief review of major potential adverse effects.

All RSI drugs are given intravenously. It does not matter how much you use as long as you use enough. With few exceptions, all RSI drug dosages are approximate—precise dosages are not necessary. Some systems have used "small/medium/large" dosing schemes. When in doubt, lean toward a higher drug dosage.

A good, safe, and universally accepted RSI drug combination to remember for a 70-kg adult patient is [etomidate 20 mg + succinylcholine 140 mg].

- **Pretreatment agents.** Pretreatment agents are not universally used. (See the section on scientific controversies.) If used, they are typically given 2 to 3 minutes before administration of the induction agent and paralytic.

   o Atropine, 0.02 mg/kg, minimum 0.1 mg. Atropine is used in pediatric patients to offset bradycardia effects of paralytic agents.

- o Lidocaine, 1 to 1.5 mg/kg. Lidocaine is believed to blunt physiologic response to intubation. However, the scientific evidence for this effect is limited. (See the section on scientific controversies.)

- o Defasciculating doses of paralytics, 0.01 mg/kg of vecuronium, pancuronium, or other nondepolarizing paralytic. These are used to eliminate fasciculations resulting from succinylcholine administration and are believed to be helpful in controlling intracranial pressure spikes in patients with head injuries. However, the benefit of this intervention is actually unknown. (See the section on scientific controversies.)

- **Induction agents and sedatives.** Rapid, deep sedation is a core component of RSI and is accomplished by the use of induction agents or sedatives. Induction agents are short-acting drugs used to induce general anesthesia. The term *sedatives* generally refers to benzodiazepines, although opioids such as fentanyl are often used in combination with benzodiazepines to accomplish sedation in RSI. Typically, induction agents are given with paralytic agents to initiate RSI, whereas sedatives are used to maintain sedation after placement of the endotracheal tube. However, some clinicians use sedatives instead of induction agents to initiate RSI.

  - o Induction agents (most commonly used agents listed as examples only—other agents are possible):

    - ■ Etomidate (Amidate), 0.3 mg/kg (20 mg in a 70-kg adult). Onset: 20 to 30 seconds. Duration: 7 to 10 minutes. This short-acting nonbarbiturate hypnotic agent is a favorite agent of emergency physicians because it causes rapid and deep sedation with little effect upon heart rate, blood pressure, or cerebral perfusion. Major adverse effects include possible adrenal suppression, although this effect is clinically insignificant in the context of emergency care.

- Thiopental (Pentothal), 3 to 5 mg/kg (200 to 350 mg in a 70-kg adult). Onset: 15 to 30 seconds. Duration: 5 to 10 minutes. Thiopental is commonly used in the operating room to induce general anesthesia. It reduces cerebral metabolism and thus is good for head injury. Its major adverse effects include clinically significant hypotension.

- Ketamine (Ketalar), 1 to 2 mg/kg (70 to 140 mg in a 70-kg adult). Onset: 15 to 30 seconds. Duration: 10 to 15 minutes. Ketamine is a dissociative anesthetic—the patient seems to be awake and to feel pain but does not seem to care. Related to phencyclidine (PCP), ketamine is commonly used for intubating patients in status asthmaticus because it causes bronchodilation. Major adverse effects include increased secretions (offset by atropine) and postemergency reaction (adults awaken with an agitated mental status).

o Sedatives (most commonly used agents listed as examples only—other agents are possible):

- Midazolam (Versed). Dosage: Varies—0.05 to 0.1 mg/kg typically given in 1- to 2-mg boluses. Onset: 30 to 60 seconds. Duration: 15 to 20 minutes.Midazolam is a short-acting, rapid-onset benzodiazepine commonly used for conscious sedation in the emergency department. Major adverse effects include hypotension. The effect of midazolam is difficult to predict—20 mg may have no appreciable effect on a young football player, whereas 1 mg may induce apnea in an elderly nursing-home patient. Some hold the opinion that midazolam (like all benzodiazepines) is not useful in the induction phase of RSI because it has a relatively slow onset. Midazolam also has unpredictable hemodynamic effects.

- Lorazepam (Ativan). Dosage: Varies.—0.05 to 0.1 mg/kg typically given in 1- to 2-mg boluses. Onset: 60 to 120 seconds. Duration: 30 to 40 minutes. Lorazepam is a long-acting benzodiazepine commonly used for long-term sedation in the ED and intensive care unit (ICU). It is generally reserved for postintubation sedation in RSI. Major adverse effects include hypotension.

- Diazepam (Valium). Dosage: Varies—0.05 to 0.1 mg/kg typically given in 1- to 2-mg boluses. Onset: 45 to 90 seconds. Duration: 30 to 40 minutes. Diazepam is a long-acting benzodiazepine commonly used for long-term sedation in the ED and ICU. It is generally reserved for postintubation sedation in RSI. Major adverse effects include hypotension and local irritation from glycol diluent.

- **Paralytics.** The most commonly used agents are listed as examples only—other agents are possible:

  o Succinylcholine (Anectine). Depolarizing agent—causes fasciculations (muscle twitching). Dosage: 1.5 to 2 mg/kg IV (100 to 140 mg in a 70-kg patient). Onset: 30 to 60 seconds. Duration: 3 to 8 minutes. Succinylcholine is a first-line, short-acting, short-duration paralytic. Considered the mainstay of RSI, it is the best agent for this application. It causes fasciculations (muscle twitching)—when twitching terminates, neuromuscular blockade has been achieved. Major contraindications include suspected hyperkalemia—suspect this in potassium overdoses, patients experiencing kidney failure or undergoing dialysis, musculoskeletal diseases (rhabdomyolysis), or prolonged entrapment (several hours of entrapment cause rhabdomyolysis, muscle breakdown, and increased potassium levels). Patients with old burns (more than 2 days old) may have elevated potassium, but use of succinylcholine on patients with acute burns is acceptable. Major adverse effects include fasciculations, hyperkalemia (may be life-threatening), and malignant hyperthermia.

o Vecuronium (Norcuron). Nondepolarizing agent—does not cause muscle twitching. Dosage: 0.08 to 0.15 mg/kg (5 to 10 mg in a 70-kg patient). Onset: 2 to 4 minutes. Duration: 25 to 40 minutes. Vecuronium, generally used to maintain prolonged paralysis after successful ETI. However, it may also be used as a first-line agent. Caution: This agent lasts a long time.

o Rocuronium (Zemuron). Rapid-acting nondepolarizing agent. Dosage: 0.6 to1.0 mg/kg (40 to 70 mg in a 70-kg patient). Onset: 1 to 3 minutes. Duration: 30 to 45 minutes. Rocuronium was touted as having as rapid an onset as succinylcholine but without the defasciculating side effects. However, rocuronium still has too long of a duration to be an ideal RSI agent. It is probably best left for post-ETI maintenance of paralysis.

PROCEDURE

1. Assess patient and the need for RSI. RSI is a dangerous procedure. Rapidly examine the patient and obtain pertinent history so that you can determine whether you can safely carry out the procedure.

   o Attach patient to a cardiac monitor and pulse oximeter.

   o Obtain vital signs.

   o RSI can result in significant physiologic effects. Make sure the patient is on a monitor before proceeding with RSI.

2. Position and prepare.

   o Establish a large-bore, proximal intravenous line.

- o Place patient in desired position (supine, flat).

- o Prepare intubation equipment.

- o Asssemble BVM device, oxygen, and oral/nasal airway.

- o Estimate dosages and draw up RSI drugs

- o Prepare and test laryngoscopes and endotracheal tubes.

- o Prepare suction.

- o Prepare tube confirmation devices.

- o Make sure rescue airway is immediately available.

3. Preoxygenate. This allows the lungs and body to serve as an oxygen reservoir, filled with almost 100% O_2 rather than 21% O_2.

- o Give 100% oxygen by nonrebreather (NRB) mask.

- o Avoid BVM ventilation unless oxygen saturation cannot be raised to 95% by NRB. Excessive BVM ventilation can result in gastric insufflation.

- o Ideally, preoxygenation should occur for 5 minutes. If this is not possible, have the patient rapidly take eight maximally deep breaths while breathing 100% O_2.

4. Have assistant apply cricoid pressure and continue until tube placement is confirmed.

5. If elected, give pretreatment agents and wait 2 to 3 minutes to ensure effectiveness.

6. Induce deep sedation and paralysis by giving the induction agent, immediately followed by paralytic agent in a rapid bolus over 10 to 20 seconds each.

- o A universally useful combination is etomidate, 0.3 mg/kg (20 mg in a 70-kg patient) plus succinylcholine, 1.5 mg/kg (100 mg in a 70-mg patient).

SECTION 3

o Watch patient and clock—fasciculations (muscle twitches) should occur from succinylcholine immediately before onset of paralysis. Onset of paralysis should occur in 30 to 60 seconds. Verify by examining flaccidity of jaw.

7. Perform laryngoscopy and place endotracheal tube. Remember common-sense ETI rules:

o Each laryngoscopy attempt should take no longer than 30 to 45 seconds (for insertion of blade).

o Abandon attempt if oxygen saturation drops below 90%.

o Re-oxygenate with BVM device before each attempt.

o If ventilating with BVM device is not possible after three attempts, go immediately to rescue-airway plan.

8. Confirm tube placement using multiple methods—primary and secondary.

o Recommended secondary methods

■ Esophageal detector device

■ End-tidal CO_2 detection

■ Waveform end-tidal capnography—strongly recommended for RSI (see section on scientific controversies)

o Cricoid pressure may be released once tube placement is confirmed.

9. Secure tube. Use tape or commercial tube holder.

10. Give postintubation sedation/paralysis. The patient will wake up as soon as the drugs wear off. You must be

prepared to administer continued sedation and paralysis agents.

o A typical regimen may include lorazepam, 2 to 4 mg or diazepam, 5 to 10 mg, for sedations and vecuronium, 10 mg for continued paralysis.

PITFALLS AND COMPLICATIONS

Can't intubate/can't ventilate. This is a rapidly fatal situation. Recognize this situation and act quickly.

o Option 1: Let RSI drugs wear off. This is why short-acting agents are good for RSI. This may restore enough airway and breathing reflex to make use of the BVM device easier.

o Option 2: Go immediately to a rescue-airway plan.

Cardiac arrest on administration of drugs or on intubation attempts. Begin CPR and immediately consider the following:

o **Hypoxia** from prolonged intubation effort or misplaced tube. Verify location of tube. If in doubt, pull tube out and use BVM/rescue-airway device. Ventilate aggressively using the BVM device.

o **Pneumothorax.** Assess breath sounds. Needle decompress as needed.

o **Hyperkalemia** from succinylcholine. Hyperkalemia may present as wide-complex tachycardia, bradycardia, or asystole. In addition to standard ACLS, give sodium bicarbonate, calcium chloride (1 amp of each). Consider also giving insulin (regular, 10 units IV) and dextrose (D50W, 1 amp) if available.

Avoid giving paralytic agents without sedative. Paralytics do not provide sedation—the patient can see, hear, and feel everything.

SECTION 3

SCIENTIFIC CONTROVERSIES

Should I pretreat with lidocaine? Maybe. The intention of intravenous lidocaine is to blunt the "pressor response" to intubation. Although this is a commonly performed procedure, the data supporting this practice are relatively limited and based primarily on nonemergency patients. Physicians in the ED often omit this step. Bottom line recommendation: Exclude this step. It adds unnecessary delay to RSI without clear benefit.

Should I give a defasciculating dose of paralytic to patients with head injuries before using succinylcholine? Maybe. It is reasoned that muscular fasciculations from succinylcholine can increase intracranial pressure and thus worsen a traumatic head injury. Although succinylcholine does increase intracranial pressure, no data indicate that this adversely affects the course or outcome of patients with head trauma. Bottom line recommendation: Exclude this step. It adds unnecessary delay to RSI without clear benefit.

Should I pretreat pediatric patients with atropine? Yes. Children can develop bradycardia from the vagal effects of paralytic agents.

Which drug should I use as my first-line RSI paralytic? We recommend succinylcholine only as a first-line paralytic. The short duration of action will be beneficial if the patient cannot be intubated. All other paralytic agents have durations that are too long. Longer-acting agents should be reserved for use after successful endotracheal tube placement. If the patient has contraindications to succinylcholine, consider performing a "sedation-only" intubation before resorting to the risky use of a long-acting paralytic.

Which induction/sedative agent should I use? The optimal induction/sedative agent is powerful and predictable, with minimal effects on cerebral perfusion and hemodynamic stability. We believe etomidate meets these criteria. It rapidly causes deep sedation without causing hemodynamic instability. Studies have demonstrated that it is cardioprotective and neuroprotective. Growing evidence suggests that it is safe for use in pediatric patients. Benzodiazepines, such as midazolam, have a slower, less predictable onset of action and are best used for postintubation sedation.

Is there a simple and reliable RSI drug combination? Remember etomidate (20 mg) + succinylcholine (140 mg)—this combination is appropriate for the vast majority of RSIs in the typical 70-kg patient.

Can succinylcholine be used in children? Yes. The Federal Drug Administration (FDA) has issued warnings regarding the use of succinylcholine in children. This caution is based on operating room case reports of succinylcholine causing hyperkalemia in children with undiagnosed, occult muscular myopathies. However, these cases are exceedingly rare. The FDA warning applies primarily to elective surgical cases, not emergency situations.

Can succinylcholine be used in patients with head injuries? Yes. As previously discussed, although fasciculations from succinylcholine may increase intracranial pressure, no evidence suggests that this phenomenon worsens outcome.

Can succinylcholine be used in patients with burns? Yes. The concern of inducing hyperkalemia in patients with major burns applies only 24 to 48 hours after the onset of injury. Succinylcholine may be safely used in patients with acute burns.

What are the fundamental differences between RSI and sedation-only intubation? RSI is the use of a paralytic agent to chemically paralyze the patient. The danger of this technique is that all protective airway reflexes and respiratory muscles are inhibited. Therefore the patient's only link to life (or death) is your ability to quickly and properly insert an endotracheal tube—or to salvage the situation with another method of ventilation, such as a BVM device. In patients with very difficult airway anatomy, a BVM device and other nonintubation techniques may be extremely difficult (or outright impossible) to perform, especially with the airway and breathing reflexes completely paralyzed. Sedation-only intubation puts the patient into a deep sleep. Although the patient's airway reflexes and respiratory drive may be ablated to the point where it is possible to perform intubation, the protective reflexes may still be intact—thus the patient may still be able to provide a small portion of his or her own airway and ventilatory management. Note that with sufficiently high dosages, it may be possible to completely ablate airway and breathing reflexes with any sedative agent.

Do I have to give a paralytic agent? No. Many intubations can be accomplished using deep sedation with an induction or sedative agent only. (Hence, sedation-only intubation.) In cases of an anticipated difficult airway, it is acceptable to give the induction or sedative agent first, attempt intubation, then proceed to give the paralytic if you are unsuccessful.

Why should I use a waveform end-tidal capnographer? Most medical directors believe that waveform end-tidal capnography is the best way to verify endotracheal tube placement. Continuous tube placement is extremely important with a chemically paralyzed patient because it may be particularly difficult to detect tube misplacement or dislodgment. Waveform capnography is one of the few ways available to continuously verify correct tube placement.

What is a good success rate for RSI? 99+%. The intention of RSI is to remove all protective airway reflexes so that only anatomic barriers are left. If you use RSI, you should be such a good intubator that you can intubate any patient (and his/her anatomic barriers) once the protective reflexes are abolished. If you use RSI, you should also be such a good clinician that you recognize when you will have trouble overcoming a patient's anatomic barriers—and thus elect not to give the paralytic agent in these situations.

Is RSI appropriate for use by all paramedics in all EMS systems? Perhaps not. RSI should be reserved for the most highly trained prehospital rescuers because of the potential risk of mismanaging a paralyzed airway. The EMS system and its medical director must acquire and study the important information about every intubation attempt. A rigorous quality management program must be in place. There is growing consensus that RSI may be safe only when performed by the most highly trained personnel in small EMS services with close medical direction and oversight. Personnel who use RSI must be exceptional at both endotracheal intubation and nonintubation airway management options, skills that many medical directors feel can be mastered only through operating room training and close supervision. Recent scientific data suggest that increased mortality may occur as a result of prehospital RSI.

BIBLIOGRAPHY

Orebaugh, S. L. (2002). Difficult airway management in the emergency department. *Journal of Emergency Medicine 1,* 3–48.

Walls, R., R. C. Luten, M. F. Murphy, & R. E. Schneider (Eds.). (2000). *The manual of emergency airway management.* Philadelphia: Lippincott Williams & Wilkins.

SECTION 3

NOTES

_____

_____

_____

CHAPTER 71

TRANSCUTANEOUS PACING

Thomas J. Rahilly, Ph.D.

Transcutaneous pacing is the initial pacing method of choice in emergency cardiac care because of the speed with which it can be instituted and because it is the least invasive pacing technique available.

INDICATIONS

EMERGENT PACING

Emergent pacing is indicated in the following situations:

- Hemodynamically compromising bradycardias (systolic BP less than 80 mm Hg, change in mental status, myocardial ischemia, pulmonary edema)

- Bradycardia with malignant escape rhythms (unresponsive to pharmacologic therapy)

- Overdrive pacing of refractory tachycardia (supraventricular or ventricular [currently indicated only in special situations refractory to pharmacologic therapy or cardioversion])

- Bradyasystolic cardiac arrest

- Not routinely recommended in patients with asystol; if used at all, should be used as early as possible after onset of arrest

STANDBY MODE

Standby mode is indicated in the following situations:

- Stable bradycardias (BP greater than 80 mm Hg, no evidence of hemodynamic compromise, or hemodynamic compromise responsive to initial drug therapy)

- Symptomatic sinus node dysfunction

- Mobitz II second-degree heart block

- Third-degree heart block

- Newly acquired left bundle-branch block, right bundle-branch block, alternating bundle-branch block, or bifascicular block

CONTRAINDICATIONS

There are no contraindications in the presence of indicators.

EQUIPMENT

The following equipment is necessary: monitor and defibrillator equipped with transcutaneous pacing option, pacing cable, and electrodes.

PROCEDURE

NOTE: Not all transcutaneous pacing-equipped monitors and defibrillators operate in the same way. Follow the manufacturer's operating guide for the one in use by your service.

ELECTRODE PLACEMENT

- Anteroposterior (AP) preferred

    o Anterior electrode (negative)—left anterior chest at the level of nipple midway between xiphoid and left nipple

    o Posterior electrode (positive)—left posterior chest beneath scapula

- Anteroanterior acceptable if AP placement is not possible

  o Apical electrode (negative)—fourth intercostal space midaxillary line

  o Sternal electrode (positive)—right anterior chest mid-clavicular line

PACING FOR BRADYARRHYTHMIAS

1. Explain the procedure to the patient (if alert), and obtain the patient's consent. Consider sedation.

2. Turn monitor and defibrillator power on.

3. Prepare the skin at electrode sites.

4. Attach monitor electrodes (lead II).

5. Connect the pacing cable.

6. Attach and apply the pacing electrodes.

7. Turn pacer on.

8. Set the desired rate, usually 60 to 80 bpm.

9. Adjust QRS size until R wave is sensed if the patient's native QRS complexes are not identified.

10. Increase current until capture occurs (start at zero).

11. Verify pulse, run rhythm strip, and monitor vital signs.

PACING FOR ASYSTOLE OR BRADYASYSTOLIC ARREST

1. Turn monitor and defibrillator power on.

2. Prepare the skin at electrode sites.

3. Attach monitor electrodes (lead II).

4. Connect the pacing cable.

5. Attach and apply the pacing electrodes.

6. Turn pacer on.

7. Set the rate at 80 bpm.

8. Increase current to maximum output.

9. Verify pulse, run rhythm strip, and monitor vital signs.

EVIDENCE OF CAPTURE

• Wide QRS complex: tall, wide T indicates electrical capture

The following indicate mechanical capture:

• Palpable pulse at "set" rate

• Improved BP reading

• Improved level of consciousness

• Improved skin color and temperature

SIDE EFFECTS

• Skeletal muscle contractions

• Chest muscle discomfort (use lowest current possible)

BIBLIOGRAPHY

Bledsoe, B. E., R. S. Porter, & R. A. Cherry (Eds.). (2003). *Essentials of paramedic care.* Englewood Cliffs, NJ: Prentice-Hall.

Roberts, J. R. & J. R. Hedges (Eds.). (2004). *Clinical procedures in emergency medicine* (4th ed.) Philadelphia: W.B. Saunders.

NOTES

_____

_____

_____

_____

SECTION 3

SECTION 4

APPENDICES

APPENDIX A

ACLS SUMMARY

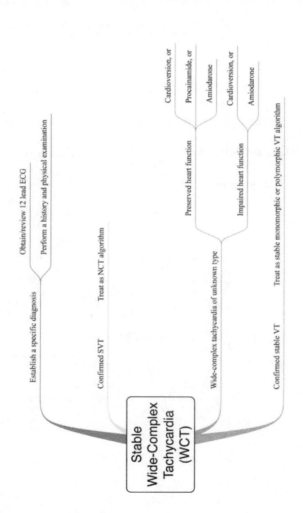

Stable Wide-Complex Tachycardia (WCT)

- Establish a specific diagnosis
  - Obtain/review 12 lead ECG
  - Perform a history and physical examination

- Confirmed SVT
  - Treat as NCT algorithm

- Wide-complex tachycardia of unknown type
  - Preserved heart function
    - Cardioversion, or
    - Procainamide, or
    - Amiodarone
  - Impaired heart function
    - Cardioversion, or
    - Amiodarone

- Confirmed stable VT
  - Treat as stable monomorphic or polymorphic VT algorithm

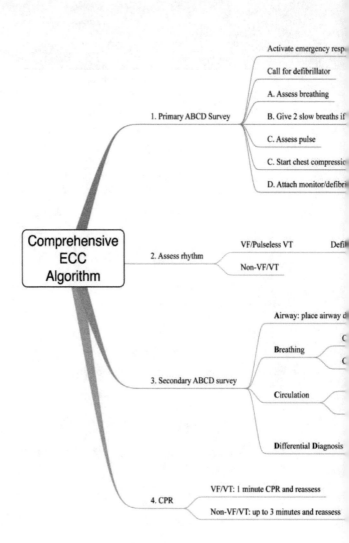

Comprehensive ECC Algorithm

1. Primary ABCD Survey
- Activate emergency resp
- Call for defibrillator
- A. Assess breathing
- B. Give 2 slow breaths if
- C. Assess pulse
- C. Start chest compressio
- D. Attach monitor/defibri

2. Assess rhythm
- VF/Pulseless VT — Defi
- Non-VF/VT

3. Secondary ABCD survey
- Airway: place airway d
- Breathing
  - C
  - C
- Circulation
- Differential Diagnosis

4. CPR
- VF/VT: 1 minute CPR and reassess
- Non-VF/VT: up to 3 minutes and reassess

tem

thing

pulse

hen available.

200 j

200-300j

360j

May use biphasic equivalent energies

possible

secure airway device

ventilation/oxygenation

h IV access

	Vasopressin 40 U IV, single dose, or
VF/VT patients	Epinephrine 1 mg IV q 3-5 minutes
	May be given after vasopressin, if no response

ster adrenergic agents

Non-VF/VT patients   Epinephrine 1 mg IV q 3-5 minutes

Search for and treat reversible causes

Tachycardia Overview

1 Evaluate patient
- Stable vs unstable?
- Are serious signs or symptoms present?
- Is the tachycardia the cause of the serious signs or symptoms?

2 Unstable patient
- Establish the rapid HR as the cause of signs/symptoms
- HR < 150 are seldom the cause of serious signs/symptoms
- Prepare for immediate cardioversion

3 Stable patient
- Atrial fibrillation or flutter
- Narrow-complex tachycardias (NCT)
- Stable wide-complex tachycardias of unknown type
- Stable monomorphic VT and/or polymorphic VT

PEA

1 Primary ABCD Survey
- Check responsiveness
- Activate the emergency response system
- Call for defibrillator
- A. Airway: open the airway
- B. Breathing: provide positive pressure ventilations
- C. Circulation: start chest compressions
- D. Defibrillation: assess for and shock VF/pulseless VT

2 Secondary ABCD Survey
- A. Airway: place airway device ASAP
- B. Breathing: confirm airway device placement using primary secondary confirmation
- B. Breathing: secure airway device
- B. Breathing: ensure effective ventilation and oxygenation
- C. Circulation: establich IV access
- C. Circulation: identify and monitor rhythm
- C. Circulation: administer meds for rhythm and condition
- C. Circulation: assess for occult blood flow ("pseudo-EMD")
- D. Differential diagnosis: Search for and treat reversible cause

3 Review for most frequent causes of PEA
- Hypovolemia
- Hypoxia
- Hydrogen ion—acidosis
- Hyper-/hypokalemia
- Hypothermia
- "Tablets" (drug OD, accidents)
- Tamponade, cardiac
- Tension pneumothorax
- Thrombosis, coronary (ACS)
- Thrombosis, pulmonary embolism

4 Medications
- Epinephrine 1 mg IV q 3-5 minutes
- Atropine 1 mg IV q 3-5 minutes prn bradycaria   Total dose 0.4 mg/kg

SECTION 4

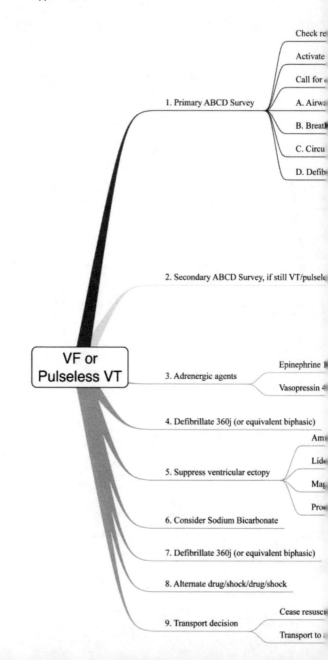

VF or Pulseless VT

1. Primary ABCD Survey
   - Check re
   - Activate
   - Call for
   - A. Airwa
   - B. Breath
   - C. Circu
   - D. Defib

2. Secondary ABCD Survey, if still VT/pulsele

3. Adrenergic agents
   - Epinephrine
   - Vasopressin 4

4. Defibrillate 360j (or equivalent biphasic)

5. Suppress ventricular ectopy
   - Am
   - Lide
   - Mag
   - Pro

6. Consider Sodium Bicarbonate

7. Defibrillate 360j (or equivalent biphasic)

8. Alternate drug/shock/drug/shock

9. Transport decision
   - Cease resusc
   - Transport to a

ness

cy response system

tor

the airway

itive pressure ventilations

art chest compressions

200j, 200-300j, 360 j or equivalent biphasic, prn

	A. Airway: insert airway device ASAP	
B. Breathing	Confirm/secure airway device	
	Confirm ventilation/oxygenation	
	Establish IV access	
C. Circulation	Identify ECG rhythm	
	Administer appropriate meds	
D. Differential Diagnosis	Search for and treat reversible causes	

3-5 minutes, or

l   may use epi as above if vasopressin is not effective

te ED

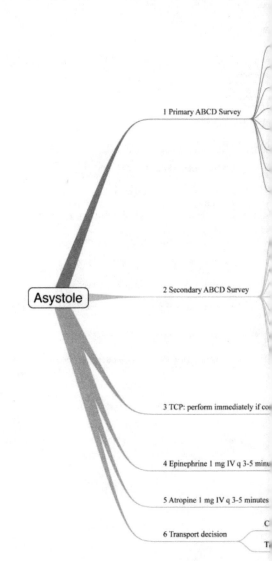

Asystole

1 Primary ABCD Survey

2 Secondary ABCD Survey

3 TCP: perform immediately if co

4 Epinephrine 1 mg IV q 3-5 minu

5 Atropine 1 mg IV q 3-5 minutes

6 Transport decision

C

T

Responsiveness

the emergency response system

defibrillator

ay: open the airway

thing: provide positive pressure ventilations

lation: give chest compressions

brillation: assess for and shock VF/pulseless VT

cene survey: is there evidence that resuscitation should not be initiated?

rway: place airway device ASAP

eathing: confirm airway device placement using primary and secondary confirmation

eathing: secure airway device

eathing: ensure effective ventilation and oxygenation

rculation: establich IV access

rculation: identify and monitor rhythm

rculation: administer meds for rhythm and condition

rculation: assess for occult blood flow ("pseudo-EMD")

fferential diagnosis: Search for and treat reversible causes

Total dose 0.4 mg/kg maximum

itation   No response to satisfactory trial of BLS/ALS

Atypical clinical features present

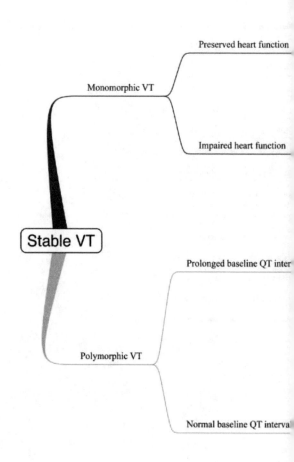

Preserved heart function

Monomorphic VT

Impaired heart function

Stable VT

Prolonged baseline QT inter

Polymorphic VT

Normal baseline QT interva

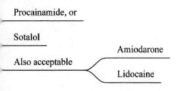

Procainamide, or

Sotalol

Also acceptable
— Amiodarone
— Lidocaine

1.1 Amiodarone 150 mg IV over 10 minutes, or

1.1 Lidocaine 0.5 -0.75 mg/kg IV, then

1.2 Synchronized cardioversion

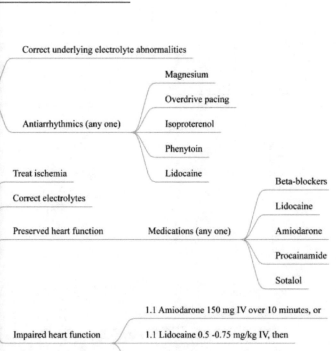

Correct underlying electrolyte abnormalities

Antiarrhythmics (any one)
— Magnesium
— Overdrive pacing
— Isoproterenol
— Phenytoin
— Lidocaine

Treat ischemia

Correct electrolytes

Preserved heart function   Medications (any one)
— Beta-blockers
— Lidocaine
— Amiodarone
— Procainamide
— Sotalol

Impaired heart function
— 1.1 Amiodarone 150 mg IV over 10 minutes, or
— 1.1 Lidocaine 0.5 -0.75 mg/kg IV, then
— 1.2 Synchronized cardioversion

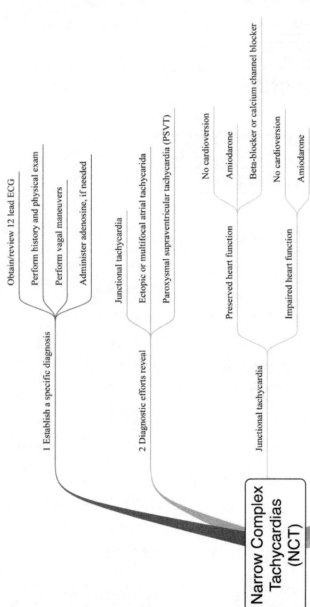

Narrow Complex Tachycardias (NCT)

1 Establish a specific diagnosis
- Obtain/review 12 lead ECG
- Perform history and physical exam
- Perform vagal maneuvers
- Administer adenosine, if needed

2 Diagnostic efforts reveal
- Junctional tachycardia
- Ectopic or multifocal atrial tachycardia
- Paroxysmal supraventricular tachycardia (PSVT)

Junctional tachycardia
- Preserved heart function
  - No cardioversion
  - Amiodarone
  - Beta-blocker or calcium channel blocker
- Impaired heart function
  - No cardioversion
  - Amiodarone
  - No cardioversion

Beta blocker

Amiodarone

No cardioversion

Amiodarone

Diltiazem

Impaired heart function

Ectopic or multifocal atrial tachycardia

1 Calcium channel blocker

2 Beta-blocker

3 Digoxin

4 Cardioversion

5 Consider procainamide, amiodarone, sotalol

Preserved heart function

1 No cardioversion

2 Digoxin

3 Amiodarone

4 Diltiazem

Impaired heart function

PSVT

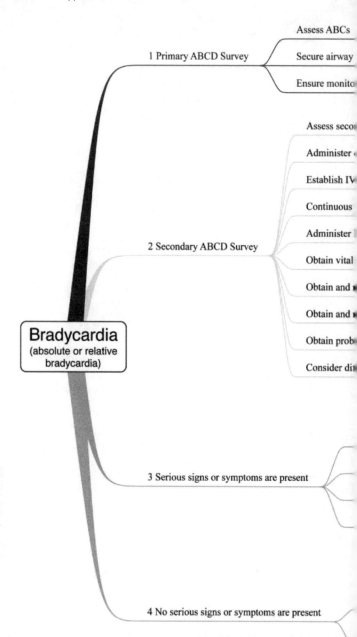

Bradycardia
(absolute or relative
bradycardia)

1 Primary ABCD Survey

Assess ABCs

Secure airway

Ensure monito

2 Secondary ABCD Survey

Assess seco

Administer

Establish IV

Continuous

Administer

Obtain vital

Obtain and

Obtain and

Obtain prob

Consider di

3 Serious signs or symptoms are present

4 No serious signs or symptoms are present

asively

illator is available

BCs (is advanced airway management needed?)

onitoring

s if needed

oxygen saturation

2 lead ECG

hest X-ray (hospital personnel only)

nted history and physical exam

l diagnosis

opine 0.5 - 1 mg IV

P

pamine 5 - 20 mcg/kg/minute

nephrine 2 - 20 mcg/kg/minute

e II second-degree AV block or   Prepare for transvenous pacer
d-degree AV block is present

    Use TCP if symptoms develop while
    awaiting transvenous pacer placement

serve for other bradycardic rhythms

SECTION 4

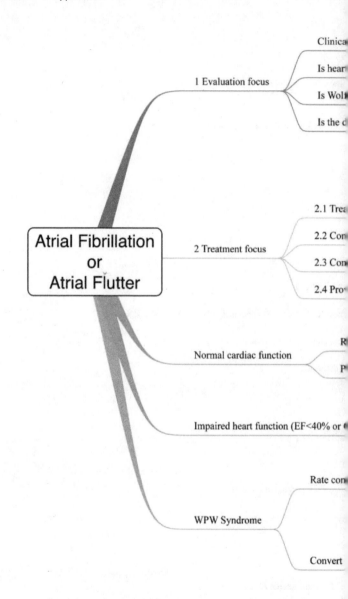

1 Evaluation focus
- Clinica
- Is hear
- Is Wol
- Is the c

2 Treatment focus
- 2.1 Trea
- 2.2 Con
- 2.3 Con
- 2.4 Pro

Normal cardiac function
- R
- P

Impaired heart function (EF<40% or

WPW Syndrome
- Rate con
- Convert

Atrial Fibrillation or Atrial Flutter

e or unstable?

on impaired (EF < 40% or CHF)

nson-White (WPW) present?

< 48 or > 48 hours?

ble patients urgently

heart rate

rhythm

icoagulation if needed

trol with calcium channel blockers, or beta blockers

tal rhythm conversion is not recommended

Rate control using digoxin, diltiazem or amiodarone

Prehospital rhythm conversion is not recommended

mpts may be dangerous

Impulses may preferentially travel down accessory pathways yielding faster HR

hm using:

amiodarone

flecainimde (not for use when the heart is impaired)

procainamide (not for use when the heart is impaired)

propafenone (not for use when the heart is impaired)

sotalol (not for use when the heart is impaired)

APPENDIX B

BASIC LIFE SUPPORT SUMMARY

	Adult (8 years old)	Child (1–8 years)	Infant (birth–1 year)
Airway technique	Head tilt–chin lift in the nontrauma patient. Jaw thrust with cervical spine precautions in the context of trauma.		
Breathing	2 breaths: 2 sec/breath initially, then 10 to 12 breaths/min	2 breaths: 1–1.5 sec/breath initially, then 20 breaths/min	
Pulse check	Carotid	Brachial or Femoral	
Compression depth	1.5–2 inches	1–1.5 inches	0.5–1 inch
Compression rate	Approx. 100/minute	100/minute	>100/minute
Ratio of compressions to ventilations	15:2	5:1	
Foreign body obstructed airway technique	Heimlich maneuver, with finger sweeps in the unconscious patient	Back blows and chest thrusts, finger sweeps only if the foreign body is visualized	

Data from Handbook for Emergency Cardiovascular Care. American Heart Association, Dallas, TX, 2000.

APPENDIX C

PALS SUMMARY

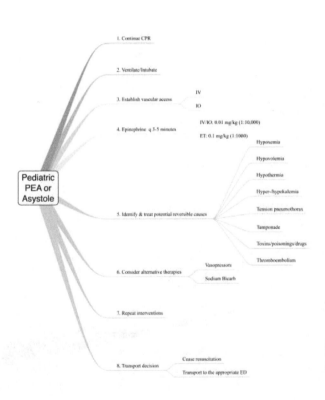

Pediatric PEA or Asystole

1. Continue CPR

2. Ventilate/Intubate

3. Establish vascular access
   - IV
   - IO

4. Epinephrine q 3-5 minutes
   - IV/IO: 0.01 mg/kg (1:10,000)
   - ET: 0.1 mg/kg (1:1000)

5. Identify & treat potential reversible causes
   - Hypoxemia
   - Hypovolemia
   - Hypothermia
   - Hyper-/hypokalemia
   - Tension pneumothorax
   - Tamponade
   - Toxins/poisonings/drugs
   - Thromboembolism

6. Consider alternative therapies
   - Vasopressors
   - Sodium Bicarb

7. Repeat interventions

8. Transport decision
   - Cease resuscitation
   - Transport to the appropriate ED

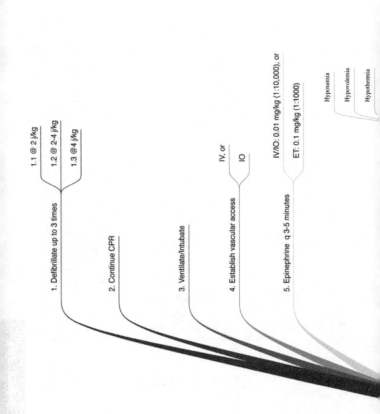

1.1 @ 2 j/kg
1.2 @ 2-4 j/kg
1.3 @ 4 j/kg

1. Defibrillate up to 3 times

2. Continue CPR

3. Ventilate/Intubate

4. Establish vascular access

IV, or
IO

5. Epinephrine q 3-5 minutes

IV/IO: 0.01 mg/kg (1:10,000), or
ET: 0.1 mg/kg (1:1000)

Hypoxemia
Hypovolemia
Hypothermia

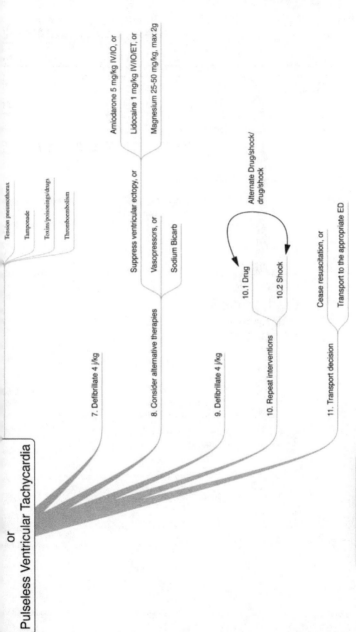

Pulseless Ventricular Tachycardia

or

Tension pneumothorax
Tamponade
Toxins/poisonings/drugs
Thromboembolism

7. Defibrillate 4 j/kg

8. Consider alternative therapies

Suppress ventricular ectopy, or

Vasopressors, or

Sodium Bicarb

Amiodarone 5 mg/kg IV/IO, or

Lidocaine 1 mg/kg IV/IO/ET, or

Magnesium 25-50 mg/kg, max 2g

9. Defibrillate 4 j/kg

10. Repeat interventions

10.1 Drug

10.2 Shock

Alternate Drug/shock/drug/shock

11. Transport decision

Cease resuscitation, or

Transport to the appropriate ED

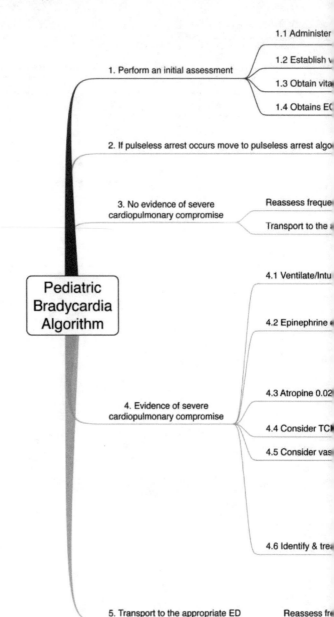

Pediatric Bradycardia Algorithm

1. Perform an initial assessment
- 1.1 Administer
- 1.2 Establish v
- 1.3 Obtain vita
- 1.4 Obtains E(

2. If pulseless arrest occurs move to pulseless arrest algo

3. No evidence of severe cardiopulmonary compromise
- Reassess freque
- Transport to the

4. Evidence of severe cardiopulmonary compromise
- 4.1 Ventilate/Intu
- 4.2 Epinephrine
- 4.3 Atropine 0.02
- 4.4 Consider TC
- 4.5 Consider vas
- 4.6 Identify & trea

5. Transport to the appropriate ED
- Reassess fre

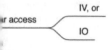

IV, or

IO

...riate ED

Start CPR for HR < 60 despite satisfactory oxygenation/ventilation

0.01 mg/kg (1:10,000) IV/IO

...inutes   0.1 mg/kg (1:1000) ET

Atropine first if there is a heart block or increased vagal tone

Minimum dose 0.1 mg

...g IV/IO/ET   Maximum dose 0.5 mg child, 1 mg adolescent

May be repeated once

Dopamine 1-20 µg/kg/min

...ors   Epinephrine 0.1 µg/kg/min

...ntial reversible causes

Hypoxemia

Hypothermia

Head injury

Heart block

Heart transplant

Toxins/poisonings/drugs

...ly

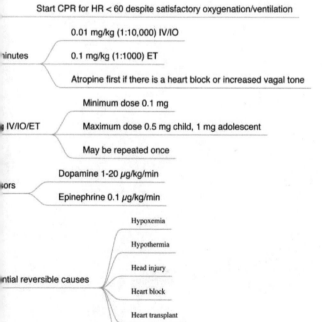

SECTION 4

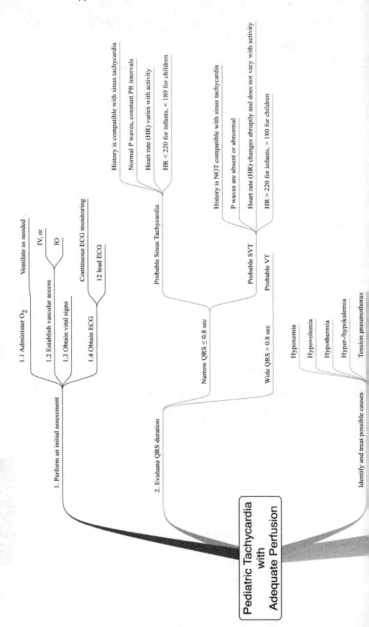

Pediatric Tachycardia with Adequate Perfusion

1. Perform an initial assessment

- 1.1 Administer O₂ — Ventilate as needed
- 1.2 Establish vascular access — IV, or / IO
- 1.3 Obtain vital signs — Continuous ECG monitoring
- 1.4 Obtain ECG — 12 lead ECG

2. Evaluate QRS duration

Narrow QRS ≤ 0.8 sec

Probable Sinus Tachycardia
- History is compatible with sinus tachycardia
- Normal P waves, constant PR intervals
- Heart rate (HR) varies with activity
- HR < 220 for infants, < 180 for children

Probable SVT
- History is NOT compatible with sinus tachycardia
- P waves are absent or abnormal
- Heart rate (HR) changes abruptly and does not vary with activity
- HR > 220 for infants, > 180 for children

Wide QRS > 0.8 sec

Probable VT

Identify and treat possible causes
- Hypoxemia
- Hypovolemia
- Hypothermia
- Hyper-/hypokalemia
- Tension pneumothorax

Toxins-poisonings/drugs

Thromboembolism

Pain

Probable Sinus Tachycardia — Treat the underlying cause of poor perfusion

Probable SVT

1. Consider vagal maneuvers

2. Adenosine 0.1 mg/kg IV/IO
   - Repeat at 0.2 mg/kg IV/IO, prn
   - Maximum first dose 6mg
   - Maximum second dose 12 mg

3. Consider cardioversion
   - 0.5 – 1j/kg, may repeat at higher energy (up to 2 j/kg)
   - Administer sedation prior to cardioversion

4. Consider antiarrhythmic agents as for probable VT

Probable VT

1. Suppress ectopy
   - Amiodarone 5 mg/kg IV over 20 to 60 minutes, or
   - Procainamide 15 mg/kg IV over 30 to 60 minutes, or
   - Lidocaine 1 mg/kg IV bolus
   - Do not routinely use amiodarone and procainamide together

2. Consider cardioversion
   - 0.5 – 1j/kg, may repeat at higher energy (up to 2 j/kg)
   - Consider sedation, but do not delay cardioversion

Transport to the Appropriate ED — Reassess frequently

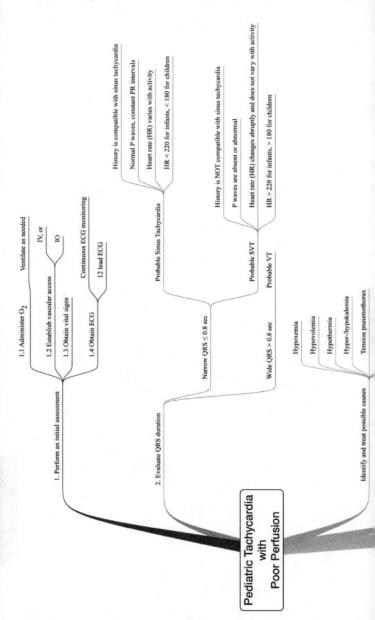

Pediatric Tachycardia with Poor Perfusion

1. Perform an initial assessment
- 1.1 Administer O₂ — Ventilate as needed
- 1.2 Establish vascular access — IV, or / IO
- 1.3 Obtain vital signs
- 1.4 Obtain ECG — Continuous ECG monitoring / 12 lead ECG

2. Evaluate QRS duration
- Narrow QRS ≤ 0.8 sec
  - Probable Sinus Tachycardia
    - History is compatible with sinus tachycardia
    - Normal P waves, constant PR intervals
    - Heart rate (HR) varies with activity
    - HR < 220 for infants, < 180 for children
  - Probable SVT
    - History is NOT compatible with sinus tachycardia
    - P waves are absent or abnormal
    - Heart rate (HR) changes abruptly and does not vary with activity
    - HR > 220 for infants, > 180 for children
- Wide QRS > 0.8 sec
  - Probable VT

Identify and treat possible causes
- Hypoxemia
- Hypovolemia
- Hypothermia
- Hyper-/hypokalemia
- Tension pneumothorax

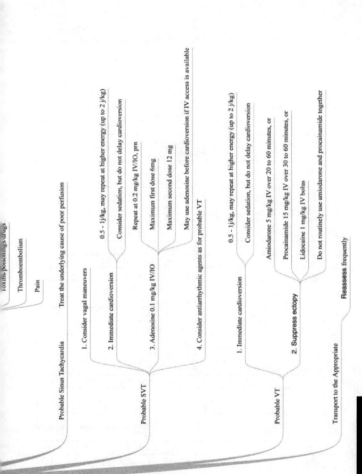

Toxins/poisonings/drugs

Thromboembolism

Pain

Probable Sinus Tachycardia — Treat the underlying cause of poor perfusion

Probable SVT

1. Consider vagal maneuvers

2. Immediate cardioversion — 0.5 - 1 j/kg, may repeat at higher energy (up to 2 j/kg)
   — Consider sedation, but do not delay cardioversion

3. Adenosine 0.1 mg/kg IV/IO — Repeat at 0.2 mg/kg IV/IO, prn
   — Maximum first dose 6mg
   — Maximum second dose 12 mg
   — May use adenosine before cardioversion if IV access is available

4. Consider antiarrhythmic agents as for probable VT

Probable VT

1. Immediate cardioversion — 0.5 - 1 j/kg, may repeat at higher energy (up to 2 j/kg)
   — Consider sedation, but do not delay cardioversion

2. Suppress ectopy — Amiodarone 5 mg/kg IV over 20 to 60 minutes, or
   — Procainamide 15 mg/kg IV over 30 to 60 minutes, or
   — Lidocaine 1 mg/kg IV bolus
   — Do not routinely use amiodarone and procainamide together

Transport to the Appropriate — Reassess frequently

APPENDIX D

COMMONLY PRESCRIBED MEDICATIONS

Trade names, GENERIC NAMES

Drug Name	Drug Type
Accolate	See Zafirlukast
Accupril	See Quinapril
Acetaminophen/Codeine	Narcotic analgesic
Aciphex	See Rabeprazole
Actonel	See Risedronate
Actos	See Pioglitazone
Acyclovir	Antiviral
Adalat CC	See Nifedipine
Adderall	Treatment for ADHD, amphetamine
Advair Diskus	See Salmeterol/Fluticasone
Albuterol	Beta agonist bronchodilator
Alesse	See Levonorgestrel/Ethinyl Estradiol
Allegra	See Fexofenadine
Allegra-D	See Fexofenadine/Pseudoephedrine
Allopurinol	Antigout treatment
Alphagan	See Brimonidine
Alprazolam	Benzodiazepine Anxiolytic agent
Altace	See Ramipril
Amaryl	See Glimepiride
Amoxicillin/Clavulanate	Antibiotic
Apri	See Desogestrel/Ethinyl Estradiol
Aricept	See Donepezil
Arthrotec	See Diclofenac/Misoprostol
Atrovent	See Ipratropium
Augmentin ES-600	See Amoxicillin/Clavulanate
Avandia	See Rosiglitazone
Aviane	See Levonorgestrel/Ethinyl Estradiol
Bextra	See Valdecoxib
Brimonidine	Antiglaucoma eye drops
Budesonide	Topical steroidal antiinflammatory agent
Bupropion	Smoking cessation agent
Buspirone	Nonbenzodiazepine antianxiety agent
Butalbital/APAP/Caffiene	Headache/migraine treatment

Drug Name	Drug Type
Calcitonin Salmon	Osteoporosis treatment
Carbidopa/Levodopa	Parkinson's disease treatment
Carvedilol	Nonselective beta–adrenergic blocking agent with alpha 1-blocking activity
Cetirizine	Antihistamine
Clarinex	See Desloratadine
Contuss-XT	See Guaifenesin/Phenylpropanolamine
Coreg	See Carvedilol
Deltasone	See Prednisone
Desloratadine	Antihistamine
Desogestrel/Ethinyl Estradiol	Oral contraceptive
Detrol LA	See Tolterodine
Diabeta	See Glyburide
Diclofenac	Nonsteroidal antiinflammatory agent
Diclofenac/Misoprostol	Nonsteroidal antiinflammatory agent/stomach protectant
Diclofenac Sodium	See Diclofenac
Digoxin	Cardiac glycoside-antiarrhythmic, CHF agent
Ditropan XL	See Oxybutynin
Donepezil	Treatment for Alzheimer's dementia
Doxepin	Antidepressant
Doxycycline	Antibiotic
Dyazide	See Hydrochlorothiazide/Triamterine
Effexor	See Venlafaxine
Estraderm	See Estradiol
Estradiol	Estrogen replacement treatment
Famotidine	Gastric acid reducer
Fexofenadine	Antihistamine
Fexofenadine/Pseudoephedrine	Antihistamine/decongestant
Furosemide	Diuretic
Gatifloxacin	Antibiotic
Gliburide	Oral hypoglycemic
Glimepiride	Oral hypoglycemic
Glipizide	Oral hypoglycemic
Glucophage	See Metformin
Glucotrol	See Glipizide
Guaifenesin/ Phenylpropanolamine	Expectorant/decongestant
Guaifenesin/PPA	See Guaifenesin/Phenylpropanolamine
Humalog	See Insulin Lispro
Human Insulin 70/30	Hypoglycemic/diabetic treatment
Human Insulin Regular	Hypoglycemic/diabetic treatment
Humulin 70/30	See Human Insulin 70/30
Humulin R	See Human Insulin Regular
Hydrochlorothiazide/Triamterine	Potassium-sparing diuretic
Hydroxyzine	Antihistamine/relaxant

Drug Name	Drug Type
Hyoscyamine	Gastrointestinal antispasmodic
Indomethacin	Nonsteroidal antiinflammatory agent
Insulin Lispro	Hypoglycemic/diabetic treatment
Ipratropium	Parasympathetic blocking bronchodilator
K-Dur-20	See Potassium Chloride
Klor-Con	See Potassium Chloride
Lamisil	See Terbinafine
Lasix	See Furosemide
Levonorgestrel/Ethinyl Estradiol	Oral contraceptive
Lisinopril	ACE inhibitor
L-Norgestrel/Ethinyl Estradiol	Oral contraceptive
Lo/Ovral 28	See Norgestrel/Ethinyl Estradiol
Loestrin Fe	See Norethindrone/Ethinyl Estradiol
Lorabid	See Loracarbef
Loracarbef	Antibiotic
Medroxyprogesterone	Hormone replacement therapy
Metformin	Oral hypoglycemic agent
Methocarbamol	See Methocarbamol
Methocarbamol	Muscle relaxant
Miacalcin Nasal	See Calcitonin Salmon
Microgestin Fe	See Norethindrone/Ethinyl Estradiol
Micronase	See Glyburide
Nifedipine	Calcium channel anthypertensive agent
Norethindrone/Ethinyl Estradiol	Oral contraceptive
Norgestrel/Ethinyl Estradiol	Oral contraceptive
Ortho-Cept	See Desogestrel/Ethinyl Estradiol
Oxybutynin	Antispasmodic bladder agent
Oxycodone/Acetaminophen	See Oxycodone/APAP
Oxycodone/APAP	Narcotic analgesic
Phenergan	See Promethazine
Pioglitazone	Oral hypoglycemic
Potassium Chloride	Potassium replacement
Prandin	See Repaglinide
Prednisone	Steroidal antiinflammatory
Promethazine	Antinausea agent
Promethazine/Codeine	Cough suppressant
Propacet	See Propoxyphene N/APAP
Propoxyphene N/APAP	Narcotic analgesic
Propranolol LA	Beta adrenergic antagonist
Proventil	See Albuterol
Provera	See Medroxyprogesterone
Quetiapine	Antipsychotic treatment
Quinapril	ACE Inhibitor
Rabeprazole	Proton pump inhibitor/reduces stomach acid
Ramipril	ACE inhibitor
Ranitidine	Gastric acid reducer
Repaglinide	Oral hypoglycemic

Drug Name	Drug Type
Retin-A	See Tretinoin
Rhinocort	See Budesonide
Risedronate	Agent to treat osteoporosis
Rosiglitazone	Oral hypoglycemic agent—reduces insulin resistance
Salmeterol/Fluticasone	Combination beta agonist/inhaled steroid; Asthma treatment
Seroquel	See Quetiapine
Sumycin	See Tetracycline HCl
Tequin	See Gatifloxacin
Terbinafine	Antifungal agent
Tetracycline HCl	Antibiotic
Theophylline	Methylxanthine bronchodilator
Timolol	Nonselective beta adrenergic blocking agent
Timolol Maleate	Ophthalmic beta adrenergic antagonist/ glaucoma
Timoptic XE	See Timolol
Tolterodine	Antispasmodic bladder agent
Topamax	See Topiramate
Topiramate	Seizure treatment
Tramadol	Analgesic
Tretinoin	Dermatologic agent
Triamcinolone	Steroidal antiinflammatory agent
Tri-Levlen	See L-Norgestrel/Ethinyl Estradiol
Trimeth/Sulfameth	Antibiotic
Trimethoprim/Sulfamethoxazole	See Trimeth/Sulfameth
Ultracet	See Tramadol/Acetaminophen
Valdecoxib	Nonsteroidal antiinflammatory agent
Venlafaxine	Antidepressant
Xanax	See Alprazolam
Zafirlukast	Leukotriene inhibitor/asthma
Zantac	See Ranitidine
Zestril	See Lisinopril
Zyban	See Bupropion HCl SR
Zyrtec	See Cetirizine

EMS MEDICATIONS

ACETYLSALICYLIC ACID (ASPIRIN, ASA)

CLASS

- Antiplatelet agent.

MODE OF ACTION

- Irreversibly inhibits platelet aggregation.

INDICATIONS

- Suspected acute coronary syndrome.

- Kawasaki's syndrome in pediatric patients.

CONTRAINDICATIONS

- Prior hypersensitivity to ASA or NSAIDS.

- Recent gastrointestinal bleeding or bleeding disorder such as hemophilia.

- Use with caution in patients taking anticoagulants.

- Pediatric patients (may develop Reye's syndrome).

SIDE EFFECTS/PRECAUTIONS

- Increased risk of bleeding or bruising.

- Gastritis.

ADULT DOSAGE

- 160 to 365 mg by mouth once daily.

PEDIATRIC DOSAGE

- No prehospital indication.

ACTIVATED CHARCOAL

CLASS

- Chemical-binding agent.

MODE OF ACTION

- Activated charcoal binds to, or absorbs to, various chemical agents, limiting their absorption from the gastrointestinal tract.

INDICATIONS

- Certain overdoses and poisonings in the alert patient.

CONTRAINDICATIONS

- None.

SIDE EFFECTS/PRECAUTIONS

- May cause vomiting, constipation, or diarrhea.

ADULT DOSAGE

- 25 to 50 g by mouth (PO) or via nasogastric (NG) tube.

PEDIATRIC DOSAGE

- 10 to 25 g PO or via NG tube.

CLASS

- Antiarrhythmic agent.

MODE OF ACTION

- Adenosine is a naturally occurring nucleoside that slows conduction through the atrioventricular (AV) node.

INDICATIONS

- As an aid in diagnosis of narrow complex tachycardias.

- For the treatment of narrow complex tachycardias, except atrial fibrillation and atrial flutter.

CONTRAINDICATIONS

- Avoid in patients with known adenosine hypersensitivity.

- Avoid in patients with bradycardias or second- or third-degree AV block.

SIDE EFFECTS/PRECAUTIONS

- May cause transient chest discomfort, palpitations, flushing, headache, nausea, and bronchoconstriction.

- May procure transient arrhythmias, such as second- or third-degree AV block, asystole, sinus bradycardia, premature atrial contractions (PACs), or premature ventricular contractions (PVCs).

ADULT DOSAGE

- 6 mg rapid IV bolus. Drug may be repeated in 1 to 2 minutes at 12 mg rapid IV bolus. If unsuccessful, it may be repeated a second time at 12 mg IV bolus. Dosage may need to be increased if patient is using theophylline preparations. Dosage may need to be reduced in the presence of dipyridamole (Persantine).

PEDIATRIC DOSAGE

- 0.1 mg/kg rapid IV bolus initially, then repeated at 0.2 mg/kg rapid IV bolus in 1 to 2 minutes. If unsuccessful, drug may be repeated a second time at 0.2 mg/kg IV bolus. Maximum single dose is 12 mg.

ALBUTEROL (PROVENTIL, VENTOLIN)

CLASS

- Beta$_2$-sympathetic agonist.

MODE OF ACTION

- Albuterol dilates smooth muscle in the bronchial tree through beta$_2$ stimulation. Also has some adrenergic effects on the heart and central nervous system (CNS) when given in high doses.

INDICATIONS

- For treatment of reversible bronchoconstriction, such as asthma, chronic bronchitis, emphysema, or other reactive airway disease.

- For treatment of hyperkalemia.

CONTRAINDICATIONS

- Avoid in patients with known hypersensitivity.

- Use with caution in patients with hypertension and in patients with a heart rate (HR) greater than 150 bpm.

SIDE EFFECTS/PRECAUTIONS

- May cause tachycardias, hypertension, chest pain, nervousness, tremor, headache, nausea, or vomiting.

ADULT DOSAGE

- 2.5 mg in 3 mL normal saline (0.9% NaCl) via nebulizer. Dose may be repeated every 6 hours; however, in cases of severe bronchospasm, it may be given as frequently as back to back. More frequent dosing may result in greater incidence of side effects.

PEDIATRIC DOSAGE

- Age younger than 12 years: one half of the adult dose (1.25 mg); age older than 12 years: use adult dosing. Dose may be repeated every 6 hours; however, in cases of severe bronchospasm, it may be given as frequently as back to back.

AMIODARONE

CLASS

- Antiarrhythmic agent.

MODE OF ACTION

- Effects on sodium, potassium, and calcium channels as well as alpha and beta adrenergic blocking effects.

INDICATIONS

- Controlling ventricular rate in rapid atrial arrhythmias and preexcitation syndromes.

- After failed defibrillation in persistent VF or pulseless VT.

- Stable VT, polymorphic VT, and wide complex tachycardia (WCT) of unknown origin.

- Adjunct to electrical cardioversion of refractory PSVTs and atrial tachycardias.

- Conversion of atrial fibrillation.

CONTRAINDICATIONS

- Known hypersensitivity to amiodarone.

- Hypotensive patients.

- Bradycardic patients.

SIDE EFFECTS/PRECAUTIONS

- Acute side effects include hypotension and bradycardia.

- May prolong QT interval—avoid concurrent use with other agents, such as procainamide, that prolong the QT interval.

ADULT DOSAGE

- Cardiac arrest: 300 mg IV push. May repeat 150 mg IV bolus in 3 to 5 minutes. Maximum total dose is 2.2 g IV over 24 hours.

- Tachycardias: 150 mg IV over 10 minutes, followed by an infusion of 1 mg/min for 6 hours, then 0.5 mg/min for 18 hours. Alternatively may repeat 150 mg bolus every 10 minutes as needed. Maximum total daily dose is 2.2 g. Repeat boluses at 150 mg IV have been used instead of continuous infusions.

PEDIATRIC DOSAGE

- Cardiac arrest: 5 mg/kg rapid bolus either IV/IO. Repeat dose of 5 mg/kg may be given to a maximum daily dose of 15 mg/kg.

ATROPINE SULFATE

CLASS

- Parasympathetic blocker.

MODE OF ACTION

- Atropine sulfate increases the HR by blocking the action of the parasympathetic nervous system on the sinoatrial (SA) node and the AV node.

INDICATIONS

- Symptomatic bradycardias and heart blocks.

- Asystole.

- Organophosphate insecticide poisoning.

SECTION 4

CONTRAINDICATIONS

- None when used in emergency situations.

SIDE EFFECTS/PRECAUTIONS

- May cause tachycardia, palpitations, seizures, hypertension, respiratory failure, and anticholinergic symptoms (i.e., blurred vision, dilated pupils, confusion, fever, decreased gastrointestinal motility).

- May worsen narrow-angle glaucoma.

- Slow administration or a low dose (less than 0.4 mg) may cause a paradoxic slowing of the HR.

ADULT DOSAGE

- 0.5 to 1.0 mg IV for symptomatic bradycardias and heart blocks. Drug may be repeated every 3 to 5 minutes up to a maximum dosage of 3 mg (0.04 mg/kg).

- 1 mg IV for asystole. Drug may be repeated every 3 to 5 minutes up to a maximum dosage of 3 mg (0.04 mg/kg).

- 2 mg IV for organophosphate poisoning. Drug may be repeated as necessary.

- Drug may be given via endotracheal tube (ET) if IV unavailable.

PEDIATRIC DOSAGE

- 0.02 mg/kg IV for bradycardias, heart blocks, and asystole.

CALCIUM CHLORIDE

CLASS

- Electrolyte solution.

MODE OF ACTION

- Stabilizes membrane potentials in muscle and nerve tissue.

INDICATIONS

- Hyperkalemia.

- Treatment of side effects of calcium channel blockade.

- Prophylaxis of calcium channel blocker side effects.

CONTRAINDICATIONS

- Do not mix with sodium bicarbonate.

SIDE EFFECTS/PRECAUTIONS

- Necrosis if extravasated.

- Hypotension, bradycardia.

ADULT DOSAGE

- Hyperkalemia and calcium channel overdose: 8 to 16 mg/kg (usually 500 to 1000 mg) IV.

- Prophylaxis before calcium channel blockers: 2 to 4 mg/kg IV.

PEDIATRIC DOSAGE

- Hyperkalemia and calcium channel overdose: 20 mg/kg (not to exceed 500 mg) IV.

CIMETIDINE (TAGAMET)

CLASS

- H_2 blocker.

MODE OF ACTION

- The addition of an H_2 blocker adds to the effectiveness of H_1 blockers in anaphylaxis.

INDICATIONS

- Anaphylaxis or severe allergic reactions.

SECTION 4

CONTRAINDICATIONS

- Known hypersensitivity to cimetidine.

SIDE EFFECTS/PRECAUTIONS

- There are few acute side effects. Important ones include headache and confusion. Rapid IV administration may cause cardiac arrhythmias and hypotension.

ADULT DOSAGE

- 300 mg IV/IM. May be repeated in 6 hours.

PEDIATRIC DOSAGE

- 5 to 10 mg/kg IV/IM. May be repeated in 6 hours.

DEXAMETHASONE (DECADRON)

CLASS

- Glucocorticoid steroid.

MODE OF ACTION

- Dexamethasone suppresses the body's immune system and thereby decreases the severity of the inflammatory response.

INDICATIONS

- Croup.
- Anaphylaxis.
- Cerebral edema.

CONTRAINDICATIONS

- Hypersensitivity to dexamethasone.

SIDE EFFECTS/PRECAUTIONS

- May cause euphoria, hypertension, hyperglycemia, fluid retention, nausea, and vomiting.

- Use with caution in patients with CHF, diabetes mellitus, renal disease, and hypertension.

ADULT DOSAGE

- Allergic reaction: 1 to 10 mg IM/IV.

PEDIATRIC DOSAGE

- Croup: 0.6 mg/kg IM.

DIAZEPAM [VALIUM]

CLASS

- Benzodiazepine.

MODE OF ACTION

- Diazepam possesses CNS depressant, antiepileptic, anxiolytic, and skeletal muscle relaxant properties.

INDICATIONS

- Prehospital indication is for the treatment of status epilepticus.

CONTRAINDICATIONS

- Avoid in patients with known hypersensitivity.

- No prehospital contraindications when used in the case of status epilepticus.

SIDE EFFECTS/PRECAUTIONS

- May cause CNS depression, respiratory depression, and increased intraocular pressure in patients with narrow-angle glaucoma.

ADULT DOSAGE

- 5 to 10 mg IV bolus (or IM). Drug may be repeated every 10 minutes to maximum total dose of 30 mg.

PEDIATRIC DOSAGE

- Younger than 5 years: 0.2 to 0.5 mg IV every 2 to 5 minutes to a maximum dose of 5 mg.

- Older than 5 years: 1 mg IV every 2 to 5 minutes to a maximum dose of 10 mg.

DEXTROSE 50% (D_{50})

CLASS

- Carbohydrate.

MODE OF ACTION

- D_{50} elevates blood glucose levels.

INDICATIONS

- Hypoglycemia.

- Diagnostic test for hypoglycemia in patients with an altered mental state of unknown etiology.

CONTRAINDICATIONS

- None when used in emergency situations.

SIDE EFFECTS/PRECAUTIONS

- Infiltration of D_{50} may cause local tissue necrosis.

- A sample of blood should be drawn before the administration of D_{50} to determine premedication serum glucose levels.

ADULT DOSAGE

- 25 g D_{50} (50 mL) IV.

PEDIATRIC DOSAGE

- 0.5 mL/kg of D_{50} IV or 1 mL/kg of dextrose 25% (D_{25}) IV.

NOTE: It is preferable to use an infusion of dextrose 10% (D_{10}) IV in pediatric patients whose symptoms of hypoglycemia are not serious (coma or seizures) to avoid overshoot hyperglycemia.

DILTIAZEM (CARDIZEM)

CLASS

- Calcium channel blocker.

MODE OF ACTION

- Diltiazem blocks the calcium channel found in the myocardium, in the cardiac conduction system, and the vascular bed, decreasing calcium's entry into the cells, resulting in decreased cardiac contractility, decreased conduction through the AV node, and vasodilation. Diltiazem's most powerful effect is on AV node conduction. It is far less likely to decrease contractility or to vasodilate than verapamil.

INDICATIONS

- Symptomatic supraventricular tachycardias, including rapid atrial fibrillation and rapid atrial flutter.

CONTRAINDICATIONS

- Hypersensitivity to diltiazem.

- Diltiazem is contraindicated under the following circumstances: bradycardias, second- and third-degree AV block, and WPW with rapid atrial fibrillation and severe CHF.

SIDE EFFECTS/PRECAUTIONS

- The most significant side effects are hypotension, bradycardias, the development of AV blocks, asystole, and CHF.

ADULT DOSAGE

- SVT and rapid atrial fibrillation/flutter: 0.25 mg/kg (15 to 20 mg typically). May repeat in 15 minutes at 0.35 mg/kg

(20 to 25 mg typically). Follow with an infusion at 5 to 15 mg/hour, titrating to ventricular response.

PEDIATRIC DOSAGE

- No dosing established.

DIPHENHYDRAMINE (BENADRYL)

CLASS

- Antihistamine (H_1 histamine blocker).

MODE OF ACTION

- Competitive blocker of H_1 histamine receptors, preventing histamine from causing vasodilation, hypotension, tachycardia, and increased gastrointestinal secretions. Histamine plays a significant role in allergic reactions. Diphenhydramine also has anticholinergic effects.

INDICATIONS

- Severe allergic reactions, such as anaphylaxis.

CONTRAINDICATIONS

- Avoid in patients with known hypersensitivity.

- Should be used with caution in asthmatic patients; may thicken bronchial secretions and thereby worsen mucus plugging.

- May worsen narrow-angle glaucoma.

- Use with caution in patients with hypertension.

SIDE EFFECTS/PRECAUTIONS

- Side effects are largely due to the anticholinergic effects and include drowsiness, dry mouth, urinary retention, hypotension, thickened bronchial secretions, wheezing, and gastrointestinal symptoms.

ADULT DOSAGE

- 25 to 50 mg slow IV bolus, or deep IM injection.

PEDIATRIC DOSAGE

- 2 to 5 mg/kg IV or deep IM injection. Usual dose is 10 to 30 mg.

DOPAMINE

CLASS

- Adrenergic vasopressor.

MODE OF ACTION

- Dopamine is an epinephrine precursor with dose-dependent dopaminergic, alpha-adrenergic, and beta-adrenergic effects.

- 0.5 to 2 µg/kg per minute IV infusion for dopaminergic effects: vasodilation of renal and mesenteric vessels without affecting heart rate or blood pressure.

- 2 to 10 µg/kg per minute IV infusion for predominantly beta-adrenergic effects: increasing HR and contractility and some vasodilation.

- Greater than 10 µg/kg per minute IV infusion for predominantly alpha-adrenergic effects: vasoconstriction, increasing peripheral vascular resistance and HR.

INDICATIONS

- Significant hypotension.

CONTRAINDICATIONS

- Avoid in patients with known hypersensitivity.

- Avoid in patients with hypovolemic hypotension, unless patient has failed aggressive IV fluid resuscitation, including resuscitation with blood products.

SECTION 4

- Contraindicated in hypotensive patients who have hypotension that is caused by a tachyarrhythmia.

SIDE EFFECTS/PRECAUTIONS

- May cause tachyarrhythmias, hypotension (at low doses), chest pain, palpitations, nausea, and vomiting.

- May also cause tissue necrosis if IV infiltrates (hospital treatment of site with phentolamine if this occurs).

ADULT DOSAGE

- 2 to 5 µg/kg minute IV infusion, titrating upward until desired effect is achieved.

PEDIATRIC DOSAGE

- 1 µg/kg minute IV infusion, titrating upward until desired effect is achieved.

ENALAPRILAT (VASOTEC)

CLASS

- Angiotensin converting enzyme (ACE) inhibitor.

MODE OF ACTION

- Enalaprilat reduces afterload through suppression of the renin-angiotensin-aldosterone system.

INDICATIONS

- Cardiogenic acute pulmonary edema.

CONTRAINDICATIONS

- Known hypersensitivity to enalapril.

- ACE inhibitors should not be used during pregnancy or in patients with hypotension.

SIDE EFFECTS/PRECAUTIONS

- The most common side effects are orthostatic hypotension, syncope, chest pain, dizziness, and cough.

- Angioneurotic edema of the face and larynx has occurred with enalaprilat use.

ADULT DOSAGE

- 1.25 mg IV. May be repeated in 6 hours. Lower doses are recommended in patients with renal failure.

PEDIATRIC DOSAGE

- Not recommended for pediatric use.

EPINEPHRINE

CLASS

- Sympathetic agonist possessing both alpha and beta properties.

MODE OF ACTION

- Its alpha effects are primarily vasoconstriction, which increases peripheral vascular resistance (PVR) and perfusion. Its beta effects are increased automaticity, increased HR, increased contractility, increased cardiac output, increased myocardial oxygen demand, and bronchodilation. It also decreases the threshold for successful defibrillation.

INDICATIONS

- Cardiac arrest.

- Asthma.

- Anaphylaxis.

- Bradycardia that failed to respond to TCP, atropine.

CONTRAINDICATIONS

- None when used during cardiac arrest.

- Use with caution in patients who are elderly, hypertensive, or pregnant or in patients who have a cardiovascular or hyperthyroid disease.

SIDE EFFECTS/PRECAUTIONS

- May cause tachycardia, palpitations, hypertension, ventricular irritability, increased myocardial oxygen demand, cerebrovascular accident (CVA), and myocardial infarction.

ADULT DOSAGE

- Cardiac arrest: 1 mg epinephrine (1:10,000) IV; dose may be repeated every 3 to 5 minutes. If given via endotracheal tube, use 5 to 2.5 times IV dose.

- Anaphylaxis: 0.3 to 0.5 mg epinephrine (1:10,000) IV if poor perfusion. 0.3 to 0.5 mg epinephrine (1:1000) SC if adequate perfusion.

- Asthma: 0.3 mg to 0.5 mg epinephrine (1:1000) SC; dose may be repeated every 20 minutes.

- Bradycardia: 2–10 µg/min, titrated to desired effect.

PEDIATRIC DOSAGE

- Cardiac arrest: 0.01 to 0.1 mg/kg epinephrine (1:10,000) IV; dose may be repeated every 3 to 5 minutes. If given via ET, use 0.1 mg/kg.

- Anaphylaxis: 0.01 mg/kg epinephrine (1:10,000) IV if poor perfusion; maximum single dose: 0.3 mg 0.01 mg/kg epinephrine (1:1000) SC if adequate perfusion; maximum single dose 0.3 mg.

- Asthma: 0.01 mg/kg epinephrine (1:1000) SC; maximum single dose: 0.3 mg. Dose may be repeated twice at 20 minute intervals.

ETOMIDATE

CLASS

- Short-acting sedative-hypnotic agent.

MODE OF ACTION

- Etomidate's mode of action may be due to its effects on the GABA-adrenergic system in the brain. It does decrease cerebral blood flow and cerebral oxygen demand without decreasing cerebral perfusion. It does not cause hemodynamic instability.

INDICATIONS

- Etomidate may be used as part of a rapid sequence intubation (RSI) algorithm.

CONTRAINDICATIONS

- Known hypersensitivity to etomidate.

SIDE EFFECTS/PRECAUTIONS

- May cause hypotension in hypovolemic patients.

- Laryngospasm, myoclonic muscle activity, hiccoughs, nausea and vomiting, and possible suppression of cortisol and aldosterone production.

- Some patients may complain of pain at the IV site during injection.

ADULT DOSAGE

- 0.3 mg/kg IV bolus. Use 0.15 mg/kg IV in hypovolemic patients.

PEDIATRIC DOSAGE

- Age > 10 years: 0.3 mg/kg IV bolus. Use 0.15 mg/kg IV in hypovolemic patients.

FAMOTIDINE (PEPCID)

CLASS

- H_2 blocker.

MODE OF ACTION

- The addition of an H_2 blocker adds to the effectiveness of H_1 blockers in anaphylaxis.

INDICATIONS

- Anaphylaxis or severe allergic reactions.

CONTRAINDICATIONS

- Known hypersensitivity to famotidine.

SIDE EFFECTS/PRECAUTIONS

- There are few acute side effects. Important ones include headache and confusion. Rapid IV administration may cause cardiac arrhythmias and hypotension.

ADULT DOSAGE

- 20 mg IV/IM. May be repeated in 12 hours.

PEDIATRIC DOSAGE

- 0.25 mg/kg IV. May be repeated in 8 hours.

FENTANYL

CLASS

- Narcotic analgesic agent.

MODE OF ACTION

- Fentanyl binds to opiate receptors in the CNS.

INDICATIONS

* Treatment of moderate to severe pain.

CONTRAINDICATIONS

* Known hypersensitivity to midazolam.

* Use with caution in patients with COPD because narcotics may cause respiratory depression.

* Use with caution in patients with a history of a seizure disorder because narcotics may lower the seizure threshold.

SIDE EFFECTS/PRECAUTIONS

* May cause CNS depression, respiratory depression, depression of the seizure threshold, hypotension, nausea, and vomiting.

ADULT DOSAGE

* 1 to 2 µg/kg IV every 30 to 60 minutes as needed.

PEDIATRIC DOSAGE

* 0.5 to 2 µg/kg IV. May repeat in 30 to 60 minutes as needed.

FUROSEMIDE (LASIX)

CLASS

* Diuretic.

MODE OF ACTION

* Furosemide is a potent diuretic, acting within 5 to 30 minutes. In addition to its diuretic action, it produces a vasodilatative effect.

INDICATIONS

* Acute pulmonary edema.

CONTRAINDICATIONS

- Avoid in patients with known hypersensitivity.

- Avid in anuric patients.

- Use with caution in patients with hepatic failure or renal failure.

SIDE EFFECTS/PRECAUTIONS

- May cause hypokalemia, hypovolemia, orthostatic hypotension, and ototoxicity.

ADULT DOSAGE

- 40 mg to 80 mg furosemide IV.

PEDIATRIC DOSAGE

- 1 to 3 mg/kg furosemide IV.

GLUCAGON

CLASS

- Antihypoglycemic agent.

MODE OF ACTION

- Glucagon converts glycogen, a stored form of glucose found in the liver and muscles, into glucose. It also inhibits glycogen synthesis and elevates blood glucose levels. Glucagon is only effective if the patient has sufficient stores of glycogen in the liver. The administration of glucagon should be followed by glucose as soon as possible. The onset of action is within 5 to 20 minutes.

- In addition, glucagon enhances myocardial contractility and increases HR and AV conduction through a cellular receptor-mediated pathway distinct from the adrenergic receptor pathway. It is, therefore, able to stimulate the myocardium during beta blockade.

INDICATIONS

- Hypoglycemia, especially when IV access in unavailable and D_{50} has not been given.

- Beta blocker overdose.

CONTRAINDICATIONS

- None when used in an emergency.

SIDE EFFECTS/PRECAUTIONS

- May cause nausea and vomiting.

ADULT DOSAGE

- Hypoglycemia: 1 mg IM or SC; dose may be repeated twice.

- Beta blocker overdose: 3 to 10 mg IV bolus, followed by a 2 to 5 mg per hour infusion.

PEDIATRIC DOSAGE

- Not recommended for prehospital use in pediatrics.

HALOPERIDOL (HALDOL)

CLASS

- Antipsychotic agent.

MODE OF ACTION

- Haloperidol decreases agitation and psychotic behavior through blockade of post-synaptic dopaminergic receptors in the prefrontal and mesolimbic cortices.

INDICATIONS

- Haloperidol may be used to decrease agitation. It may be indicated as a form of chemical restraint to prevent violent behavior.

CONTRAINDICATIONS

- Known hypersensitivity to haloperidol.

- Decreased mental status, hypotension.

SIDE EFFECTS/PRECAUTIONS

- Common side effects include sedation, extrapyramidal effects (dystonias, akithesia, and dyskinesias), dry mouth, blurred vision, urinary retention, and postural hypotension.

ADULT DOSAGE

- 5 mg IM/IV. May repeat at 5 to 10 mg IM/IV in 15 to 30 minutes. Elderly patients start at 1 mg IM/IV. Repeat at 1 to 2 mg IM/IV in 15 to 30 minutes.

PEDIATRIC DOSAGE

- Age 6 to 12 years: 1 to 3 mg IM.

- Age > 12 years: 2 to 5 mg IM.

IPRATROPIUM BROMIDE (ATROVENT)

CLASS

- Anticholinergic bronchodilator.

MODE OF ACTION

- Inhibits vagally mediated effects on bronchial smooth muscle.

INDICATIONS

- Acute bronchospasm.

CONTRAINDICATIONS

- Hypersensitivity to ipratroprium or atropine.

SIDE EFFECTS/PRECAUTIONS

- Use with caution in narrow angle glaucoma.

- Should not be used alone in patients with acute bronchospasm.

ADULT DOSAGE

- Acute bronchospasm: 1 unit dose (2.5 mL (500 µg) of a 0.2% solution) nebulized. May be repeated in 4 to 6 hours.

PEDIATRIC DOSAGE

- Acute bronchospasm: age < 12 years: 1/2 unit dose (1.25 mL (250 µg) of a 0.2% solution) nebulized. Repeated in 4 to 6 hours, if needed.

- Acute bronchospasm: age >12 years: 1/2 to 1 unit dose (1.25 mL (250 µg) to 2.5 mL (500 µg) of a 0.2% solution) nebulized. Repeated in 4 to 6 hours, if needed.

ISOPROTERENOL (ISUPREL)

CLASS

- Sympathetic agonist possessing 100% beta effects.

MODE OF ACTION

- Isoproterenol is a 100% beta agent, and its effects are increased automaticity, increased HR, increased contractility, decreased PVR, increased cardiac output, increased myocardial oxygen demand, and bronchodilation.

INDICATIONS

- Symptomatic bradycardias, heart blocks, or both that are unresponsive to atropine therapy.

CONTRAINDICATIONS

- None when used emergently as indicated.

SIDE EFFECTS/PRECAUTIONS

- May cause tachydysrhythmias, ventricular ectopy, PACs, hypotension, angina pectoris, and headache.

  NOTE: Isoproterenol has been implicated in causing cellular damage to the myocardium. It also increases the myocardial workload and myocardial oxygen demand. This may extend the area of an infarction.

ADULT DOSAGE

- 2 µg per minute to 10 µg per minute IV infusion (1 mg in 250 mL of D_5W, to a concentration of 4 µg/mL).

Infusion Amount	Drip Rate
2 µg/min	30 gtts/min
4 µg/min	60 gtts/min
6 µg/min	90 gtts/min
8 µg/min	120 gtts/min
10 µg/min	150 gtts/min

PEDIATRIC DOSAGE

- 0.1 to 0.2 µg per minute IV infusion. Dose may be titrated to desired effect.

LIDOCAINE

CLASS

- Antiarrhythmic agent.

MODE OF ACTION

- Lidocaine suppresses ventricular ectopic activity by decreasing the irritability of the heart muscle and the conduction system and raises the fibrillatory threshold.

INDICATIONS

- Significant ventricular ectopy.

- VT and recurrent VF.

CONTRAINDICATIONS

- Avoid in patients with known hypersensitivity.

- Avoid in patients with bradydysrhythmias, heart blocks, and idioventricular escape rhythms.

SIDE EFFECTS/PRECAUTIONS

- May cause hypotension, numbness, drowsiness, confusion, respiratory depression, and seizures.

ADULT DOSAGE

- 1 to 1.5 mg per kg IV bolus, which may be repeated at 0.5 to 0.75 mg/kg every 5 to 10 minutes until a maximum dose of 3 mg/kg or 225 mg has been administered.

- 2 to 4 mg per minute (1 g of lidocaine in 250 mL of D_5W or 2 g in 500 mL in concentration of 4 mg/mL). Lidocaine infusion should be begun if lidocaine is effective.

  NOTE: Give the typical loading dose, and reduce the maintenance dose by 50% in adults older than 70 years of age who have CHF, liver disease, or impaired hepatic blood flow to prevent toxicity.

Infusion Amount	Drip Rate
2 mg/min	30 gtts/min
3 mg/min	45 gtts/min
4 mg/min	60 gtts/min

PEDIATRIC DOSAGE

- 1 mg/kg IV bolus (maximum dose of 50 mg), followed by an infusion of 20 to 50 µg/kg per minute.

LORAZEPAM (ATIVAN)

CLASS

- Benzodiazepine.

MODE OF ACTION

- Lorazepam possesses CNS depressant, antiepileptic, anxiolytic, and skeletal muscle relaxant properties.

INDICATIONS

- Prehospital indication is for status epilepticus and sedation.

CONTRAINDICATIONS

- Known hypersensitivity to lorazepam.

- May precipitate acute glaucoma in patients with acute narrow angle glaucoma.

- Some benzodiazepines have been associated with birth defects when used during pregnancy.

SIDE EFFECTS/PRECAUTIONS

- May cause respiratory depression and respiratory arrest.

- Hypotension.

- Concomitant use with other CNS depressants increases the risk of side effects.

ADULT DOSAGE

- Seizure control: 0.1 mg/kg IV at 1 to 2 mg/min, up to 10 mg total dose.

- Sedation: 0.044 mg/kg IV. Typical maximum dose is 2 mg.

PEDIATRIC DOSAGE

- Seizure control: 0.05 to 0.1 mg/kg. Administer over 2 to 5 minutes. Maximum 2 mg per dose. May repeat in 10 minutes to a cumulative dose of 0.4 mg/kg.

- Sedation: 0.05 mg/kg IV. May be repeated every 4 to 8 hours.

MEPERIDINE (DEMEROL)

CLASS

- Narcotic analgesic agent.

MODE OF ACTION

- Meperidine binds to opiate receptors in the CNS.

INDICATIONS

- Treatment of moderate to severe pain.

CONTRAINDICATIONS

- Avoid in patients with known hypersensitivity.

- Should be used with caution in patients with chronic obstructive pulmonary disease (COPD) because narcotics may cause respiratory depression.

- Use with caution in patients with a history of a seizure disorder because narcotics may lower the seizure threshold.

SIDE EFFECTS/PRECAUTIONS

- May cause CNS depression, respiratory depression, depression of the seizure threshold, hypotension, nausea, and vomiting.

ADULT DOSAGE

- 50 to 100 mg IM every 3 to 4 hours.

SECTION 4

PEDIATRIC DOSAGE

- 1.1 to 1.8 mg/kg IM every 3 to 4 hours. Maximum single dose: 100 mg.

MAGNESIUM SULFATE

CLASS

- CNS depressant, anticonvulsant, and antiarrhythmic.

MODE OF ACTION

- Magnesium sulfate depresses the CNS.

- Improves muscle cell membrane stability.

- Relaxes smooth and cardiac muscle.

INDICATIONS

- Convulsions associated with eclampsia and pre-eclampsia.

- Polymorphic VT.

CONTRAINDICATIONS

- Avoid in patients with heart block.

- Avoid in patients with a history of renal disease.

SIDE EFFECTS/PRECAUTIONS

- May cause respiratory distress or failure.

- May cause cardiac arrest.

ADULT DOSAGE

- Eclampsia: 2 to 4 g slow IV over a minimum of 3 minutes.

- Polymorphic VT: 1 to 2 g IV over 1 minute.

PEDIATRIC DOSAGE

- Not recommended for prehospital use.

METHYLPREDNISOLONE (SOLUMEDROL)

CLASS

- Glucocorticoid steroid.

MODE OF ACTION

- Methylprednosolone suppresses the body's immune system and thereby decreases the severity of the inflammatory response.

INDICATIONS

- Treatment of anaphylaxis.

- Treatment of severe bronchospasm.

- Treatment of spinal cord injury.

CONTRAINDICATIONS

- None when used in the emergent treatment of anaphylaxis.

SIDE EFFECTS/PRECAUTIONS

- May cause euphoria, hypertension, hyperglycemia, fluid retention, nausea, and vomiting.

- Use with caution in patients with CHF, diabetes mellitus (DM), renal disease, and hypertension.

ADULT DOSAGE

- Anaphylaxis or bronchospasm regimen: 100 to 200 mg IV bolus or IM. Drug must be reconstituted.

- Spinal cord injury regimen: 30 mg/kg IV infusion given over 15 minutes.

SECTION 4

PEDIATRIC DOSAGE

- Anaphylaxis or bronchospasm regimen: 2 mg/kg IV bolus or IM. Drug must be reconstituted.

- Spinal cord injury regimen: 30 mg/kg IV infusion given over 15 minutes. This is controversial.

METOPROLOL (LOPRESSOR)

CLASS

- Beta$_1$ sympathetic antagonist.

MODE OF ACTION

- Reduces the work of the heart and its oxygen demand by decreasing heart rate.

INDICATIONS

- Acute myocardial infarction.

CONTRAINDICATIONS

- Beta blockade is contraindicated in patients with myocardial infarction who are bradycardic; have second- or third-degree heart blocks; are hypotensive, and those who are in moderate to severe heart failure.

- Known hypersensitivity to metoprolol or other beta blockers.

SIDE EFFECTS/PRECAUTIONS

- Use with caution in patients with bronchospasm and in patients with myocardial infarctions and first-degree AV blocks.

- Common side effects include bradycardia, hypotension, dizziness, headache, fatigue, and wheezing.

ADULT DOSAGE

- 5 mg IV every 5 minutes for a total of 3 doses, if needed to achieve a heart rate of approximately 60 bpm.

PEDIATRIC DOSAGE

- Not recommended for pediatric use.

MIDAZOLAM (VERSED)

CLASS

- Benzodiazepine.

MODE OF ACTION

- Midazolam possesses CNS depressant, antiepileptic, anxiolytic, and skeletal muscle relaxant properties.

INDICATIONS

- Prehospital indication is for sedation.

CONTRAINDICATIONS

- Known hypersensitivity to midazolam.

- May precipitate acute glaucoma in patients with acute narrow angle glaucoma.

- Some benzodiazepines have been associated with birth defects when used during pregnancy.

SIDE EFFECTS/PRECAUTIONS

- May cause respiratory depression and respiratory arrest.

- Hypotension.

- Concomitant use with other CNS depressants increases the risk of side effects.

SECTION 4

ADULT DOSAGE

- Sedation: 0.5 to 2 mg IV every 2 to 3 minutes up to 0.1 to 0.15 mg/kg.

PEDIATRIC DOSAGE

- Sedation: age 6 months to 5 years: 0.05 to 0.1 mg/kg IV (maximum total dose is 6 mg). Age 6 to 12 years: 0.025 to 0.05 mg/kg IV (maximum total dose is 10 mg). Repeat every 3 to 5 minutes as needed.

MORPHINE SULFATE

CLASS

- Narcotic analgesic agent.

MODE OF ACTION

- Morphine sulfate binds to opiate receptors in the CNS.

INDICATIONS

- Treatment of moderate to severe pain.

- Treatment of cardiogenic acute pulmonary edema.

CONTRAINDICATIONS

- Avoid in patients with known hypersensitivity.

- Contraindicated for use in patients with a depressed level of consciousness or respiratory depression.

- Should be used with caution in patients with COPD because narcotics may cause respiratory depression.

- Use with caution in patients with a history of a seizure disorder because narcotics may lower the seizure threshold.

SIDE EFFECTS/PRECAUTIONS

- CNS depression, respiratory depression, depression of the seizure threshold, hypotension, nausea, and vomiting.

ADULT DOSAGE

- 2 to 5 mg IV every 5 to 30 minutes until desired effect is achieved.

PEDIATRIC DOSAGE

- Not recommended for prehospital use in pediatric patients.

NALOXONE (NARCAN)

CLASS

- Narcotic antagonist.

MODE OF ACTION

- Naloxone reverses the effects of narcotics.

INDICATIONS

- Known or suspected narcotic overdose with respiratory depression.

- Diagnostic test for narcotic overdose.

CONTRAINDICATIONS

- Avoid in patients with known hypersensitivity.

SIDE EFFECTS/PRECAUTIONS

- May cause an acute withdrawal syndrome in the narcotic-dependent patient. The duration of naloxone is, in general, less than that of the narcotic. Therefore patients who initially respond well to naloxone may fall back into coma as the naloxone wears off. Naloxone is not effective against nonopiates such as cocaine and marijuana.

ADULT DOSAGE

- 0.4 mg to 2 mg IV, IM, or SC. Dose may be repeated as necessary. Therapeutic goal is improved ventilation.

SECTION 4

- May be given as a continuous infusion (2.0 mg naloxone in 500 mL of 0.9% NaCl or D_5W in a concentration of 0.004 mg/mL), titrating the dose to clinical response. Usual dose is 0.4 mg per hour.

PEDIATRIC DOSAGE

- 0.01 mg/kg IV, IM, or SC; dose may be repeated as necessary. If no response is achieved, dose may be increased to 0.1 mg/kg. Therapeutic goal is improved ventilation.

NITROGLYCERIN

CLASS

- Antianginal analgesic.

MODE OF ACTION

- Nitroglycerin dilates coronary arteries, thus increasing myocardial oxygenation. Peripheral vasculature dilates as well, promoting pooling of the blood, thereby reducing preload.

INDICATIONS

- Relief of the pain of angina pectoris, myocardial infarction, or both.

- Treatment of cardiogenic pulmonary edema.

CONTRAINDICATIONS

- Avoid in patients with known hypersensitivity.

- Avoid in patients with hypotension.

- Avoid in patients using phosphodiesterase inhibitors for erectile dysfunction within the last 24 to 36 hours.

SIDE EFFECTS/PRECAUTIONS

- May cause hypotension, headache, dizziness, reflex tachycardia, syncope, and a burning sensation in the mouth.

- Be sure to remove topical nitroglycerin preparations from patients when giving additional nitroglycerin to avoid overdosing. Topical nitroglycerin preparations should be removed from the chest before defibrillation or cardioversion to avoid electrical arcing.

ADULT DOSAGE

- Nitroglycerin comes in several forms, each with its own dosing regimen.

- 1/150 g (0.4 mg) sublingual. Dose may be repeated every 5 minutes.

- 1 to 2 metered dose sprays (0.4 mg/dose) of translingual nitroglycerin onto oral mucosa. Dose may be repeated every 5 minutes. Higher doses (i.e., 2 to 4 metered dose sprays) may be given every 3 to 5 minutes for acute pulmonary edema when the patient's blood pressure is elevated.

- 1/2 to 2 inches of 2% nitroglycerin ointment (1 inch equals 15 mg nitroglycerin). Duration is approximately 6 hours.

- 0.2 to 0.4 mg per hour transdermal nitroglycerin (patches in 0.1 to 0.6 mg per hour dosing). Duration is approximately 12 to 24 hours.

- 5 to 20 µg/min IV, titrated to effect.

NITROUS OXIDE-OXYGEN 50:50 MIXTURE (NITRONOX)

CLASS

- Medicinal gas.

MODE OF ACTION

- Nitrous oxide produces rapid onset and readily reversible analgesia and CNS depression when inhaled.

INDICATIONS

- Relief of moderate to severe pain.

CONTRAINDICATIONS

- Avoid in patients with known hypersensitivity.

- Contraindicated under the following conditions:

  o Decreased level of consciousness

  o Patient unable to follow simple commands

  o Concurrent use of CNS depressants

  o Pregnancy

  o Abdominal distension or trauma (nitrous oxide may accumulate in gas-filled spaces, worsening abdominal obstruction)

  o Chest trauma (nitrous oxide may accumulate in gas-filled spaces, worsening chest injuries)

  o Respiratory compromise

  o Hypoxia

SIDE EFFECTS/PRECAUTIONS

- May cause lightheadedness, respiratory depression, nausea, and vomiting.

- Patient must be monitored during administration. Use of a pulse oximeter is helpful.

ADULT DOSAGE

- Patient self-administers the drug until pain is relieved or patient is unable to self-administer.

PEDIATRIC DOSAGE

- Patient self-administers the drug until pain is relieved or patient is unable to self-administer.

OXYGEN

CLASS

- Medicinal gas.

MODE OF ACTION

- Oxygen diffuses across membranes to act as a necessary agent for aerobic metabolism. Hypoxia, anoxia, or both leads inevitably to death.

INDICATIONS

- Suspected hypoxia or anoxia, be it local, as in patients with ischemia, or systemic, as in patients with cardiac arrest.

CONTRAINDICATIONS

- None when used emergently.

SIDE EFFECTS/PRECAUTIONS

- May cause respiratory depression in patients with a hypoxic drive.

- Although oxygen toxicity may occur after prolonged ventilatory support with a high-oxygen concentration, even 100% oxygen is not hazardous to the patient's lungs during the time frame that prehospital care is rendered. Oxygen should never be withheld from anyone who needs it.

- May worsen the pulmonary injury in patients poisoned by paraquat. Use only if patient is hypoxic.

ADULT DOSAGE/PEDIATRIC DOSAGE

- 85% to 100% via nonrebreather mask.

- 24% to 40% via Venturi mask.

- 24% to 40% via nasal cannula.

- Bag-valve-mask (BVM) devices fitted with reservoirs and liter flow of 15 liters per minute supply approximately 85% to 100% oxygen. Use of a BVM device allows continuous assessment of pulmonary compliance. Pop-off valves are not recommended for use in pediatric patients.

- Intermittent positive-pressure devices supply approximately 100% oxygen.

OXYTOCIN (PITOCIN, SYNTOCINON)

CLASS

- Hormone.

MODE OF ACTION

- Oxytocin causes the uterus to contract after delivery of a fetus, thereby decreasing uterine bleeding.

INDICATIONS

- Control of postpartum bleeding after delivery of the placenta.

CONTRAINDICATIONS

- None when used emergently; however, ensure that there is no undelivered fetus.

SIDE EFFECTS/PRECAUTIONS

- May cause nausea and vomiting.
- May cause cardiac dysrhythmias.

ADULT DOSAGE

- 10 to 40 units in 1000 mL of 0.9% NaCL IV, titrated to patient's response (1 to 2 mL per minute initially).

PEDIATRIC DOSAGE

- Not recommended for prehospital use in pediatric patients.

PRALIDOXIME (PROTOPAM CHLORIDE, 2-PAM)

CLASS

- Nerve agent antidote.

MODE OF ACTION

- Pralidoxime reactivates acetylcholinesterase that has been reversibly phosphorylated by nerve agents or pesticides. Irreversible phosphorylation or "aging" is a time-dependent phenomenon that cannot be treated by pralidoxime.

INDICATIONS

- Poisoning with organophophates and nerve agents that inactivate acetylcholinesterase.

CONTRAINDICATIONS

- None in the presence of nerve agent or organophosphate poisoning.

- Caution in patients with myasthenia gravis.

SIDE EFFECTS/PRECAUTIONS

- Hypertension.

- Muscular rigidity with rapid infusion, respiratory arrest, nausea and vomiting, and blurred vision may occur.

ADULT DOSAGE

- 1 to 2 g IV over 10 to 30 minutes. May be given via IM or SC, if IV is not available. Various protocols are recommended. Some recommend the use of maintenance infusions.

- The Mark I kit contains a 600 mg dose of pralidoxime in an autoinjector.

PEDIATRIC DOSAGE

- 20 to 50 mg/kg IV over 30 minutes. May be given via IM or SC.

PROCAINAMIDE (PROCAN, PRONESTYL)

CLASS

- Antiarrhythmic agent.

MODE OF ACTION

- Procainamide increases the refractory period of the atria and to a lesser extent the AV node, bundle of His, and the Purkinje system. It slows conduction velocity throughout the conduction system. Its actions on the AV node are variable—a direct slowing action coexists with a mild vagolytic effect (slightly increasing AV conduction). It also decreases automaticity. The net effects make this drug effective for the treatment of both atrial and ventricular arrhythmias.

INDICATIONS

- Treatment of PVCs and monomorphic VT when lidocaine is contraindicated or fails to control ventricular ectopy.

- Treatment of wide-complex monomorphic tachycardias that cannot be distinguished from VT.

CONTRAINDICATIONS

- Avoid in patients with known hypersensitivity.

- Do not use in the presence of prolonged QT interval or torsades de pointes.

SIDE EFFECTS/PRECAUTIONS

- May cause hypotension, nausea, vomiting, and ventricular arrhythmias such as torsades de pointes, AV block, and asystole.

- May depress cardiac contractility; therefore, use with caution in the context of an acute myocardial infarction.

ADULT DOSAGE

- 20 mg per minute IV infusion until arrhythmia is suppressed, patient becomes hypotensive, QRS complex widens by 50%, or a maximum dose of 17 mg/kg has been given. If the patient is unstable, procainamide may be given at a rate of 30 mg per minute. Maintenance infusion rate of 1 to 4 mg per minute.

PEDIATRIC DOSAGE

- Not recommended for prehospital use in pediatric patients.

PROMETHAZINE (PHENERGAN)

CLASS

- Phenothiazine derivative antiemetic agent.

MODE OF ACTION

- The antiemetic effects result from dopaminergic receptor blockade on the chemotactic trigger zone (CTZ) in the medulla. Promethazine also possesses sedative and anticholinergic properties.

INDICATIONS

- Moderate to severe nausea and vomiting.

CONTRAINDICATIONS

- Known sensitivity to promethazine or other phenothiazines.

- Patients with altered mental status, those with compromised respiratory status.

- Pregnancy is a relative contraindication.

SECTION 4

SIDE EFFECTS/PRECAUTIONS

- Sedation and drowsiness are the most common reactions.

- Other CNS reactions include dystonias and akithesias. Dystonic reactions are more common in dehydrated, elderly, pediatric, or severely ill patients.

- Promethazine can reduce the seizure threshold. Neuroleptic malignant syndrome, a rare syndrome involving muscle rigidity, hyperthermia, tachycardia, and altered mental status, can be caused by promethazine.

- Patients may report dry mouth, urinary retention, blurred vision, and photosensitivity.

- Alterations in vital signs, tachycardias and bradycardias, hypotension and hypertension.

- May cause vasospasm if injected subcutaneously or intraarterially

ADULT DOSAGE

- 12.5 to 25 mg IM or slow IV push. May be repeated in 4 hours.

PEDIATRIC DOSAGE

- Age > 2 years: 0.25 to 1 mg/kg IM or slow IV. Maximum dose 25 mg. May be repeated in 4 hours.

RANITIDINE (ZANTAC)

CLASS

- H_2 blocker.

MODE OF ACTION

- The addition of an H_2 blocker adds to the effectiveness of H_1 blockers in anaphylaxis.

INDICATIONS

- Anaphylaxis or severe allergic reactions.

CONTRAINDICATIONS

- Known hypersensitivity to ranitidine.

SIDE EFFECTS/PRECAUTIONS

- There are few acute side effects. Important ones include headache and confusion. Rapid IV administration may cause cardiac arrhythmias and hypotension.

ADULT DOSAGE

- 50 mg IV/IM. May be repeated in 6 to 8 hours.

PEDIATRIC DOSAGE

- 0.5 to 1 mg/kg IV. May be repeated in 6 hours.

RETEPLASE (RETAVASE)

CLASS

- Thrombolytic agent.

MODE OF ACTION

- Reteplase is a recombinant DNA human tissue-type plasminogen activator that activates the conversion of plasminogen into plasmin, helping to dissolve thrombi.

INDICATIONS

- Patients with acute myocardial infarction presenting within 6 hours of the onset of symptoms.

  o ECG criteria include ST segment elevation of ≥ 0.1 mm in 2 or more leads.

  o Patients with posterior myocardial infarction also qualify if there is ST depression in leads V1 to 4.

o Patients with new or presumably new left bundle branch block (BBB).

• Early administration of thrombolytic agents yields the greatest benefit.

CONTRAINDICATIONS

• Absolute contraindications include:

o Known hypersensitivity to Reteplase.

o Prior history of a hemorrhagic CVA.

o Prior history of cerebral arteriovenous malformation or aneurysm.

o History of an ischemic CVA or TIA in the past year.

o Intracranial neoplasm.

o Active internal bleeding.

o Suspected aortic dissection.

• Relative contraindications:

o Recent (≤ 10 days) puncture of a noncompressible blood vessel.

o Prior history of poorly controlled hypertension, or acute severe hypertension (SBP > 180 mm Hg, DBP > 110 mm Hg).

o Diabetic retinopathy or other hemorrhagic eye condition.

o Bleeding diathesis.

o Anticoagulation with Coumadin.

o Pregnancy.

o Recent trauma or major surgery at a noncompressible site.

o History of ischemic CVA > 1 year ago.

o Prolonged (> 5 minutes) or traumatic CPR.

o Any other condition associated with bleeding.

SIDE EFFECTS/PRECAUTIONS

- The chief side effect is bleeding. Intracranial bleeding, reperfusion arrhythmias, and allergic reactions have been reported.

ADULT DOSAGE

- 10 units IV over 2 minutes. Repeat 10 units IV in 30 minutes.

PEDIATRIC DOSAGE

- Not recommended for pediatric use.

SODIUM BICARBONATE

CLASS

- Alkalinizing agent.

MODE OF ACTION

- Sodium bicarbonate reacts with hydrogen to form water and carbon dioxide to buffer metabolic acidosis. Sodium bicarbonate's high carbon dioxide content readily diffuses into cells, causing a paradoxical worsening of intracellular hypercarbia and acidosis. Bicarbonate diffuses into cells more slowly.

INDICATIONS

- During cardiac arrest resuscitation (if at all), only after the use of more definitive and better substantiated interventions, such as prompt defibrillation, effective CPR, ET intubation, ventilation with 100% oxygen, and the use of drugs such as epinephrine and lidocaine. The administration of sodium bicarbonate has not been demonstrated to improve ventricular defibrillation or survival in cardiac arrest.

- Hyperkalemia.

- Tricyclic antidepressant overdose.

SECTION 4

CONTRAINDICATIONS

- Pulmonary edema.

SIDE EFFECTS/PRECAUTIONS

- The performance of the ischemic heart is depressed by the high levels of carbon dioxide that result from the administration of sodium bicarbonate. Sodium bicarbonate administration may inhibit hemoglobin release of oxygen to the tissues. Sodium bicarbonate forms a precipitate when mixed with calcium chloride and deactivates epinephrine.

ADULT DOSAGE/PEDIATRIC DOSAGE

- 1 mEq/kg IV initial dose.

- Drug may be repeated at 0.5 mEq/kg, which should not be given more frequently than every 10 minutes.

SUCCINYLCHOLINE

CLASS

- Depolarizing neuromuscular blocking agent.

MODE OF ACTION

- Succinylcholine binds to acetylcholine receptors in the neuromuscular junction, causing depolarization. Fasciculations result from the depolarization and is followed by paralysis.

INDICATIONS

- Rapid sequence intubation (RSI).

CONTRAINDICATIONS

- Known hypersensitivity to succinylcholine.
- Personal or family history of malignant hyperthermia.

- Succinylcholine is also contraindicated when hyperkalemia is suspected (renal failure patients who have not been dialyzed, patients who are 24 hours or more post burn, ≥ 7 days post crush injury, or patients with progressive neuromuscular disease).

SIDE EFFECTS/PRECAUTIONS

- Succinylcholine's adverse reactions include fasciculations, hyperkalemia, and increased intracranial and intraocular pressure.

ADULT DOSAGE

- 1.5 to 2 mg/kg IV bolus.

PEDIATRIC DOSAGE

- Newborn: 3 mg/kg IV.

- Age < 10 years: 2 mg/kg IV.

SYRUP OF IPECAC

CLASS

- Emetic agent.

MODE OF ACTION

- Syrup of ipecac stimulates the chemotactic (emetic) area of the brain and irritates the gastrointestinal mucosa to stimulate vomiting.

INDICATIONS

- To induce vomiting in the alert patient with a suspected or known poisoning or overdose.

CONTRAINDICATIONS

- Avoid patients with known hypersensitivity.

- Contraindicated in patients with a decreased level of consciousness, without an intact gag reflex, or who have ingested caustic or petroleum-based products.

SIDE EFFECTS/PRECAUTIONS

- May cause CNS depression, arrhythmias, hypotension, and diarrhea.

- Take care to use only syrup of ipecac and not ipecac extract, which is several-fold more concentrated.

ADULT DOSAGE

- 15 to 30 mL by mouth, followed by several glasses of warm water. Dose may be repeated once in 20 minutes.

PEDIATRIC DOSAGE

- 6 months to 1 year: 5 to 10 mL by mouth followed by warm water.

- Older than 1 year: 15 to 25 mL by mouth followed by warm water.

TENECTEPLASE (TNKASE)

CLASS

- Thrombolytic agent.

MODE OF ACTION

- Tenecteplase is a recombinant DNA human tissue-type plasminogen activator that activates the conversion of plasminogen into plasmin, helping to dissolve thrombi.

INDICATIONS

- Patients with acute myocardial infarction presenting within 6 hours of the onset of symptoms.

  o ECG criteria include ST segment elevation of ≥ 0.1 mm in 2 or more leads.

- o Patients with posterior myocardial infarction also qualify if there is ST depression in leads V1 to 4.

- o Patients with new or presumably new left bundle branch block (BBB).

- Early administration of thrombolytic agents yields the greatest benefit.

CONTRAINDICATIONS

- Absolute contraindications include:

- o Known hypersensitivity to Tenecteplase.

- o Prior history of a hemorrhagic CVA.

- o Prior history of cerebral arteriovenous malformation or aneurysm.

- o History of an ischemic CVA or TIA in the past year.

- o Intracranial neoplasm.

- o Active internal bleeding.

- o Suspected aortic dissection.

- Relative contraindications:

- o Recent (≤ 10 days) puncture of a noncompressible blood vessel.

- o Prior history of poorly controlled hypertension, or acute severe hypertension (SBP > 180 mm Hg, DBP > 110 mm Hg).

- o Diabetic retinopathy or other hemorrhagic eye condition.

- o Bleeding diathesis.

- o Anticoagulation with Coumadin.

- o Pregnancy.

- o Recent trauma or major surgery at a noncompressible site.

- o History of ischemic CVA > 1 year ago.

SECTION 4

o Prolonged (> 5 minutes) or traumatic CPR.

o Any other condition associated with bleeding.

SIDE EFFECTS/PRECAUTIONS

- The chief side effect is bleeding. Intracranial bleeding, reperfusion arrhythmias, and allergic reactions have been reported.

ADULT DOSAGE

- A single weight-based bolus is given over 5 seconds.

Patient weight (kg)	Patient weight (lbs)	Tenecteplase (mg)	Volume of Tenecteplase (mL)
< 60	< 132	30	6
≥ 60 to < 70	≥ 132 to < 154	35	7
≥ 70 to < 80	≥ 154 to < 176	40	8
≥ 80 to < 90	≥ 176 to < 198	45	9
≥ 90	≥ 198	50	10

PEDIATRIC DOSAGE

- Not recommended for pediatric use.

TERBUTALINE

CLASS

- $Beta_2$ sympathetic agent.

MODE OF ACTION

- Terbutaline dilates smooth muscle in the bronchial tree through $beta_2$ stimulation. It has some adrenergic effects on the heart and central nervous system (CNS) when used in high doses.

- The $beta_2$ sympathetic action on the uterine smooth muscle causes relaxation.

INDICATIONS

- For treatment of reversible bronchoconstriction, such as asthma, chronic bronchitis, emphysema, or other reactive airway disease.

- Treatment of preterm labor.

CONTRAINDICATIONS

- Avoid in patients with known hypersensitivity to terbutaline.

- Use with caution in patients with heart rates > 150 bpm and those with hypertension.

- Do not use during an acute myocardial infarction.

SIDE EFFECTS/PRECAUTIONS

- May cause tachycardias, hypertension, chest pain, nervousness, tremor, headache, nausea or vomiting.

ADULT DOSAGE

- Bronchospasm: 0.25 mg SC. May be repeated once in 15 to 30 minutes if insufficient improvement. Maximum total dose 0.5 mg in a 4-hour period.

- Preterm labor: (various protocols exist) 0.25 mg SC. May be repeated in 25 to 30 minutes if insufficient improvement. Maximum total dose 1 mg in a 4-hour period.

PEDIATRIC DOSAGE

- Bronchospasm, age > 6 years: 5 to 10 μg/kg SC. May be repeated once in 15 to 50 minutes if insufficient improvement. Maximum single dose 0.4 mg.

THIAMINE (VITAMIN B1)

CLASS

- Vitamin.

MODE OF ACTION

- Thiamine is a necessary co-enzyme in the metabolism of glucose. Thiamine deficiency may cause Wernicke's syndrome. Signs and symptoms of Wernicke's syndrome include an altered mental state, involuntary muscular contractions, and ophthalmoplegia (most commonly bilateral nystagmus).

INDICATIONS

- Known or suspected thiamine deficiency.

- Altered mental state of unknown etiology, especially if alcohol abuse or malnourishment is suspected.

- The administration of D_{50} may precipitate Wernicke's syndrome in the thiamine-deficient patient, and therefore thiamine is often administered whenever D^{50} is administered.

CONTRAINDICATIONS

- None when used emergently.

SIDE EFFECTS/PRECAUTIONS

- IV Thiamine has been associated with anaphylaxis; administer slowly IV.

ADULT DOSAGE

- 100 mg (1 mL) IM or IV.

PEDIATRIC DOSAGE

- Thiamine is rarely used for pediatric patients.

VECURONIUM (NORCURON)

CLASS

- Competitive, nondepolarizing neuromuscular blocking agent.

MODE OF ACTION

- Vecuronium competes with acetylcholine and blocks its action at the neuromuscular junction receptor sites. This causes paralysis without fasciculations.

INDICATIONS

- Postintubation paralysis.

- Pretreatment of succinylcholine-induced fasciculations.

- RSI when succinylcholine is contraindicated.

CONTRAINDICATIONS

- Known hypersensitivity to vecuronium.

SIDE EFFECTS/PRECAUTIONS

- Vecuronium has a slower onset and a significantly prolonged action compared with succinylcholine.

- Side effects can also include bronchospasm, tachycardia, and hypotension.

ADULT DOSAGE

- Defasciculation dose: 0.01 mg/kg IV.

- Paralytic dose: 0.1 mg/kg IV.

- Postintubation paralysis: 0.1 mg/kg IV. Repeat at 0.01 to 0.015 mg/kg IV in 25 to 40 minutes.

PEDIATRIC DOSAGE

- Defasciculation dose, only age > 5 years: 0.01 mg/kg IV.

- Paralytic dose: 0.1 mg/kg IV.

- Postintubation paralysis: 0.1 mg/kg IV. Repeat at 0.01 to 0.015 mg/kg IV in 25 to 40 minutes.

SECTION 4

VERAPAMIL (CALAN, ISOPTIN)

CLASS

- Calcium channel blocker.

MODE OF ACTION

- Verapamil blocks the calcium channel found in the myo-cardium, in the cardiac conduction system, and in the vascular bed, decreasing calcium's entry into the cells, resulting in decreased cardiac contractility, decreased conduction through the AV node, and vasodilation.

INDICATIONS

- Symptomatic supraventricular tachycardias, including rapid atrial fibrillation and rapid atrial flutter.

CONTRAINDICATIONS

- Verapamil is contraindicated under the following circum-stances: bradycardias, second- and third-degree AV block, Wolf-Parkinson-White syndrome with rapid atrial fibrillation or atrial flutter, severe CHF.

SIDE EFFECTS/PRECAUTIONS

- The most significant side effects are hypotension, brady-cardias, development of AV blocks, asystole, and CHF.

ADULT DOSAGE

- 2.5 to 5 mg IV bolus over 1 minute: drug may be repeated at 5 to 10 mg IV bolus in 15 to 30 minutes.

PEDIATRIC DOSAGE

- Younger than 1 year: 0.1 to 0.2 mg/kg IV bolus over 2 minutes. Typical dose: 0.75 to 2 mg.

- 1 year to 15 years: 0.1 to 0.3 mg/kg IV bolus over 2 min-utes. Typical dose: 2 to 5 mg.

BIBLIOGRAPHY

Beck, R. (2003). *Pharmacology for prehospital emergency care.* (3rd ed.) Clifton Park, NY: Thomson Delmar Learning.

Deglin, J. H. & A. H. Vallerand (2004). *Davis' Drug Guide for Nurses* (9th ed.) Philadelphia, PA: F. A.Davis Co.

APPENDIX
F

EYE OPENING

Spontaneous	4
To voice	3
To pain	2
None	1

VERBAL RESPONSE
(PATIENT'S BEST VERBAL RESPONSE)

Oriented	5
Confused	4
Inappropriate words	3
Incomprehensible sounds	2
None	1

MOTOR RESPONSE
(PATIENT'S BEST MOTOR
RESPONSE)

Obeys command	6
Localizes pain	5
Withdraw (pain)	4
Flexion (pain)	3
Extension (pain)	2
None	1
Total GCS Score	(3 to 15)

Pediatric Glasgow Coma Score

	Infant	Child	
Eye Opening			
4	Spontaneous	Spontaneous	4
3	To speech	On command	3
2	To pain	To pain	2
1	None	None	1
Best Verbal Response			
5	Coos, babbles, smiles	Oriented	5
4	Irritable, cries	Confused	4
3	Cries, screams to pain	Inappropriate words	3
2	Moans, grunts	Incomprehensible	2
1	None	None	1
Best Motor Response			
6	Spontaneous	Obeys command	6
5	Withdraws from touch	Localizes pain	5
4	Withdraws from pain	Withdraws from pain	4
3	Flexion	Flexion	3
2	Extension	Extension	2
1	None	None	1
(3 to 15)	**Total GCS Score**		**(3 to 15)**

LUND AND BROWDER
RULE OF NINES CHARTS

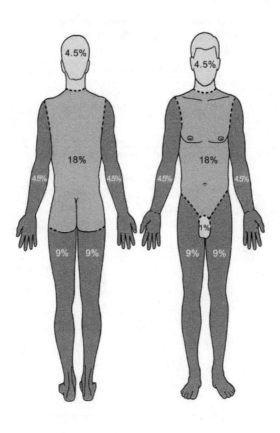

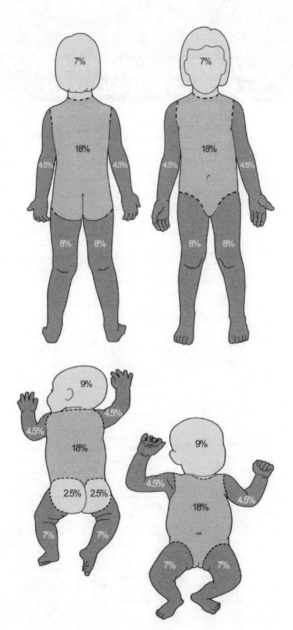

APPENDIX H

PEDIATRIC AIRWAY SIZES AND DRUG POSING

Drug doses are in mls except as noted.

Age	Preemie	Newborn	6 mo
Weight lbs	2.2-4.4	7.7	15.4
Weight kg	1-2	3.5	7
Airway			
ET Size uncuffed; c=cuffed	2.5 -3.0	3.0-3.5	3.5-4.0
Laryngoscope blade s=straight, c=curved	0 s	1 s	1 s
Allergy & Anaphylaxis			
Diphenhydramine 1 mg/kg, max 50 mg	1-2 mg	3.5 mg	7 mg
Epinephrine 0.01 mg/kg 1:1000 SC, max 0.5 in ml	.01-.02	0.03	0.07
Solumedrol 2 mg/kg, max 125 in mg	2-4 mg	7 mg	15 mg
Pulseless Arrest			
Amiodarone 5 mg/kg IV/IO, max 150 mg	5-10 mg	17.5 mg	35 mg
Atropine 0.02 mg/kg (minimum 0.1 mg)	0.1 mg	0.1 mg	0.14 mg
Defib @ 2j/kg	2-4 j	7 j	14 j
Defib @ 4j/kg	4-8 j	14 j	28 j
Epi ET 0.1 mg/kg (1:1000; 0.1 mL/kg) in ml	0.1-0.2	0.25	0.7
Epi IV/IO 0.01 mg/kg (1:10,000; 0.1 mL/kg) in ml	0.1-0.2	0.25	0.7
Lidocaine 2% 1 mg/kg IV/IO/PT in ml	0.05-0.1	0.175	0.35
Magnesium 25-50 mg/kg IV/IO (max 2g) in g	25-50	87.5-175	175-350
Altered LOC & Seizures			
Diazepam 0.1-0.3 mg/kg IV/IO, max 10 mg	0.1-0.3 mg	0.35-1 mg	0.7-2.1 mg
Diazepam 0.5 mg/kg rectal initial dose, repeat @ 0.25 mg/kg, maximum 10 mg	0.5-1 mg	1.75 mg	3.5 mg
Dextrose 0.5 g/kg in ml	5-10 (D10)	17.5 (D10)	14 (D25)
Lorazepam 0.05-0.1 mg/kg IV, max 2 mg	0.05 –0.1 mg	0.18 mg	0.35 mg
Naloxone 1 mg/ml 0.1 mg/kg; 2 mg max	0.1-0.2 mg	0.35 mg	0.7 mg
Bradycardia Algorithm			
Atropine 0.02 mg/kg (minimum 0.1 mg)	0.1 mg	0.1 mg	0.14 mg
Epi ET 0.1 mg/kg (1:1000; 0.1 mL/kg) in ml	0.1-0.2	0.25	0.7
Epi IV/IO 0.01 mg/kg (1:10,000; 0.1 mL/kg) in ml	0.1-0.2	0.25	0.7
Tachycardia Algorithm			
Adenosine 0.1 mg/kg IV/IO max 6 mg; in ml	.3-7	0.12	0.23
Adenosine 0.2 mg/kg IV/IO max 12 mg; in ml	0.07-0.13	0.23	0.47
Amiodarone 5 mg/kg IV/IO, max 150 mg	5-10 mg	17.5 mg	35 mg
Cardioversion 0.5 J/Kg	0.5-1 j	2 j	4 j
Cardioversion 1 J/Kg	1-2 j	4 j	7 j
Lidocaine 2% 1 mg/kg IV/IO/PT in ml	0.05-0.1	0.175	0.35
Procainamide 15 mg/kg IV over 30-60 minutes (dilute desired total in 50 ml if < 400 mg, 400-800 in 100 ml, 800-2000 in 250 ml D5W) in mg	15-30 mg	50 mg	105 mg

1 yr	3 yr	6 yr	8 yr	10 yr	12 yr	15 yr	18 yr
22	33	44	55	66	88	110	143
10	15	20	25	30	40	50	65
4.0-4.5	4.5-5.0	5.0-5.5	6.0-6.5	6.5-7.0	7.0 c	7.0-7.5c	7.0-8.0 c
2 s	2 s	2 s	2 s/c	3 s/c	3 s/c	3 s/c	3 s/c
10 mg	15 mg	20 mg	25 mg	30 mg	40 mg	50 mg	50 mg
0.1	0.15	0.20	0.25	0.3	0.4	0.5	0.5
22 mg	33 mg	44 mg	55 mg	66 mg	88 mg	110 mg	125 mg
50 mg	75 mg	100 mg	125 mg	150 mg	150` mg	150 mg	150 mg
0.2 mg	0.3 mg	0.4 mg	0.5 mg	0.5 mg	0.8 mg	1 mg	1 mg
20 j	30 j	40 j	50 j	60 j	80 j	100 j	130 j
40 j	60 j	80 j	100 j	120 j	160 j	200 j	260 j
1	1.5	2	2.5	3	4	5	6.5
1	1.5	2	2.5	3	4	5	6.5
0.5	0.75	1	1.25	1.5	2	2.5	3.25
250-500	375-750	500-1000	625- 1250	750-1500	1000-2000	1250-2000	1650-2000
1-3 mg	1.5-4.5 mg	2-6 mg	2.5-7.5 mg	3-9 mg	4-10 mg	5-10 mg	5-10 mg
5 mg	7.5 mg	10 mg	10 mg	10 mg	10 mg	10 mg	10 mg
20 (D25)	30 (D25)	40 (D25)	50 (D25)	30 (D50)	40 (D50)	50 (D50)	50 (D50)
0.5 mg	0.75 mg	1 mg	1.25 mg	1.5 mg	2 mg	2 mg	2 mg
1 mg	1.5 mg	2 mg	2 mg	2 mg	2 mg	2 mg	2 mg
0.2 mg	0.3 mg	0.4 mg	0.5 mg	0.5 mg	0.8 mg	1 mg	1 mg
1	1.5	2	2.5	3	4	5	6.5
1	1.5	2	2.5	3	4	5	6.5
0.33	0.5	0.7	0.8	1	1.3	1.7	2
0.7	1	1.3	1.7	2	2.7	3.3	4
50 mg	75 mg	100 mg	125 mg	150 mg	150` mg	150 mg	150 mg
5 j	8 j	10 j	13 j	15 j	20 j	25 j	33 j
10 j	15 j	20 j	25 j	30 j	40 j	50 j	65 j
0.5	0.75	1	1.25	1.5	2	2.5	3.25
150 mg	225 mg	300 mg	375 mg	450 mg	600 mg	750 mg	975 mg

Age-based estimates for weight and vital signs. The blood pressures are mean BPs ± 2 standard deviations.

Age	Weight (kg)	Heart Rate	Resp Rate	SBP	DBP
Premature	1	145	≈ 40	42±10	21±8
Premature	1-2	135	≈ 40	50±10	28±8
Newborn	2-3	125	≈ 40	60±10	37±8
1 month	4	120	24-35	80±16	46±16
6 months	7	130	24-35	89±29	60±10
1 year	10	120	20-30	96±30	66±25
2-3 years	12-14	115	20-30	99±25	64±25
4-5 years	16-18	100	20-30	99±20	65±20
6-8 years	20-26	100	12-25	100±15	60±10
10-12 years	32-42	75	12-25	110±17	60±10
> 14 years	> 50	70	12-18	118±20	60±10

Rothrock SG. Tarascon Pediatric Emergency Pocketbook, 4th edition, Mako Publishing Inc, Winter Park, FL, 2003.

TRAUMA SCORE

Trauma Score

Glasgow Coma Scale (GCS)	Systolic Blood Pressure (SBP)	Respiratory Rate (RR)	Coded Value
13-15	> 89	10-29	4
9-12	76-89	> 29	3
6-8	50-75	6-9	2
4-5	1-49	1-5	1
3	0	0	0

Add up the coded values for GCS, SBP, and RR. Maximum score is 12, minimum score is 0.

Pediatric Trauma Score

Component	+2	+1	-1
Weight	> 20 kg	10-20 kg	< 10 kg
Airway	Normal	Maintenance without invasive procedures	Requires invasive procedures
CNS	Alert, no LOC	Responds to verbal or painful stimuli	Unresponsive
Systolic BP/ pulses	> 90/ radial pulse	50-90/carotid or femoral pulse	< 50/No pulse
Wounds	None	Minor	Major/ penetrating or burns
Fractures	None	Closed fracture	Open or multiple fractures

Add up the point values for each component. Maximum score is 12, minimum –6.

Biological Agents

Agent Names	Bacteria		Viruses		Toxins		
	Anthrax	Plague	Smallpox	Viral Hemorrhagic Fevers (Ebola)	Botulinum	Ricin	Staphylococcal Enterotoxin B
Incubation period	1–7 days	2–3 days	7–17 days	3–21 days	1–3 days	1–7 days	
Contagious	NO	Pneumonic – YES Bubonic – NO	YES	YES	NO	NO	YES
Signs/ symptoms	Chills, fever, fatigue, cough, nausea, swollen lymph nodes	Chills, high fever, headache, hemoptysis, severe dyspnea	Fever, rigors, vomiting, headache, pustules	Fever, vomiting, diarrhea, mottled/ blotchy skin, coagulation disorders	Weakness, dizziness, dry mouth & throat, blurred vision, paralysis	Nausea, vomiting, bloody diarrhea, cough, SOB, death in 36–72 hours of S&S	Fever, chills, body aches, SOB, nonproductive cough
Personal protection	BSI	BSI	BSI	BSI	BSI	BSI Respiratory	BSI Respiratory
Emergency decontamination	Wet Strip Flush Cover	Wet Strip Flush Cover	Wet Strip Flush Cover	Wet Strip Flush Cover	Wet Strip Flush Cover	Wet Strip Flush Cover	Wet Strip Flush Cover
Treatment	ABCs Supportive care	ABCs Supportive care	ABCs Supportive care	ABCs Treat for shock Supportive care	ABCs Airway control & ventilatory support Supportive care	ABCs Supportive care	ABCs Supportive care

Chemical Agents

Agent Names	Signs/Symptoms	Onset of Signs/Symptoms	Unique Characteristics	Decontamination	Initial Treatment
Nerve Agents Tabun (GA) Sarin (GB) Soman (GD) Cyclohexyl Sarin (GF) VX Organophosphate poisons	*Moderate exposure* Miosis Salivation Lacrimation Urination Defecation *Severe exposure* Gastrointestinal distress (nausea, pain, gas, diarrhea) Emesis Convulsions	Vaporized (G) agents: seconds to minutes Liquids: minutes to hours	G agents are liquids that vaporize readily VX has a motor oil quality	Remove clothing Gently wash skin with soap & water Thorough flush of eyes with water or saline	Ventilatory support Atropine 2 mg IV or Mark I kit Pralidoxime (2 PAM) chloride 600–1000 mg IV or Mark I kit; repeat according to severity of S&S
Cyanides (blood agents) Hydrogen cyanide Cyanogens chloride	Confusion, dizziness Palpitations Headache Hyperventilation Nauseal vomiting Cherry red or cyanotic skin	Seconds to minutes	Cyanide may have bitter almond odor	Remove clothing Gently wash skin with soap & water Thorough flush of eyes with water or saline	Ventilatory support Inhalation of 0.2 ml of amyl nitrate Administer 300 mg sodium nitrate slow IV (5–10 minutes) & 12.5 mg sodium thiosulfate IV
Vesicants/ Blister Agents Mustard/sulfur mustard Mustard gas Lewisite Phosgene oxime	Irritation, burning and blistering of skin Tearing, conjunctivitis and corneal damage Respiratory distress, pulmonary edema	Mustard–hours to days Lewisite–minutes	Mustard may smell of garlic, horseradish or mustard Lewisite may smell like geraniums Phosgene oxime may have a pepper-like smell	Remove clothing Gently wash skin with soap & water Thorough irrigation of eyes with water or saline	Ventilatory support & supportive care, eye care. Thermal burn care No antidote for mustard Lewisite antidote – British antilewisite (BAL)
Pulmonary (choking) Agents Phosgene Chlorine Hydrogen chloride Nitrogen oxides	Respiratory distress, pulmonary edema Eye & skin irritation Sore throat Tightness in chest Wheezing Laryngeal spasms	1 to 24 hours	Chlorine gas is greenish-yellow, pungent smell Phosgene smells like newly-mown hay or grass	Remove clothing Gently wash skin with soap & water Thorough irrigation of eyes with water or saline	Ventilatory support with PEEP No antidote
Incapacitating/Riot Control Agents Pepper gas Mace®	Burning, tearing eyes Burning airway, coughing, difficulty breathing Burning, reddened skin	On contact with agent	Usually short acting, "tear gas" agents incapacitate by producing eye, mouth, nose, skin & airway irritation	Thorough irrigation of eyes with water or saline; remove contact lenses For severe exposure wash with soap & water	Supportive care If patient is wheezing, treat with bronchodilators

note: Unless they have been properly trained and equipped with personal protective equipment appropriate for the identified agent, EMS responders should treat only decontaminated patients.

Acute Radiation Syndrome
1 Gray (Gy) = 100 rads   1 centiGray (cGy) = 1 rad

Phase of syndrome	Feature	Whole body radiation from external radiation or internal absorption					
		Subclinical range	Sublethal range			Lethal range	
		0 – 100 rad or 1 Gy	100 – 200 rad 1-2 Gy	200 – 600 rad 2-6 Gy	600 – 800 rad 6-8 Gy	800 – 3000 rad 8-30 Gy	>3000 rad >30 Gy
Prodromal phase	Nausea, vomiting	None	5%50%	50% – 100%	75%-100%	90%-100%	100%
	Time of onset		3-6 hrs	2-4hrs	1-2 hrs	<1 hr	Minutes
	Duration		<24 hrs	<24 hrs	<48 hrs	<48 hrs	NA
	Lymphocyte count	Unaffected	Minimally decreased	< 1000 at 24 h	< 500 at 24h	Decreases within hours	Decreases within hours
	CNS function	No impairment	No impairment	Routine task performance Cognitive impair-ment for 6-20 hrs	Simple and routine task performance Cognitive impairment for >24 hrs	Rapid incapacitation, may have a lucid interval of several hours	
Latent phase (subclinical)	Absence of symptoms	> 2 wks	7-15 days	0-7 days 0-2 days		None	
Acute radiation illness or "Manifest illness" phase	Signs and symptoms	None	Moderate leuko-penia	Severe leukopenia, purpura, hemorrhage Pneumonia Hair loss after 300 rad/3 Gy		Diarrhea Fever Electrolyte disturbance	Convulsions, Ataxia, Tremor, Lethargy
	Time of onset		> 2 wks	2 days – 2 wks		1-3 days	1-48 hrs
	Critical period	None		4-6 wks – Most potential for effective medical intervention		2-14 days	1-48 hrs
	Organ system	None		Hematopoietic and respiratory (mucosal) systems		GI tract Mucosal systems	CNS
Hospitalization	% Duration	0	<5% 45-60 days	90% 60-90 days	100% 90+ days	100% weeks to months	100% days to weeks
Mortality		None	Minimal	Low with aggressive therapy	High	Very high, significant neurological symptoms indicate lethal dose	

Cite: Armed Forces Radiobiology Research Institute, United States Department of Defense, Pocket Guide for Responders to Ionizing Radiation Terrorism, pg. 2, 2003.

APPENDIX L

CIWA SCALE, REVISED

Clinical Institute Withdrawal Assessment of Alcohol Scale, Revised (CIWA-Ar)

Patient:_____   Date:_____ Time:_____

Heart rate, taken for 1 minute:____   Blood Pressure: _____

Nausea & Vomiting—Ask "Do you feel sick to your stomach? Have you vomited?"
Observation
0: no nausea and no vomiting
1: mild nausea with no vomiting
2:
3:
4: intermittent nausea with dry heaves
5:
6:
7: constant nausea, frequent dry heaves and vomiting

Tactile Disturbances—Ask "Have you any itching, pins and needles sensations, any burning, any numbness, or do you feel bugs crawling on or under your skin?"
Observation
0: none
1: very mild itching, pins and needles, burning or numbness
2: mild itching, pins and needles, burning or numbness
3: moderate itching, pins and needles, burning or numbness
4: moderately severe hallucinations
5: severe hallucinations
6: extremely severe hallucinations
7: continuous hallucinations

Tremor—Arms extended and fingers spread apart.
Observation
0: no tremor
1: not visible, but can be felt fingertip to fingertip
2
3
4: moderate, with patient's arms
5
6
7: severe, even with arms not extended

Auditory Disturbances—Ask "Are you more aware of the sounds around you? Are they harsh? Do they frighten you? Are you hearing anything that is disturbing you? Are you hearing things you know are not there?"
Observation
0: not present
1: very mild harshness or ability to frighten
2: mild harshness or ability to frighten
3: moderate harshness or ability to frighten
4: moderately severe hallucinations
5: severe hallucinations
6: extremely severe hallucinations
7: continuous hallucinations

Paroxysmal Sweats
Observation.
0: no sweat visible
1: barely perceptible sweating, palms moist
2
3
4: beads of sweat obvious on forehead
5
6
7: drenching sweats

Anxiety
Ask "Do you feel nervous?"
Observation
0: no anxiety, at ease
1: mildly anxious
2:
3:
4: moderately anxious, or guarded, so anxiety is inferred
5:
6:
7: equivalent to acute panic states as seen in severe delirium or acute schizophrenic reactions

Agitation
Observation
0: normal activity
1: somewhat more than normal activity
2:
3:
4: moderately fidgety and restless
5:
6:
7: paces back and forth during most of the interview, or constantly thrashes about

Visual Disturbances—Ask "Does the light appear to be too bright? Is its color different? Does it hurt your eyes? Are you seeing anything that is disturbing you? Are you seeing things you know are not there?"
Observation
0: not present
1: very mild sensitivity
2: mild sensitivity
3: moderate sensitivity
4: moderately severe hallucinations
5: severe hallucinations
6: extremely severe hallucinations
7: continuous hallucinations

Headache, Fullness in Head—Ask "Does your head feel different? Does it feel like there is a band around your head?" Do not rate for dizziness or lightheadedness. Otherwise, rate severity.
Observation
0: not present
1: very mild
2: mild
3: moderate
4: moderately severe
5: severe
6: very severe
7: extremely severe

Orientation and Clouding of Sensorium— Ask "What day is this? Where are you? Who am I?"
Observation
0: oriented and can do serial additions
1: cannot do serial additions or is uncertain about date
2: disoriented for date by no more than 2 calendar days
3: disoriented for date by more than 2 calendar days
4: disoriented for place/or person

Maximum possible score 67

Patients scoring < 10 do not usually need additional medication for withdrawal.

Total CIUWA-Ar Score

Rater's Initials: _____

The CIWA-Ar is not copyrighted and may be reproduced freely.
Sullivan, J. T., Sykora, K., Schneiderman, J., Naranjo, C. A., & Sellers, E. M. (1989). Assessment of alcohol withdrawal: The revised Clinical Institute Withdrawal Assessment for Alcohol scale (CIWA-Ar). *British Journal of Addiction*, 84, 1353–1357.

INDEX

SECTION 4

SECTION 4